Recent Results in Cancer Research 180

AF858847

Rüdiger Liersch · Wolfgang E. Berdel
Torsten Kessler (Eds.)

Angiogenesis Inhibition

Springer

Editors
Dr. Rüdiger Liersch
Department of Medicine
Hematology/Oncology
University Hospital Münster
Albert-Schweitzer-Str. 33
48129 Münster
Germany
rliersch@uni-muenster.de

Prof. Dr. Wolfgang E. Berdel
Department of Medicine
Hematology/Oncology
University Hospital Münster
Albert-Schweitzer-Str. 33
48129 Münster
Germany
berdel@uni-muenster.de

Dr. Torsten Kessler
Department of Medicine
Hematology/Oncology
University Hospital Münster
Albert-Schweitzer-Str. 33
48129 Münster
Germany
torstenkessler@uni-muenster.de

ISBN: 978-3-642-26143-5 e-ISBN: 978-3-540-78281-0

DOI: 10.1007/978-3-540-78281-0

Springer Heidelberg Dordrecht London New York

Cover design: eStudioCalamar Figueres/Berlin

Printed on acid-free paper

Springer is part of Springer Science+Business Media (www.springer.com)

Contents

Contributors

Gian Carlo Alghisi
Division of Experimental Oncology
Centre Pluridisciplinaire d'Oncologie
Lausanne Cancer Center
University of Lausanne
Lausanne
Switzerland

Iris Appelmann
Department of Medicine
Hematology and Oncology
University of Münster
Albert-Schweitzer-Strasse 33
48129 Münster
Germany
Iris.Appelmann@ukmuenster.de

Michael Bayer
Department of Medicine
Hematology and Oncology
University of Münster
Albert-Schweitzer-Strasse 33
48129 Münster
Germany

Wolfgang E. Berdel
Department of Medicine
Hematology/Oncology
University of Münster
Albert-Schweitzer-Strasse 33
48129 Münster, Germany
berdel@uni-muenster.de

Christoph Biermann
Department of Medicine
Hematology and Oncology
University Hospital Münster
Albert-Schweitzerstrasse 33
48129 Münster
Germany

Urban Emmenegger
Department of Medicine
Division of Medical Oncology, and
Department of Medical Biophysics
Division of Molecular and Cellular Biology
Sunnybrook Health Sciences Centre
University of Toronto
2075 Bayview Avenue Toronto ON
Canada M4N3M5
urban.emmenegger@sri.utoronto.ca

Giulio Francia
Department of Medical Biophysics
Division of Molecular and Cellular Biology
Sunnybrook Health Sciences Centre
University of Toronto
2075 Bayview Avenue
Toronto, ON
Canada M4N3M5

Hans-Peter Gerber
Sr Dir Discovery Tumor Prog
Pharma, Research & Development
Pearl River, NY
gerberh@wyeth.com

Iqbal S. Grewal
Department of Preclinical Therapeutics
Seattle Genetics Inc.
Bothell
Washington 98021
USA

C.-H. Heldin
Ludwig Institute for Cancer Research
Uppsala University
S-751 24 Uppsala
Sweden
C-H.Heldin@LICR.uu.e

Carina Hellberg
Ludwig Institute for Cancer Research
Uppsala University
S-751 24 Uppsala
Sweden
Carina.Hellberg@LICR.uu.se

Andreas Hippe
Department of Dermatology
Heinrich-Heine-University
Moorenstrasse 5
40225 Düsseldorf
Germany
ahippe@gmail.com

Bernhard Homey
Department of Dermatology
Heinrich-Heine-University
Moorenstrasse 5
40225 Düsseldorf
Germany
Bernhard.Homey@uni-duesseldorf.de

Robert S. Kerbel
Department of Medical Biophysics
Division of Molecular and Cellular Biology
Sunnybrook Health Sciences Centre
University of Toronto
2075 Bayview Avenue
Toronto, ON,
Canada M4N3M5

Torsten Kessler
Department of Medicine
Hematology/Oncology
University Hospital Münster
Albert-Schweitzer-Str. 33
48129 Münster
Germany
torstenkessler@uni-muenster.de

Mei Yee Koh
Department of Experimental Therapeutics
M.D. Anderson Cancer Center
Houston, TX 77030
USA

Rüdiger Liersch
Department of Medicine
Hematology/Oncology
University Hospital Münster
Albert-Schweitzer-Str. 33
48129 Münster
Germany
rliersch@uni-muenster.de

Kerri A. Massey
Sidney Kimmel Cancer Center
10905 Road to the Cure
San Diego, CA 92121
USA

Rolf M. Mesters
Department of Medicine
Hematology and Oncology
University of Münster
Albert-Schweitzer-Strasse 33
48129 Münster
Germany

Anja Mueller-Homey
Department of Radiation Therapy
and Radiation Oncology
Heinrich-Heine-University
Moorenstrasse 4
40225 Düsseldorf
Germany
A.Mueller@uni-duesseldorf.de

Dario Neri
Institute of Pharmaceutical Sciences
Department of Chemistry and
Applied Biosciences
Swiss Federal Institute of Technology Zürich
Wolfgang-Pauli-Strasse 10
CH-8093 Zürich
Switzerland
dario.neri@pharma.ethz.ch

Ezogelin Olazoglu
Department of Preclinical Therapeutics
Seattle Genetics Inc.
Bothell
Washington, DC 98021
USA

Arne Östman
Department of Pathology-Oncology
Cancer Center Karolinska
Karolinska Institute
171 76, Stockholm
Sweden
Arne.Ostman@cck.ki.se

Garth Powis
MD Anderson Cancer Center
1400 Holcombe Blvd.
FC6.3044
Unit 422
Houston, TX 77030
USA
gpowis@mdanderson.org

Yvonne Reiss
Institute of Neurology/Edinger Institute
Frankfurt University Medical School
Heinrich-Hoffmann-Strasse
760528 Frankfurt
Germany
Yvonne.Reiss@kgu.de

Curzio Rüegg
Division of Experimental Oncology
Centre Pluridisciplinaire d'Oncologie
155 Chemin des Boveresses
CH1066 Epalinges
Switzerland
curzio.ruegg@unil.ch

Christoph Schliemann
Institute of Pharmaceutical Sciences,
Department of Chemistry and Applied
Biosciences
Swiss Federal Institute of Technology Zürich
Wolfgang-Pauli-Strasse 10
CH-8093 Zürich
Switzerland
Christoph.schliemann@pharma.ethz.ch

Jan E. Schnitzer
Proteogenomics Research Institute
for Systems Medicine,
11107 Roselle St,
San Diego, CA 92121
USA
jschnitzer@prism-sd.org

Christian Schwöppe
Department of Medicine
Hematology and Oncology
University of Münster
Albert-Schweitzer-Strasse 33
48129 Münster
Germany

Yuval Shaked
Department of Medical Biophysics
Division of Molecular and Cellular Biology
Sunnybrook Health Sciences Centre
University of Toronto
2075 Bayview Avenue
Toronto
ON, Canada M4N3M5

Taly R. Spivak-Kroizman
Department of Experimental Therapeutics
M.D. Anderson Cancer Center
Houston, TX 77030
USA

Introduction 1

Judah Folkman

Judah Folkman agreed to write an introductory overview on the field of angiogenesis and cancer for this book. The topic was his field of research, indeed his passion, and he put it into the center of interest for a whole generation of researchers and clinicians working to combat and treat cancer. Judah Folkman died suddenly on January 14, 2008 at age 74, on the way to a scientific conference on angiogenesis. He could not finish his chapter. This day witnessed the loss of a scientific pioneer and humanitarian.

Born in 1933, Dr. Folkman was trained at Ohio State University and Harvard Medical School. During his time of serving in the U.S. Navy, he began studying tumors and soon concentrated on the dependence of tumor growth and spread from the formation of new blood vessels. In 1971 the *New England Journal of Medicine* published his ground-breaking hypothesis on angiogenesis and antiangiogenic therapy. Initially met with skepticism, this paper opened the field of neoangiogenesis and cancer for a growing community of scientists and physician–scientists working on biological mechanisms of the connections between the vascular systems and cancer and on the development of antiangiogenic therapy against cancer. Judah Folkman and his team of scientists were always on the forefront of this research. He and his team isolated the first proangiogenic factor bFGF, identified multiple angiogenic inhibitors such as endostatin, angiostatin, and fumagillin, and made numerous other discoveries that moved the field forward. His laboratory also studied molecular pathways of angiogenesis and helped to develop numerous antiangiogenic drugs.

Today antiangiogenic therapy, as envisaged by Judah Folkman, has made a difference for many patients with cancer. This book will provide the reader with an overview of the field of antiangiogenic therapy for cancer, but because of the large scope of the field, it concentrates on certain aspects as well. The editors hope that it contains interesting and stimulating information for scientists and physicians alike working on aspects of the vascular systems and cancer. In a very real sense, we hope this book will commemorate the tremendous influence Judah Folkman's farsighted thinking and pioneering work has had on all of us.

Germany Wolfgang E. Berdel

R. Liersch et al. (eds.), *Angiogenesis Inhibition,* Recent Results in Cancer Research,
DOI: 10.1007/978-3-540-78281-0_1, © Springer Verlag Berlin Heidelberg 2010

Angiopoietins

2

Yvonne Reiss

Abstract The formation of new blood vessels plays an important role during the development and progression of a disease. In recent years, there has been a tremendous effort to uncover the molecular mechanisms that drive blood vessel growth in adult tissues. Angiopoietins belong to a family of growth factors that are critically involved in blood vessel formation during developmental and pathological angiogenesis. The importance of Angiopoietin signaling has been recognized in transgenic mouse models as the genetic ablation of Ang-1, and its primary receptor Tie2 has led to early embryonic lethality. Interesting and unusual for a family of ligands, Ang-2 has been identified as an antagonist of Ang-1 in endothelial cells as evidenced by a similar embryonic phenotype when Ang-2 was overexpressed in transgenic mice. In this review, we focus on the functional consequences of autocrine Angiopoietin signaling in endothelial cells.

Y. Reiss
Institute of Neurology/Edinger Institute,
Frankfurt University Medical School,
Heinrich-Hoffmann-Strasse,
760528, Frankfurt,
Germany
e-mail: Yvonne.Reiss@kgu.de

2.1 Introduction

Angiogenesis involves the complex signaling between multiple angiogenic growth factors, and requires the coordinated interaction between endothelial and adjacent cells. Vascular endothelial growth factor (VEGF) possesses a dominant role in mediating endothelial cell sprouting, migration, and network formation as indicated by the early lethality of VEGF-deficient mice (Carmeliet et al. 1996; Ferrara et al. 1996; for review see Ferrara et al. 2003; Conway et al. 2001; Risau 1997). The Angiopoietin (Ang) family has primary roles in the latter stages of vascular development and in the adult vasculature, where it controls vessel remodeling and stabilization. Ang-1 has the capability to stimulate Tie2 receptor activation while Ang-2 has been identified as an antagonizing ligand (Suri et al. 1998; Maisonpierre et al. 1997). Ang-2 overexpression in transgenic mice led to embryonic death with a phenotype similar to Ang-1 or Tie2 deletion (Maisonpierre et al. 1997). Thus, genetic evidence suggests that signaling through Tie2 appears to depend on the balance between Ang1 and Ang2. In the quiescent vasculature in adults, Ang1 provides a basal signal to maintain the integrity of the endothelial cells (Brindle et al. 2006). In contrast, Ang-2 induced by VEGF or hypoxia suppresses these effects

R. Liersch et al. (eds.), *Angiogenesis Inhibition,* Recent Results in Cancer Research,
DOI: 10.1007/978-3-540-78281-0_2, © Springer Verlag Berlin Heidelberg 2010

and leads to vessel destabilization. Consequently, effects mediated by Ang-2 allow vessel growth or regression, depending on the presence of additional growth factors (Hanahan 1997).

2.2 Importance of the Angiopoietin/Tie System During Developmental Angiogenesis

Ang-1 and Ang-2 (Davis et al. 1996; Maisonpierre et al. 1997) are best characterized among the Angiopoietin family. Additional members are designated as Ang-3 and Ang-4, and represent diverging counterparts in mice and humans (Valenzuela et al. 1999). Ang-1 and Ang-2 are ligands for the receptor *t*yrosine kinase with *i*mmunoglobulin and *e*pidermal growth factor homology domains 2 (Tie2; Maisonpierre et al. 1997; Davis et al. 1996; Sato et al. 1995; Dumont et al. 1995) with predominant expression in endothelial cells. They share approximately 60% of aminoacid identity (Maisonpierre et al. 1997). Ang-1 has initially been discovered as the primary Tie2 ligand (Davis et al. 1996). Although Ang-1 and Ang-2 act as antagonizing molecules, they bind to Tie2 with similar affinities. They share the same binding domains of the Tie2 receptor, including the first Ig-like loop and the epidermal growth factor-like repeats (Barton et al. 2006; Fiedler et al. 2003). The two highly related members of the Tie receptor tyrosine kinase family, Tie1 and Tie2, display unique extracellular domains: epidermal growth factor repeats, immunoglobulin-like domains, fibronectin-type III repeats, and a separated tyrosine kinase domain in the cytoplasmic region (Dumont et al. 1993; Sato et al. 1993; Schnurch and Risau 1993; Partanen et al. 1992). Although Tie2 is the best established receptor for Ang-1, there are emerging data showing that the ligand may also signal through the related tyrosine kinase Tie1 (Saharinen et al. 2005).

Engagement of Tie2 by Ang-1 is responsible for receptor phosphorylation and the induction of survival signals in endothelial cells (Jones et al. 1999; Papapetropoulos et al. 2000). There is additional evidence that Ang-1 plays an active role in vessels sprouting as Ang-1 overexpression in mice increased vessel density and branching (Suri et al. 1998). Ang-1-mediated endothelial cell sprouting and migration has also been proven in in vitro models (Audero et al. 2004; Hayes et al. 1999; Koblizek et al. 1998). Consistent with these findings, interactions between endothelial and pericytes/smooth muscle cells are stabilized only in the presence of Ang-1, and decreased association of endothelial cells with support cells is evident in Ang-1 mutant mice (Suri et al. 1996). In the adult vasculature, Ang-1 binding to Tie2 is constitutive and essential to maintain endothelium in the quiescent state (Wong et al. 1997; Saharinen et al. 2008; Fukuhara et al. 2008). By contrast, opposing functions have been described for Ang-2. Binding of Tie2 by Ang-2 antagonizes receptor phosphorylation in transgenic animals (Maisonpierre et al. 1997; Reiss et al. 2007), thereby disrupting contacts between endothelial- and periendothelial support cells. Ang-2 also disrupts endothelial monolayer interaction with smooth muscle cells in culture (Scharpfenecker et al. 2005). This process is fundamental for the initiation of vessel sprouting or regression.

Evidence for the importance of the Angiopoietin/Tie2 system for the vascular development is derived from genetic experiments following the ablation of Ang-1 or Tie2 in transgenic mice (Suri et al. 1996; Sato et al. 1995; Dumont et al. 1995). A summary of genetic mouse models available of Angiopoietins and Tie receptors are displayed in Table 2.1. Embryos lacking Tie2 receptor tyrosine kinase or Ang-1 ligand display aberrant vascular development and die around embryonic day E11 as a consequence of insufficient remodeling of the primary capillary plexus. Analysis of the vasculature of mice deficient for Tie2 or Ang-1 has indicated abnormal interactions between endothelial cells and peri-endothelial support cells (Suri et al. 1996; Sato et al. 1995; Dumont et al. 1995). Contrary to these findings, mice with targeted expression of Ang-1 in the skin exhibit larger and

Table 2.1 Transgenic mice resulting from Angiopoietin/Tie deletion and overexpression

Ang-1	
Ang-1$^{-/-}$	Lethal at E11–12.5, defective vessel remodeling, enlarged vessels, and poor endothelial cell interaction with perivascular cells, complementary to Tie2$^{-/-}$ phenotype (Suri et al. 1996)
Ang-1 overexpression	Overexpression in skin increases number, size and branching of vessels (hypervascularization), vessel sealing, anti-inflammatory (Suri et al. 1998; Thurston et al. 1999)
Ang-2	
Ang-2$^{-/-}$	Lethal at postnatal day 14 (depending on genetic background), normal embryonic vascular development, defects in postnatal angiogenic remodeling (disturbed hyaloid vessel regression), and defects in the lymphatic vasculature (disorganization/hypoplasia in dermal and intestinal lymphatics) (Gale et al. 2002)
Ang-2 overexpression	Ang-2 overexpression in the vasculature, lethal at E9.5–10.5. complementary to Ang-1 and Tie2 mutant phenotypes but more severe, rounded endothelial cells, poor interaction with matrix, endocardial defects (Maisonpierre et al. 1997)
Inducible Ang-2 overexpression in endothelial cells	Tie1 promoter driven, Tet-inducible expression of Ang-2 in endothelial cells, embryonic lethality during gestation, defective collateral artery growth, and smooth muscle cell coverage during pathological angiogenesis (limb ischemia) (Reiss et al. 2007)
Tie receptors	
Tie1$^{-/-}$	Die embryonic day >13.5 (E13.5), vessel hemorrhage, edema, rupture, endocardial defects (Sato et al. 1995; Puri et al. 1995; Puri et al. 1999)
Tie2$^{-/-}$	Lethal E9.5–10.5, complementary phenotype to Ang-1$^{-/-}$, defective vessel remodeling, dilated vessels, decreased branching, rounded endothelial cells lacking pericytes, hemorrhage, vessel rupture (Dumont et al. 1994; Sato et al. 1995)
Tie1 and Tie2$^{-/-}$	Similar to Tie2$^{-/-}$ but more severe. Tie1$^{-/-}$embryos sensitive to Tie2 gene dosage, Tie1$^{-/-}$/Tie2$^{-/-}$endothelial cells absent from capillaries of adult chimeric wildtype/double knockout mice (Puri et al. 1999)
	Tie1$^{-/-}$/Tie2$^{-/-}$cells have reduced capacity to contribute to hematopoiesis in the adult, but not in the fetus (Puri and Bernstein 2003)

more numerous branched vessels that are resistant to vascular leakage induced by permeability factors, such as VEGF (Suri et al. 1998). These findings support the present concept that the Angiopoietin/Tie2 system plays an important role in the interaction between endothelial and mural cells. Angiogenic remodeling of the mature vasculature requires a progressive disengagement of endothelial cells from the surrounding support cells, and this destabilization can result in vessels sprouting or regression. The distinct expression pattern of Ang-2 at sites of active vascular remodeling (Maisonpierre et al. 1997) and in highly vascularized tumors (Holash et al. 1999; Stratmann et al. 1998) has implicated Ang-2 in the blockade of the Ang-1 stabilizing function to facilitate angiogenesis. In addition, transgenic overexpression in embryonic endothelial cells resulted in a similar phenotype as the deletion of the Tie2 gene, supporting the view that Ang-2 is an antagonistic ligand (Maisonpierre et al. 1997). However, genetic ablation of Ang-2 in mice resulted in a less severe phenotype, which is compatible with life, as such providing evidence that Ang-2 is not redundant with Ang-1 (Gale et al. 2002). Ang-2 is selectively upregulated in tumor vessels before the onset of VEGF in adjacent tumor cells, and can synergize with VEGF to enhance neovascularization. This indicated that Ang-2 might be antagonist in particular environments, such as in postnatal remodeling or pathological angiogenesis (Gale et al. 2002; Holash et al. 1999).

2.3 Angiopoietins and Tumor-Associated Angiogenesis

The essential role of angiogenesis for the expansion of solid tumors is demonstrated by the observation that avascular tumors are not able to grow beyond a certain size unless they acquire new blood vessels for the supply of nutrients and oxygen (Folkman 1971; Hanahan and Folkman 1996; Yancopoulos et al. 2000). Co-option of existing vessels from the neighboring tissue thereby displays one possible mechanism to promote tumor growth (Holash et al. 1999). In addition, tumor cells provide endothelium-specific growth factors such as VEGF and Angiopoietins for the recruitment of new blood vessel.

During development, Tie2 expression is present on virtually all endothelial cells (Dumont et al. 1995; Sato et al. 1995). In addition, Tie2 expression is increased during physiological and pathological angiogenesis in the adult. However, endothelial cells of the vasculature remain quiescent during adult life. Numerous studies have demonstrated altered expression patterns for Angiopoietin ligands and corresponding Tie receptors in a variety of tumors. This clearly indicated important roles for Angiopoietin/Tie signaling beyond development in experimental models of tumor growth (Reiss et al. 2005; Tait and Jones 2004). Tumor vessels are known to have abnormal phenotypes that include changes in the architecture and assembly of the vessel wall (Morikawa et al. 2002; Ward and Dumont 2002). These vessel abnormalities are likely the cause for increased vascular permeability within the tumor. With respect to potential targeted interventions of angiogenesis in tumors, it is required to decipher the mechanisms that promote or inhibit the vessel growth. Regarding the current knowledge of Angiopoietin biology during tumor angiogenesis, results are controversial and include pro- and antiangiogenic functions for both, Ang-1 and Ang-2. In detail, overexpression of Ang-1 in experimental tumors induced stabilization by the recruitment of pericytes and smooth muscle cells to recently formed vessels (for review see (Reiss et al. 2005; Tait and Jones 2004)). Consequently, reduced tumor growth or tumor stasis has been reported by a number of research laboratories in experimental tumors, such as colon-, lung-, mammary- and squamous cell carcinoma (Stoeltzing et al. 2003; Hawighorst et al. 2002; Tian et al. 2002; Stoeltzing et al. 2002; Ahmad et al. 2001; Yu and Stamenkovic 2001; Hayes et al. 2000). However, findings derived from certain tumor types, including our own results, indicate proangiogenic functions when overexpressing Ang-1 (Shim et al. 2002; Machein et al. 2004). These controversial findings may be related to differences in the presence of growth factors within the tumor types investigated. Although effector functions of Ang-1 on the outcome of tumor growth are not completely resolved, an improved vessel architecture in the presence of Ang-1 is typically observed. This is mainly exerted by a higher degree of pericyte coverage. Ang-2 in contrast, is necessary to initiate vessel sprouting and is associated with pericyte loss of the host tumor vasculature (Reiss et al. 2009; Cao et al. 2007; Machein et al. 2004; Zhang et al. 2003; Hu et al. 2003; Ahmad et al. 2001; Yu and

Stamenkovic 2001; Etoh et al. 2001; Tanaka et al. 1999). This is achieved through the destabilizing actions on the previously quiescent vasculature. At present, findings that have been reported for the role of Ang-2 during tumor progression are not well understood. However, what can be concluded from the literature with regard to Ang-2 functions in tumors is a shift in the balance of Ang-1 and Ang-2 in favor of Ang-2. Consequently, instability of the host vasculature and aberrant, nonfunctional vessels were often observed (Reiss et al. 2009; Reiss et al. 2005). Furthermore, Lewis lung carcinoma, mammary carcinoma, gastric and brain tumors overexpressing Ang-2 display increased frequencies of metastatic dissemination and are highly invasive (Hu et al. 2003; Yu and Stamenkovic 2001; Etoh et al. 2001). In summary, evidence from the literature implies that vessel destabilizing defects of Ang-2 might be caused by the disengagement of pericytes from the tumor vessels, and the defective cellular linings caused by openings between endothelial cells might to some extent explain increased permeabilities within tumor vessels (Hashizume et al. 2000). Ang-2-mediated functions during tumor angiogenesis are illustrated in Fig. 2.1.

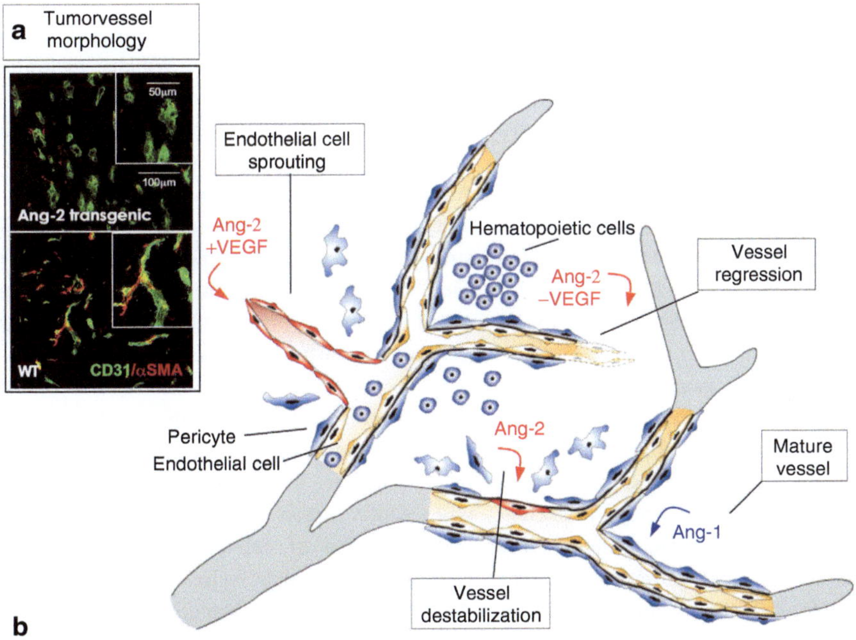

Fig. 2.1 Influence of the Angiopoietin/Tie system on the formation of new blood vessels in tumors. Inducible Ang-2 expression in the vasculature of transgenic animals (adapted from Reiss et al. 2007) leads to increased vascular densities (*green*: αCD31 immunohistochemistry) in subcutaneous Lewis lung tumors, indicative for excessive vessel sprouting (**a**). Furthermore, reduced in red pericyte coverage (**a**, indicated by αSMA labeling) in red is prominent within the tumor vasculature (insets: higher magnification). A schematic drawing of Angiopoietin/Tie mediated functions in tumors is illustrated in (**b**). Ang-1 contributes to the stabilization and maturation of new blood vessels in tumors. In concert with VEGF, Ang-2 destabilizes the vasculature and leads to vessel sprouting or regression (modified after (Reiss et al. 2005)) Ang-2 additionally might be able to promote the recruitment of hematopoietic cells during tumor progression or other pathological conditions as Ang-2 deficient mice display delayed inflammatory cell recruitment (Fiedler et al., 2006)

Ang-2 is highly regulated at the transcriptional level (Hegen et al. 2004) and induced in endothelial cells in areas of active angiogenesis (Holash et al. 1999; Stratmann et al. 1998) such as in tumors, making it an attractive target for therapeutic intervention. Moreover, Ang-2 has been associated with poor prognosis and lymphnode metastasis in human tumors pointing towards a need for therapeutic intervention (Ochiumi et al. 2004; Hu et al. 2003; Sfiligoi et al. 2003; Etoh et al. 2001). Pharmacological inhibition of Angiopoietin functions by sequestration with soluble Tie2 (Siemeister et al. 1999; Lin et al. 1998; Lin et al. 1997) or by the usage of dominant-negative Tie2 mutants has earlier been shown to have a negative impact on tumor growth and progression. Furthermore, neutralization of Ang-2-Tie2 interactions (Oliner et al. 2004) or overexpression of Ang-2 (Cao et al. 2007) inhibited tumor angiogenesis and tumor growth in mice. Whether targeted intervention of Ang-2 will be applicable in human tumors as well remains to be elucidated in the future.

In spite of the intense research on Angiopoietin functions during physiological angiogenesis (Suri et al. 1998; Maisonpierre et al. 1997) and tumor angiogenesis (Holash et al. 1999; Stratmann et al. 1998), the biological actions of Angiopoietins during tumor progression have not been fully ascertained. Clearly, molecular mechanisms for a more precise understanding of Angiopoietin/Tie-mediated effector functions that may lead to increased vessel integrity or drive vascular remodeling/regression are largely missing. In detail, it is well established that tumor vessels display highly permeable vessels, but only few studies focused on the cellular basis of tumor vessel permeability (McDonald et al. 1999; Morikawa et al. 2002; Hashizume et al. 2000). For instance, it is largely unknown how Ang-1 prevents and Ang-2 increases vessel permeability, although they both seem to interfere with cell–cell interactions and junctional proteins (e.g., stabilize or destabilize EC junctions in vitro) (Gamble et al. 2000; Scharpfenecker et al. 2005). Recently, two reports provided some insight in the molecular mechanism of Ang-1-induced Tie2 signaling in regulating endothelial cell quiescence vs. angiogenic activation (Saharinen et al. 2008; Fukuhara et al. 2008). Using an in vitro system, the authors elegantly showed that Ang1-activated Tie2 assembles novel signaling complexes leading to preferential activation of different downstream signal transduction proteins in the presence vs. absence of cell–cell contacts.

In our own studies, we analyzed the cellular consequences of Angiopoietin expression on tumor vessel morphology in two mouse mammary carcinoma models which naturally displayed distinct Ang/Tie2 expression profiles and generated mammary carcinomas to express Ang-1 and Ang-2 (Reiss et al. 2009). Analysis of Angiopoietin-overexpressing mammary xenografts at the ultrastructural level strongly supported the hypothesis that Ang-1/Tie2 signaling is essential for proper vessel organization, and suggested that Ang-2 is mainly responsible for the induction of disrupted endothelial cells (Reiss et al. 2009). Furthermore, our findings supported the hypothesis that Ang-2 can trigger important signals that are decisive for a switch of vascular phenotypes within tumors. Current results also imply that disruption of cell–cell contacts between endothelial cells might be inversely regulated by Ang-1 and Ang-2. For instance, it has been shown that VEGF-mediated disruption of cell–cell interactions is attributed to the dissociation of β-catenin from VE-cadherin (Wang et al. 2004). Interestingly, this effect can be opposed by Ang-1 as it specifically counteracts the ability of VEGF to induce the phosphorylation-dependent redistribution of VE-cadherin, thereby rescueing the endothelial barrier function (Gavard et al. 2008). Our own observations in tumors of Ang-2 transgenic animals (unpublished data);

(Reiss et al. 2007) suggest that high serum levels of Ang-2 are mainly responsible for improper vessel function. Future studies will help to unravel participating cellular elements during pathological angiogenesis more precisely.

2.4 Therapeutic Implications

Clearly, the effects of Angiopoietins in vivo suggest that manipulation of this ligand could have therapeutical potential. Pharmacological inhibition of Angiopoietin functions by sequestration with soluble Tie2 (Siemeister et al. 1999; Lin et al. 1998; Lin et al. 1997), or by the usage of dominant-negative Tie2 mutants has previously been shown to have a negative impact on tumor growth and progression. Until now, novel inhibition strategies for cancer treatment are at the preclinical level in murine angiogenesis models. Possible manipulation includes neutralization of Ang-2-Tie2 interactions (Oliner et al. 2004) or overexpression of Ang-2 (Cao et al. 2007), which inhibited tumor angiogenesis and tumor growth in mice. Whether targeted intervention of Ang-2 will be favorable in human tumors needs to be determined in the future. However, interfering with Ang-2 will shift the relative level of Ang1 and Ang-2. In case of Ang-2 inhibition, increased levels of Ang-1 will be beneficial for vessel perfusion and permeability and might lead to increased angiogenesis. Thus, Angiopoietin dosage is critical for the net outcome on angiogenesis inhibition and has to be taken into account for possible therapeutic interventions. Interestingly, VEGFR2 blockage can temporarily normalize tumor vessel structure (increased pericyte coverage) and lead to vascular normalization via expression of Ang-1 (Winkler et al. 2004). As a consequence, transient stabilization of vessels and improved oxygen delivery to hypoxic zones is achieved following VEGF neutralization which may facilitate drug delivery into tumors. The delivery of drugs utilizing the Angiopoietin/Tie system as a vehicle has recently been reported by De Palma et al. (De Palma et al. 2008). In this study, the authors exploited the tumor-homing ability of proangiogenic Tie2-expressing monocytes to deliver IFN-α to tumors which inhibited tumor growth and metastasis.

The complex interplay between complementary and yet conflicting roles of both Angiopoietins during tumor angiogenesis has impeded the development of drugs interfering with this angiogenic pathway. Collectively, a better understanding of the molecular mechanisms of Ang-1 and Ang-2 signaling during pathological angiogenesis may set the stage for novel therapies targeting this pathway.

2.5 Conclusions

Angiopoietins (Ang-1 and Ang-2) and their Tie receptors have wide-ranging effects on tumor malignancy that includes angiogenesis, vascular stabilization and permeability, and the recruitment of inflammatory cells. These multifaceted pathways present a valuable opportunity in developing novel inhibition strategies for cancer treatment. Ang-1 is not significantly upregulated in the majority of tumors. In contrast, Ang-2 is highly induced in the tumor vasculature, even prior to the induction of VEGF. As such, a shift in the Ang-1:Ang-2 balance in advantage of Ang-2 is the consequence. Therefore, it is evident that Ang-2 dosage is critical in shaping the outcome of angiogenesis. However, the regulatory role of Ang-1 and Ang-2 in tumor angiogenesis remains controversial, and the complex interplay between complementary yet conflicting roles of both the Angiopoietins during adult angiogenesis need to be addressed more precisely, for example, by using Ang-2 transgenic animals. Further studies are needed to discern how Angiopoietins cooperate with other molecules and to develop new strategies for therapy targeting the Ang/Tie pathway.

Acknowledgment I gratefully acknowledge Jutta Reiss for helping with the illustrations and cartoons, and Andrea Tal for confocal images. This work is supported by the SFB/TR23 – C1 and the Excellence Cluster Cardio-Pulmonary System (ECCPS).

References

Carmeliet P, Ferreira V, Breier G et al (1996) Abnormal blood vessel development and lethality in embryos lacking a single VEGF allele. Nature 380:435–439

Ferrara N, Carver-Moore K, Chen H et al (1996) Heterozygous embryonic lethality induced by targeted inactivation of the VEGF gene. Nature 380:439–442

Ferrara N, Gerber HP, LeCouter J (2003) The biology of VEGF and its receptors. Nat Med 9:669–676

Conway EM, Collen D, Carmeliet P (2001) Molecular mechanisms of blood vessel growth. Cardiovasc Res 49:507–521

Risau W (1997) Mechanisms of angiogenesis. Nature 386:671–674

Suri C, McClain J, Thurston G et al (1998) Increased vascularization in mice overexpressing angiopoietin-1. Science 282:468–471

Maisonpierre PC, Suri C, Jones PF et al (1997) Angiopoietin-2, a natural antagonist for Tie2 that disrupts in vivo angiogenesis. Science 277:55–60

Brindle NP, Saharinen P, Alitalo K (2006) Signaling and functions of angiopoietin-1 in vascular protection. Circ Res 98:1014–1023

Hanahan D (1997) Signaling vascular morphogenesis and maintenance. Science 277:48–50

Davis S, Aldrich TH, Jones PF et al (1996) Isolation of angiopoietin-1, a ligand for the TIE2 receptor, by secretion-trap expression cloning. Cell 87: 1161–1169

Valenzuela DM, Griffiths JA, Rojas J et al (1999) Angiopoietins 3 and 4: diverging gene counterparts in mice and humans. Proc Natl Acad Sci U S A 96:1904–1909

Sato TN, Tozawa Y, Deutsch U et al (1995) Distinct roles of the receptor tyrosine kinases Tie-1 and Tie-2 in blood vessel formation. Nature 376:70–74

Dumont DJ, Fong GH, Puri MC, Gradwohl G, Alitalo K, Breitman ML (1995) Vascularization of the mouse embryo: a study of flk-1, tek, tie, and vascular endothelial growth factor expression during development. Dev Dyn 203:80–92

Barton WA, Tzvetkova-Robev D, Miranda EP et al (2006) Crystal structures of the Tie2 receptor ectodomain and the angiopoietin-2-Tie2 complex. Nat Struct Mol Biol 13:524–532

Fiedler U, Krissl T, Koidl S et al (2003) Angiopoietin-1 and angiopoietin-2 share the same binding domains in the Tie-2 receptor involving the first Ig-like loop and the epidermal growth factor-like repeats. J Biol Chem 278:1721–1727

Dumont DJ, Gradwohl GJ, Fong GH, Auerbach R, Breitman ML (1993) The endothelial-specific receptor tyrosine kinase, tek, is a member of a new subfamily of receptors. Oncogene 8:1293–1301

Sato TN, Qin Y, Kozak CA, Audus KL (1993) Tie-1 and tie-2 define another class of putative receptor tyrosine kinase genes expressed in early embryonic vascular system. Proc Natl Acad Sci U S A 90:9355–9358

Schnurch H, Risau W (1993) Expression of tie-2, a member of a novel family of receptor tyrosine kinases, in the endothelial cell lineage. Development 119:957–968

Partanen J, Armstrong E, Makela TP et al (1992) A novel endothelial cell surface receptor tyrosine kinase with extracellular epidermal growth factor homology domains. Mol Cell Biol 12:1698–1707

Saharinen P, Kerkela K, Ekman N et al (2005) Multiple angiopoietin recombinant proteins activate the Tie1 receptor tyrosine kinase and promote its interaction with Tie2. J Cell Biol 169:239–243

Jones N, Master Z, Jones J et al (1999) Identification of Tek/Tie2 binding partners. Binding to a multifunctional docking site mediates cell survival and migration. J Biol Chem 274:30896–30905

Papapetropoulos A, Fulton D, Mahboubi K et al (2000) Angiopoietin-1 inhibits endothelial cell apoptosis via the Akt/survivin pathway. J Biol Chem 275:9102–9105

Audero E, Cascone I, Maniero F et al (2004) Adaptor ShcA protein binds tyrosine kinase Tie2 receptor and regulates migration and sprouting but not

survival of endothelial cells. J Biol Chem 279: 13224–13233
Hayes AJ, Huang WQ, Mallah J, Yang D, Lippman ME, Li LY (1999) Angiopoietin-1 and its receptor Tie-2 participate in the regulation of capillary-like tubule formation and survival of endothelial cells. Microvasc Res 58:224–237
Koblizek TI, Weiss C, Yancopoulos GD, Deutsch U, Risau W (1998) Angiopoietin-1 induces sprouting angiogenesis in vitro. Curr Biol 8:529–532
Suri C, Jones PF, Patan S et al (1996) Requisite role of angiopoietin-1, a ligand for the TIE2 receptor, during embryonic angiogenesis. Cell 87: 1171–1180
Wong AL, Haroon ZA, Werner S, Dewhirst MW, Greenberg CS, Peters KG (1997) Tie2 expression and phosphorylation in angiogenic and quiescent adult tissues. Circ Res 81:567–574
Saharinen P, Eklund L, Miettinen J et al (2008) Angiopoietins assemble distinct Tie2 signalling complexes in endothelial cell-cell and cell-matrix contacts. Nat Cell Biol 10:527–537
Fukuhara S, Sako K, Minami T et al (2008) Differential function of Tie2 at cell-cell contacts and cell-substratum contacts regulated by angiopoietin-1. Nat Cell Biol 10:513–526
Reiss Y, Droste J, Heil M et al (2007) Angiopoietin-2 impairs revascularization after limb ischemia. Circ Res 101(1):88–96
Scharpfenecker M, Fiedler U, Reiss Y, Augustin HG (2005) The Tie-2 ligand angiopoietin-2 destabilizes quiescent endothelium through an internal autocrine loop mechanism. J Cell Sci 118:771–780
Holash J, Maisonpierre PC, Compton D et al (1999) Vessel cooption, regression, and growth in tumors mediated by angiopoietins and VEGF. Science 284:1994–1998
Stratmann A, Risau W, Plate KH (1998) Cell type-specific expression of angiopoietin-1 and angiopoietin-2 suggests a role in glioblastoma angiogenesis. Am J Pathol 153:1459–1466
Gale NW, Thurston G, Hackett SF et al (2002) Angiopoietin-2 is required for postnatal angiogenesis and lymphatic patterning, and only the latter role is rescued by Angiopoietin-1. Dev Cell 3:411–423
Folkman J (1971) Tumor angiogenesis: therapeutic implications. N Engl J Med 285:1182–1186
Hanahan D, Folkman J (1996) Patterns and emerging mechanisms of the angiogenic switch during tumorigenesis. Cell 86:353–364
Yancopoulos GD, Davis S, Gale NW, Rudge JS, Wiegand SJ, Holash J (2000) Vascular-specific growth factors and blood vessel formation. Nature 407:242–248
Reiss Y, Machein MR, Plate KH (2005) The role of angiopoietins during angiogenesis in gliomas. Brain Pathol 15:311–317
Tait CR, Jones PF (2004) Angiopoietins in tumours: the angiogenic switch. J Pathol 204:1–10
Morikawa S, Baluk P, Kaidoh T, Haskell A, Jain RK, McDonald DM (2002) Abnormalities in pericytes on blood vessels and endothelial sprouts in tumors. Am J Pathol 160:985–1000
Ward NL, Dumont DJ (2002) The angiopoietins and Tie2/Tek: adding to the complexity of cardiovascular development. Semin Cell Dev Biol 13:19–27
Stoeltzing O, Ahmad SA, Liu W et al (2003) Angiopoietin-1 inhibits vascular permeability, angiogenesis, and growth of hepatic colon cancer tumors. Cancer Res 63:3370–3377
Hawighorst T, Skobe M, Streit M et al (2002) Activation of the tie2 receptor by angiopoietin-1 enhances tumor vessel maturation and impairs squamous cell carcinoma growth. Am J Pathol 160:1381–1392
Tian S, Hayes AJ, Metheny-Barlow LJ, Li LY (2002) Stabilization of breast cancer xenograft tumour neovasculature by angiopoietin-1. Br J Cancer 86:645–651
Stoeltzing O, Ahmad SA, Liu W et al (2002) Angiopoietin-1 inhibits tumour growth and ascites formation in a murine model of peritoneal carcinomatosis. Br J Cancer 87:1182–1187
Ahmad SA, Liu W, Jung YD et al (2001) The effects of angiopoietin-1 and -2 on tumor growth and angiogenesis in human colon cancer. Cancer Res 61:1255–1259
Yu Q, Stamenkovic I (2001) Angiopoietin-2 is implicated in the regulation of tumor angiogenesis. Am J Pathol 158:563–570
Hayes AJ, Huang WQ, Yu J et al (2000) Expression and function of angiopoietin-1 in breast cancer. Br J Cancer 83:1154–1160
Shim WS, Teh M, Bapna A et al (2002) Angiopoietin 1 promotes tumor angiogenesis and tumor vessel plasticity of human cervical cancer in mice. Exp Cell Res 279:299–309
Machein MR, Knedla A, Knoth R, Wagner S, Neuschl E, Plate KH (2004) Angiopoietin-1 promotes tumor angiogenesis in a rat glioma model. Am J Pathol 165:1557–1570
Cao Y, Sonveaux P, Liu S et al (2007) Systemic

overexpression of angiopoietin-2 promotes tumor microvessel regression and inhibits angiogenesis and tumor growth. Cancer Res 67:3835–3844

Zhang L, Yang N, Park JW et al (2003) Tumor-derived vascular endothelial growth factor up-regulates angiopoietin-2 in host endothelium and destabilizes host vasculature, supporting angiogenesis in ovarian cancer. Cancer Res 63:3403–3412

Hu B, Guo P, Fang Q et al (2003) Angiopoietin-2 induces human glioma invasion through the activation of matrix metalloprotease-2. Proc Natl Acad Sci U S A 100:8904–8909

Etoh T, Inoue H, Tanaka S, Barnard GF, Kitano S, Mori M (2001) Angiopoietin-2 is related to tumor angiogenesis in gastric carcinoma: possible in vivo regulation via induction of proteases. Cancer Res 61:2145–2153

Tanaka S, Mori M, Sakamoto Y, Makuuchi M, Sugimachi K, Wands JR (1999) Biologic significance of angiopoietin-2 expression in human hepatocellular carcinoma. J Clin Invest 103:341–345

Hashizume H, Baluk P, Morikawa S et al (2000) Openings between defective endothelial cells explain tumor vessel leakiness. Am J Pathol 156:1363–1380

Hegen A, Koidl S, Weindel K, Marme D, Augustin HG, Fiedler U (2004) Expression of angiopoietin-2 in endothelial cells is controlled by positive and negative regulatory promoter elements. Arterioscler Thromb Vasc Biol 24:1803–1809

Ochiumi T, Tanaka S, Oka S et al (2004) Clinical significance of angiopoietin-2 expression at the deepest invasive tumor site of advanced colorectal carcinoma. Int J Oncol 24:539–547

Sfiligoi C, de Luca A, Cascone I et al (2003) Angiopoietin-2 expression in breast cancer correlates with lymph node invasion and short survival. Int J Cancer 103:466–474

Siemeister G, Schirner M, Weindel K et al (1999) Two independent mechanisms essential for tumor angiogenesis: inhibition of human melanoma xenograft growth by interfering with either the vascular endothelial growth factor receptor pathway or the Tie-2 pathway. Cancer Res 59:3185–3191

Lin P, Buxton JA, Acheson A et al (1998) Antiangiogenic gene therapy targeting the endothelium-specific receptor tyrosine kinase Tie2. Proc Natl Acad Sci U S A 95:8829–8834

Lin P, Polverini P, Dewhirst M, Shan S, Rao PS, Peters K (1997) Inhibition of tumor angiogenesis using a soluble receptor establishes a role for Tie2 in pathologic vascular growth. J Clin Invest 100:2072–2078

Oliner J, Min H, Leal J et al (2004) Suppression of angiogenesis and tumor growth by selective inhibition of angiopoietin-2. Cancer Cell 6:507–516

McDonald DM, Thurston G, Baluk P (1999) Endothelial gaps as sites for plasma leakage in inflammation. Microcirculation 6:7–22

Gamble JR, Drew J, Trezise L et al (2000) Angiopoietin-1 is an antipermeability and anti-inflammatory agent in vitro and targets cell junctions. Circ Res 87:603–607

Wang Y, Pampou S, Fujikawa K, Varticovski L (2004) Opposing effect of angiopoietin-1 on VEGF-mediated disruption of endothelial cell-cell interactions requires activation of PKC beta. J Cell Physiol 198:53–61

Gavard J, Patel V, Gutkind JS (2008) Angiopoietin-1 prevents VEGF-induced endothelial permeability by sequestering Src through mDia. Dev Cell 14:25–36

Murdoch C, Muthana M, Coffelt SB, Lewis CE (2008) The role of myeloid cells in the promotion of tumour angiogenesis. Nat Rev Cancer 8:618–631

Grunewald M, Avraham I, Dor Y et al (2006) VEGF-induced adult neovascularization: recruitment, retention, and role of accessory cells. Cell 124:175–189

De Palma M, Murdoch C, Venneri MA, Naldini L, Lewis CE (2007) Tie2-expressing monocytes: regulation of tumor angiogenesis and therapeutic implications. Trends Immunol 28:519–524

De Palma M, Venneri MA, Roca C, Naldini L (2003) Targeting exogenous genes to tumor angiogenesis by transplantation of genetically modified hematopoietic stem cells. Nat Med 9: 789–795

De Palma M, Venneri MA, Galli R et al (2005) Tie2 identifies a hematopoietic lineage of proangiogenic monocytes required for tumor vessel formation and a mesenchymal population of pericyte progenitors. Cancer Cell 8: 211–226

Machein MR, Renninger S, de Lima-Hahn E, Plate KH (2003) Minor contribution of bone marrow-derived endothelial progenitors to the vascularization of murine gliomas. Brain Pathol 13:582–597

Fiedler U, Reiss Y, Scharpfenecker M et al (2006) Angiopoietin-2 sensitizes endothelial cells to TNF-alpha and has a crucial role in the induction of inflammation. Nat Med 12:235–239

Winkler F, Kozin SV, Tong RT et al (2004) Kinetics of vascular normalization by VEGFR2 blockade governs brain tumor response to radiation: role of oxygenation, angiopoietin-1, and matrix metalloproteinases. Cancer Cell 6:553–563

De Palma M, Mazzieri R, Politi LS et al (2008) Tumor-targeted interferon-alpha delivery by Tie2-expressing monocytes inhibits tumor growth and metastasis. Cancer Cell 14:299–311

Thurston G, Suri C, Smith K et al (1999) Leakage-resistant blood vessels in mice transgenically overexpressing angiopoietin-1. Science 286: 2511–2514

Puri MC, Rossant J, Alitalo K, Bernstein A, Partanen J (1995) The receptor tyrosine kinase TIE is required for integrity and survival of vascular endothelial cells. EMBO J 14:5884–5891

Puri MC, Partanen J, Rossant J, Bernstein A (1999) Interaction of the TEK and TIE receptor tyrosine kinases during cardiovascular development. Development 126:4569–4580

Dumont DJ, Gradwohl G, Fong GH et al (1994) Dominant-negative and targeted null mutations in the endothelial receptor tyrosine kinase, tek, reveal a critical role in vasculogenesis of the embryo. Genes Dev 8:1897–1909

Puri MC, Bernstein A (2003) Requirement for the TIE family of receptor tyrosine kinases in adult but not fetal hematopoiesis. Proc Natl Acad Sci U S A 100:12753–12758

Reiss Y, Knedla A, Tal AO et al (2009) Switching of vascular phenotypes within a murine breast cancer model induced by Angiopoietin-2. J Path 217 (4):571–580

HIF-1α and Cancer Therapy

3

Mei Yee Koh, Taly R. Spivak-Kroizman, and Garth Powis

Abstract Most solid tumors develop regions of hypoxia as they grow and outstrip their blood supply. In order to survive in the stressful hypoxic environment, tumor cells have developed a coordinated set of responses orchestrating their adaptation to hypoxia. The outcomes of the cellular responses to hypoxia are aggressive disease, resistance to therapy, and decreased patient survival. A critical mediator of the hypoxic response is the transcription factor hypoxia-inducible factor 1 (HIF-1) that upregulates expression of proteins that promote angiogenesis, anaerobic metabolism, and many other survival pathways. Regulation of HIF-1α, a component of the HIF-1 heterodimer, occurs at multiple levels including translation, degradation, and transcriptional activation, and serves as a testimony to the central role of HIF-1. Studies demonstrating the importance of HIF-1α expression for tumor survival have made HIF-1α an attractive target for cancer therapy. The growing l.ist of pharmacological inhibitors of HIF-1 and their varied targets mirrors the complex molecular mechanisms controlling HIF-1. In this chapter, we summarize recent findings regarding the regulation of HIF-1α and the progress made in identifying new therapeutic agents that inhibit HIF-1α.

G. Powis (✉)
MD Anderson Cancer Center, 1400 Holcombe Blvd., FC6.3044, Unit 422, Houston, TX 77030, USA
e-mail: gpowis@mdanderson.org

3.1 Background

More than 50% of locally advanced solid tumors exhibit hypoxic tissue areas (i.e., areas with oxygen tensions of <2.5 mmHg) heterogeneously distributed within the tumor mass (Vaupel and Mayer 2007). Tumor hypoxia occurs due to the inability of the local vasculature to supply sufficient oxygen to the rapidly growing tumor. In an attempt to alleviate hypoxia, tumor cells release factors that generate new vasculature, which is itself highly irregular, tortuous, and leaky with arterio-venous shunts and blind ends (Brown and Giaccia 1998). The insufficient/intermittent oxygen supply, both from the existing vasculature and from the irregular tumor neovasculature, gives rise to a highly dynamic tumor microenvironment containing hypoxic/reoxygenation gradients (Bristow and Hill 2008). Tumor hypoxia is of major significance since it can promote both tumor progression and resistance to radiation and chemotherapy.

The tumor response to hypoxia includes the induction of angiogenesis, a switch from aerobic metabolism to anaerobic glycolysis, and the

R. Liersch et al. (eds.), *Angiogenesis Inhibition,* Recent Results in Cancer Research,
DOI: 10.1007/978-3-540-78281-0_3,

expression of a variety of stress proteins regulating cell death or survival (Table 3.1).The hypoxia-inducible factor-1 (HIF-1 or HIF) transcription factor is the master regulator of the hypoxic response, inducing the expression of a large number of genes critical for adaptation to hypoxia (Semenza and Wang 1992). Indeed, hypoxia has been recognized as a primary physiological regulator of the angiogenic switch in which HIF-1 acts as a focal point, tipping the balance of anti- and proangiogenic factors toward hypoxia-induced angiogenesis (Bergers and Benjamin 2003; Giordano and Johnson 2001). Hypoxic cells are also more genetically unstable, more resistant to treatment by ionizing radiation and chemotherapy, and generally more invasive and metastatic (Vaupel and Mayer 2007). Hence, HIF-1 is a positive factor in tumor growth and its increased expression has been correlated with poor patient prognosis, making targeting tumor hypoxia/HIF-1 an attractive approach for the development of novel anticancer therapies (Semenza 2004; Welsh et al. 2006).

3.2 Molecular and Cellular Biology of HIF-1

The HIF-1 transcription factor is a heterodimer of the oxygen-regulated HIF-α subunit, and the constitutively expressed HIF-1β subunit (also known as the aryl hydrocarbon receptor nuclear translocator (ARNT)) (Wang et al. 1995). When HIF-α is stabilized (such as during hypoxia), it enters the nucleus and heterodimerizes with HIF-1β and binds to a conserved DNA sequence known as the hypoxia responsive element (HRE) to transactivate a variety of hypoxia-responsive genes (Maxwell et al. 2001). Both subunits are basic helix-loop-helix-Per-ARNT-Sim (bHLH-PAS) domain proteins in which DNA binding and dimerization is mediated by the basic HLH domains, whilst the PAS domain is involved in dimer formation (Jiang et al. 1996) (Fig. 3.1). The HIF-α subunit also contains an oxygen-dependent degradation (ODD) domain that regulates its ODD and two transactivation domains (N-TAD and C-TAD). To date, three HIF-α isoforms (HIF-1/2/3α) have been described, of which HIF-1α and HIF-2α are the best characterized. HIF-1α is expressed ubiquitously, whereas HIF-2α displays more tissue-specific expression (Wiesener et al. 2003). Both have been shown to regulate common and unique target genes (Hu et al. 2003), and may be differentially regulated depending on the duration and severity of hypoxia exposure (Holmquist-Mengelbier et al. 2006). The least studied HIF-α isoform, HIF-3α, is regulated in a similar manner to HIF-1α and HIF-2α and can also dimerize with HIF-1β (Gu et al. 1998). HIF-3α has high similarity with HIF-1α and HIF-2α in the bHLH and PAS domains, but lacks the C-TAD found in HIF-1α and HIF-2α. HIF-3α has multiple splice variants, including the best-known, inhibitory PAS domain protein (IPAS), which is a truncated protein that acts as a dominant negative inhibitor of HIF-1 (Makino et al. 2002).

The HIF-1 heterodimer binds a conserved HIF binding sequence (HBS) within the HRE in the promoter or enhancer regions of target genes, thereby eliciting their transactivation and an adaptive hypoxic response (Semenza 2003). To date, more than 70 genes have been confirmed as HIF-1 target genes (Table 3.1). These genes regulate a diverse set of cellular processes critical for the physiological response to hypoxia important both for normal development and for the hypoxic adaptation of tumor cells.

3.3 HIF-1 Regulation

3.3.1 Regulation of HIF-1α Translation

Numerous studies support the idea that in addition to inhibition of ODD, continued translation also contributes to the accumulation of HIF-1α

Table 3.1 Role of HIF-1 in the response to hypoxia

Hypoxic response	HIF-1 target genes
Angiogenesis: HIF-1 directly activates the expression of a number of proangiogenic factors, the best characterized of which is the vascular endothelial growth factor (VEGF). This event promotes the formation of new blood vessels, thus restoring the supply of oxygen and nutrients. Increased angiogenesis is one of the key HIF-1-dependent protumorigenic events that enable continued tumor growth	Vascular endothelial growth factor (VEGF), VEGF receptor 1 (Flt-1), erythropoietin (EPO), plasminogen activator inhibitor 1 (PAI-1), adrenomedullin (ADM), endothelin-1 (EDN1), nitric oxide synthase-2 (NOS2A). leptin (LEP)
Anaerobic metabolism: HIF-1 promotes both the uptake and metabolism of glucose through anaerobic glycolysis by upregulating the expression of glucose transporters (GLUT1, GLUT3) and of glycolytic enzymes (PFKFB3). To maintain the metabolic flux through glycolysis, HIF-1 activation also leads to the inhibition of the Kreb's cycle by upregulating PDK1 and LDHA. This shift from aerobic to anaerobic metabolism is frequently observed in cancer cells, even in normoxia, and is known as the Warburg effect	Glucose transporter 1 and 3 (GLUT1, GLUT3), 6-phosphofructo-2-kinase/fructose-2,6-bisphosphatase (PFKFB3), pyruvate dehydrogenase kinase 1 (PDK1), lactate dehydrogenase A (LDHA), hexokinase 1 and 2 (HK1, HK2), glucose phosphate isomerase (AMF/GP1), enolase 1 (ENO1), glyceraldehyde-3-phosphate dehydrogenase (GAPDH), phosphofructokinase L (PFKL), phosphoglycerate kinase 1 (PGK1), pyruvate kinase M (PKM)
pH regulation: To counter the potentially toxic intracellular acidosis owing to increased production of lactic acid and CO by anaerobic glycolysis, HIF-1 also upregulates MCT4, which mediates lactic acid efflux, and CA IX, which catalyzes the conversion of extracellular CO_2 to carbonic acid (H_2CO_3)	Carbonic anhydrase 9 and 12 (CAIX, CAXII), monocarboxylic acid transporter 4 (MCT4)
Apoptosis, survival and proliferation: HIF-1 regulates a complex array of pro- and antiapoptotic genes as well as genes regulating cell cycle and proliferation. The final outcome of HIF-1 activation on cell growth and survival may be dictated by the severity and duration of hypoxia as well as the presence of other regulatory cofactors	BCL2/adenovirus E1B 19 kDa interacting protein 3 (BNIP3), BNIP3-like (BNIP3L/NIX), DNA-damage-inducible transcript 4 (DDIT4), ADM, Insulin-likegrowth factor 2 (IGF2), Insulin-like growth factor binding protein 1, 2, and 3 (IGF-BP1, IGF-BP2, IGF-BP3), NOS2, transforming growth factor α (TGF-α), cyclin G2
Invasion, metastasis, differentiation: HIF-1 promotes tumor cell invasion and metastasis and particularly when composed of the HIF-2α isoform, has been implicated in the inhibition of differentiation and maintenance of the stem cell phenotype	AMF/GP1, hepatocyte growth factor receptor (c-MET), low density lipoprotein-related protein 1 (LRP1), lysyl oxidase (LOX), TWIST1, POU class 5 homeobox 1(POU5F1/OCT4)

Poorly vascularized regions are associated with hypoxia and nutrient deprivation, thereby limiting ATP production, a requirement for cell proliferation. Hypoxia induces HIF-1, which activates a variety of genes that regulate the cellular response to hypoxia. These are summarized below. This list is by no means exhaustive and has been described in greater detail previously (Semenza 2002; Semenza 1999)

3

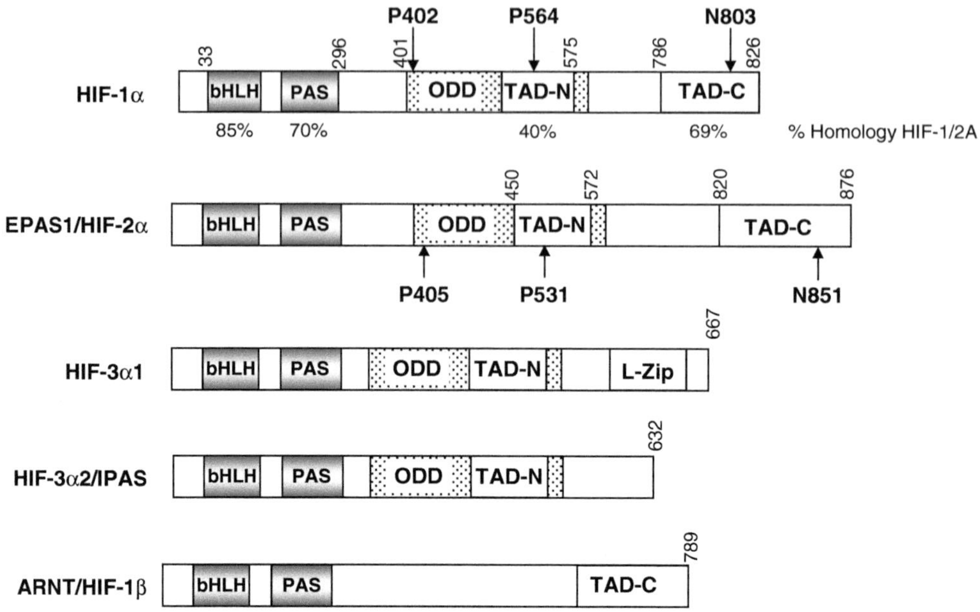

Fig. 3.1 Domain structures of HIF-1α, HIF-2α, HIF-3α and HIF-1β/ARNT. The HIF-α and HIF-β subunits are basic helix-loop-helix/Per-ARNT-Sim homology (bHLH/PAS) transcription factors. HIF-1α and HIF-2α contain two transactivation (TAD) domains, one at the amino terminal and the other at the carboxy terminal. Six splice versions of HIF-3α have been identified (only two are depicted here) and those that have been mapped contain only an N-TAD. HIF-1β/ARNT, the constitutive member of the HIF-1 heterodimer contains a C-TAD which is not required for HIF-1 transcriptional activity

protein in hypoxia (Koh et al. 2008c). However, it is well-known that hypoxia inhibits global protein translation by 20–70%, and the precise mechanism which allows sustained translation of HIF-1α as well as other stress proteins during hypoxia is unclear. Hypoxia-mediated inhibition of overall protein translation is controlled mainly by two distinct pathways that are regulated in a biphasic manner. The first pathway, the unfolded protein response (UPR) is activated rapidly by hypoxia, leading to phosphorylation of the eukaryotic initiation factor 2 (eIF2α) by PERK. This prevents the assembly of the 40S ribosome-binding eIF2-GTP-met-tRNA ternary complex required for initiation of translation. The second pathway, activated by prolonged hypoxia, inhibits the activity of the mammalian target of rapamycin (mTOR) that promotes protein synthesis by phosphorylating the inhibitory eukaryotic initiation factor 4E (eIF4E)-binding proteins (4E-BPs). Active mTOR phosphorylates 4E-BPs on multiple sites thus releasing eIF4E allowing it thus, to mediate the binding of the eIF4F complex to the 5' cap of the mRNA and engage in translation (Fig. 3.2).

Initially it was suggested that HIF-1α translation occurs through internal ribosome-entry-site (IRES) elements, which are RNA sequences that form secondary or tertiary structures and direct ribosome binding without the need for the eIF4F cap-binding complex. Several studies have reported that the 5'UTR of HIF-1α contains an IRES capable of promoting translation of a downstream reporter in bicistronic reporter assay (Lang et al. 2002; Zhou et al. 2004; Schepens et al. 2005). However, recent work convincingly disputes the role of IRES in HIF1-α translation, and suggests that the measured activity is due to cryptic

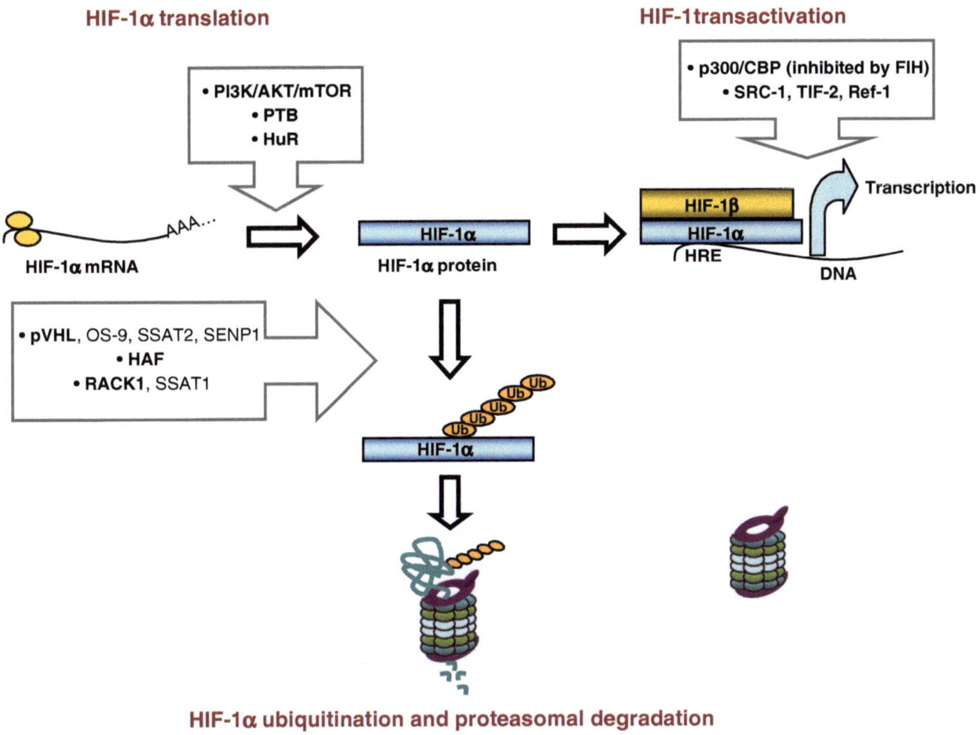

Fig. 3.2 Focal points of HIF-1 regulation. HIF-1α translation is regulated by the PI3K-AKT/mTOR pathway and the RNA binding proteins PTB and HuR. HIF-1α protein is degraded by the ubiquitin-proteasome system through either oxygen-dependent or oxygen-independent mechanisms. The mediators of HIF-1α degradation are pVHL (oxygen-dependent), HAF and RACK1 (oxygen-independent) which are themselves regulated by OS-9, SSAT2, SENP1, and SSAT1 as indicated. Stabilized HIF-1α enters the nucleus where it heterodimerizes with HIF-1β forming the HIF-1 transcription factor and initiating transcription of targets genes containing the HRE sequence. HIF-1 transactivating activity requires the cofactors p300/CBP through an interaction inhibiting by FIH. Other transcriptional cofactors recruited by HIF-1 are SRC-1, TIF-2, and Ref-1

promoter activity rather than IRES-mediated translation (Young et al. 2008; Bert et al. 2006).

The RNA-binding proteins polypyrimidine tract-binding protein (PTB) and HuR bind the HIF-1α 3'UTR and 5'UTR, respectively, and have also been proposed to enhance HIF-1α translation (Galban et al. 2008; Schepens et al. 2005). A role for calcium in the regulation of HIF-1α translation during hypoxia is receiving increased attention. Most cells respond to hypoxia with a sustained increase in cytoplasmic free calcium that results from the combined influx of extracellular calcium and the release of calcium present in the ER lumen (Seta et al. 2004). Studies addressing the role of calcium in the regulation of HIF-1α levels have been inconsistent with regard to the effect or the mechanism (Berchner-Pfannschmidt et al. 2004; Liu et al. 2007b; Hui et al. 2006; Liu et al. 2004; Metzen et al. 1999; Mottet et al. 2002; Salnikow et al. 2002; Werno et al. 2008; Zhou et al. 2006). This reflects the complexity of calcium-dependent signaling which is involved in pathways regulating degradation, translation, and transcription of HIF-1α. Further studies are needed to define the role of calcium in HIF-1α regulation.

A recent study provides a new molecular mechanism for maintaining translation of HIF-2α in hypoxia (Zimmer et al. 2008). The authors showed that in normoxia, the iron-regulatory protein 1 (IRP1) binds to an iron-responsive element (IRE) within the 5'UTR of HIF2α mRNA and represses HIF-2α translation. Hypoxia induces posttranslational changes in IRP1 that impair its ability to bind IRE, allowing translation of HIF-2α. The authors also identified small-molecule inhibitors that selectively decrease HIF-2α translation by enhancing the binding of IRP1 to IRE. Interestingly, the IRP1 mechanism does not appear to contribute to translation of HIF-1α in hypoxia despite the presence of a putative IRE sequence within the 5'UTR of HIF-1α (Zimmer et al. 2008).

Phosphorylation of eIF2α may allow preferential translation of stress proteins such as HIF-1α by creating a shift in translation, referred to as "translational reprogramming" (Ron and Walter 2007). This mechanism proposes that eIF2α phosphorylation allows resetting of the translational machinery by liberating ribosomes and translation factors from their binding to preexisting mRNA (Harding et al. 2000). Thus, HIF-1α mRNA is able to compete more effectively for the limited number of translation factors present in hypoxia, possibly through its binding to PTB and HuR (Galban et al. 2008; Schepens et al. 2005).

mTOR has been implicated as contributing to HIF-1α accumulation in both normoxia and hypoxia (Bernardi et al. 2006; Brugarolas et al. 2004; Hudson et al. 2002; Majumder et al. 2004). The mechanism that may allow translation of HIF-1α in cancer cells is through accumulation of mutations in pathways regulating mTOR activity that bypass the hypoxia-mediated mTOR inhibition. For example, loss of the tumor suppressor PTEN leads to activation of the PI3K/AKT pathway, and is associated with the induction of mTOR-dependent HIF-1α translation (Zundel et al. 2000). Another study has shown that growth of AKT-dependent prostate intraepithelial neoplasia requires mTOR-dependent activation of HIF-1α, and that clinical resistance to mTOR inhibitors may emerge through upregulation of HIF-1α activity (Majumder et al. 2004). Also, loss of the VHL gene has been found to sensitize kidney cancer cells to the mTOR inhibitor CCI-779 and correlated with inhibition of HIF-1α translation (Thomas et al. 2006). Another example of mutation that promotes HIF-1α translation was demonstrated in breast cancer where overexpressed 4E-BP1 and eIF4G function as a hypoxia-activated switch that facilitate cap-independent translation over cap-dependent translation of HIF-1α and other key proangiogenic and prosurvival mRNAs (Braunstein et al. 2007).

In addition, the antitumor activity of several mTOR inhibitors has been shown to be related to their ability to inhibit HIF-1α and its targets, again supporting the involvement of mTOR in HIF-1α translation in tumors. The antitumor activity of CCI-779 (temsirolimus, Wyeth) was attributed to its ability to inhibit HIF-1α and VEGF in both normoxia and hypoxia in the Her-2 amplified breast cancer cells, BT-747 (Del Bufalo et al. 2006), and to inhibition of mTOR/HIF-1α/VEGF pathway in human rhabdomyosarcoma xenografts (Wan et al. 2006). Similarly, the activity of another mTOR inhibitors RAD001 (everolimus, Novartis) was also shown to be dependent on HIF-1α (Majumder et al. 2004). Taken together, this information suggests that the continued translation of HIF-1α in hypoxia promotes tumorigenesis, and hence translation may be a promising therapeutic target.

3.3.2 Regulation of HIF-1α Degradation

Under aerobic conditions, HIF-1α is hydroxylated by specific prolyl hydroxylases (PHD1, PHD2, and PHD3) at two conserved proline residues (402 and 564) situated within its ODD domain in a reaction requiring oxygen, 2-oxoglutarate, and ascorbate (Jaakkola et al. 2001). A fourth PHD containing a transmembrane domain,

P4H-TM has recently been described (Koivunen et al. 2007). Under hypoxic conditions, PHD activity is inhibited, resulting in HIF-1α stabilization. In addition to the enzymatic inhibition of the PHDs, hypoxia causes perturbations in the mitochondrial electron transport chain, thus increasing the levels of cytoplasmic reactive oxygen species (ROS) which alters the oxidation state of Fe^{2+}, a cofactor for PHD activity, to Fe^{3+}, which cannot be utilized. This alteration inhibits PHD activity and promotes HIF-1α stabilization. Thus the disruption of mitochondrial function using either pharmacological or genetic inhibition/knockout of the mitochondrial electron transport chain prevents HIF-1α stabilization during hypoxia (Hagen et al. 2003; Simon 2006). In addition to mitochondrial-dependent mechanisms, the PHDs are subject to regulation by other factors including intracellular calcium concentration (Berchner-Pfannschmidt et al. 2004) and the Siah1 and Siah2 E3 ubiquitin ligases (Nakayama and Ronai 2004).

HIF-1α hydroxylation facilitates binding of pVHL to the HIF-1α ODD (Ohh et al. 2000). pVHL forms the substrate recognition module of an E3 ubiquitin ligase complex comprising elongin C, elongin B, cullin-2, and ring-box 1 (Rbx1), which directs HIF-1α poly-ubiquitylation and proteasomal degradation. The central role of pVHL in HIF-1α regulation is manifested in VHL disease where the inactivation of the *VHL* gene results in the development of highly vascularized tumors of the kidney, retina, and central nervous system (Kaelin 2007).

Although pVHL has been well established as the key player in the regulation of the ODD of HIF-1α, a number of alternative pathways have recently been described (Koh et al. 2008c). HIF-1α can be ubiquitylated and degraded in a manner mechanistically similar to the pVHL pathway through the binding of receptor of activated protein kinase C (RACK1) to HIF-1α. As RACK1 competes with Hsp90 for binding to HIF-1α, Hsp90 inhibitors such as 17-(Allylamino)-17-demethoxygeldanamycin (17-AAG) cause the oxygen-independent degradation of HIF-1α through RACK1 (Liu et al. 2007a). The hypoxia-associated factor (HAF) is a new E3 ligase specific for HIF-1α that causes HIF-1α ubiquitination and proteasomal degradation in an oxygen- and pVHL-independent manner (Koh et al. 2008a). HAF is the first HIF-1α specific E3 ligase to be identified, and may provide a mechanism for HIF-1α/HIF-2α isoform selectivity. The characterization of these novel modulators of HIF-1α degradation may provide novel approaches for HIF-1 inhibition.

3.3.3 Regulation of HIF-1 Transactivation

The transactivation activity of the HIF-1 heterodimer is mediated by the N-TAD and the C-TAD on the HIF-α subunit. Both the N-TAD and the C-TAD recruit the coactivators p300/CBP, SRC-1, and TIF-2 (Arany et al. 1996; Carrero et al. 2000). p300 and CBP are homologous transcriptional coactivators and are essential for linking HIF-1 and other transcription factors with coactivator complexes and the basal transcriptional machinery. p300/CBP, SRC-1, and TIF-2 have histone acetyltransferase activity allowing chromatin remodeling prior to transcription (Carrero et al. 2000; Lando et al. 2002). Although HIF-1β also contains a C-TAD, it appears to be dispensable for HIF-1 transcription activity. A key difference between the N-TAD and C-TAD is the oxygen-dependent regulation of the C-TAD. Under normoxic conditions, the ability of HIF-1α to activate transcription is prevented by another oxygen-regulated enzyme, factor inhibiting HIF-1 (FIH-1). FIH-1 hydroxylates asparagine 803 within the C-TAD of HIF-1α, disrupting its interaction with the transcription coactivators p300/CBP (Mahon et al. 2001). As with the PHDs, asparagine hydroxylation is inhibited under hypoxic conditions allowing the p300/CBP complex to bind to HIF-1α allowing HIF-1 transactivation.

3.4 Relationship Between HIF-1 and Other Key Oncogenic Pathways

3.4.1 HIF-1 Activation by Growth Factors

In addition to hypoxia-dependent regulation, HIF-1 may be activated by a wide range of growth-promoting stimuli and oncogenic pathways such as insulin, insulin-like growth factor-1, epidermal growth factor and mutant Ras, Src and/or PI-3K pathways (Brugarolas et al. 2004; Gray et al. 2005; Hudson et al. 2002; Zundel et al. 2000). Dysregulation of growth factors and/or their cognate receptors due to loss-of-function of tumor suppressor genes or activation of oncogenes may result in constitutive activation of HIF-1, such as through the PI3K/mTOR pathway (Zhong et al. 2000), or in increased HIF-1α activity through p42/p44 MAPK phosphorylation (Berra et al. 2000; Richard et al. 1999). Activation of these oncogenic pathways is associated with increased angiogenesis through HIF-1 activation (Jiang and Liu 2008).

3.4.2 Interplay Between HIF-1 and the p53 Tumor Suppressor

The p53 tumor suppressor is a transcription factor with an important role in the regulation of the cellular response to environmental stress and DNA damage (Giaccia and Kastan 1998). The p53 gene is one of the most frequently mutated genes in human cancer (Levine 1997). In normal, unstressed cells, p53 is present at low levels due to its association with MDM2, an E3-ubiquitin ligase that targets p53 for proteasomal degradation. Chronic hypoxia or anoxia may cause the upregulation of p53 through posttranslational modifications (including N-terminal phosphorylation) that disrupt the p53-MDM2 interaction, leading to p53 nuclear translocation and transactivation (An et al. 1998; Giaccia and Kastan 1998; Graeber et al. 1994). Hypoxia alone may be insufficient to induce p53 (Wenger et al. 1998) but may induce p53 accumulation when accompanied by acidosis and nutrient deprivation (Pan et al. 2004). Hypoxia-induced p53 protein is stabilized by a direct interaction with the ODD of HIF-1α, whereby one p53 dimer interacts with a single HIF-1α ODD domain. However, by binding to HIF-1α, p53 may also promote the ubiquitin-mediated degradation of HIF-1α via recruitment of MDM2 (Ravi et al. 2000). Consequently, loss of p53 in tumor cells results in an increase in hypoxia-induced HIF-1α and augments HIF-1-dependent transactivation. p53 may also attenuate HIF-1α signaling by competing for binding to p300/CBP. Both HIF-1α and p53 bind to p300/CBP, which is required for full activity of both transactivators (Gu et al. 1997). The repression of HIF-1α transactivation or protein levels by p53 is supported by a significant correlation between HIF-1α levels and the presence of mutant p53, suggesting that increased HIF-1α in cancer may be due at least partly, to a loss of p53 function (Zhong et al. 1999). A further link between p53 and HIF-1α is mediated by pVHL. pVHL ubiquitinates and degrades HIF-1α under normoxic conditions. Under DNA-damaging conditions, pVHL has been shown to physically associate with p53, thus stabilizing and transactivating p53, ATM, and p300 (Roe et al. 2006). Hence pVHL-deficient renal carcinoma cells (RCC), in addition to increased HIF-1 activity, also exhibit attenuated p53 activation in response to DNA damage.

3.4.3 Interplay Between HIF-1 and Myc

Myc is a transcription factor that heterodimerizes with Myc-associated protein (Max) to regulate a large number of processes important for normal biology and tumorigenesis such as growth, differentiation, apoptosis, and metabolism

(Adhikary and Eilers 2005). The Myc transcription factors contribute to almost every aspect of tumor cell biology and aberrantly high and/or deregulated Myc activity has been implicated causally in the majority of cancers (Adhikary and Eilers 2005; Shchors and Evan 2007). Myc regulates its many target genes by either promoting or inhibiting transcription. In certain scenarios, HIF-1α can act by displacing Myc from binding to its promoter. For example, hypoxia-induced HIF-1α increases the expression of the cyclin-dependent kinase inhibitors (CKIs) $p21^{cip1}$ and $p27^{kip1}$ by displacing the inhibitory Myc from their promoters (Koshiji et al. 2004). Myc displacement by HIF-1α has also been shown to account for repression of Myc activated genes including genes *hTERT* and *BRCA1*, the DNA repair genes *MSH2*, *MSH6*, and *NBS1* and the cell-cycle gene *CDC25A* (Huang 2008; Koshiji et al. 2004). Intriguingly, in contrast to the Myc-antagonizing properties of HIF-1α, HIF-2α, can enhance Myc activity by stimulating its interaction with Max (Gordan et al. 2007). Hence, HIF-2α overexpression promotes tumorigenesis in pVHL-deficient RCC, while HIF-1α inhibits RCC growth. However, both HIF-α isoforms can also act in concert to inhibit the Myc-activated gene *PPARGC1B* (encoding PGC-1β) important in mitochondria biogenesis by transcriptionally activating Mxi1, a protein that competes with Myc for binding to Max (Corn et al. 2005). Additionally severe or prolonged hypoxia results in Myc degradation via the ubiquitin-proteasome pathway in a HIF-α dependent but Mxi1-independent manner (Zhang et al. 2007). To add to the complexity, HIF-1α can also cooperate with Myc in cancer settings to enhance the expression of shared target genes such as those involved in glycolysis (*HK2*, *PDK1*) and angiogenesis (*VEGFA*) (Kim et al. 2007). Hence, although Myc may function as a critical hub for the control of normal cellular growth and proliferation, it appears that under hypoxic conditions, its activities can be usurped by HIF-α for tumor-cell adaptation and survival (Dang et al. 2008).

3.5 Hypoxia and HIF-1 Effects on Cancer Stem Cells

A new concept of "cancer stem cells" has emerged over the past 10 years (Pardal et al. 2003) defined as a subset population of cancer cells endowed with extensive potential for cell division. Experimentally, it has been shown that cancer stem cells have an increased potential to form tumors and only relatively few cells are required to initiate tumors in mice. How cells acquire properties such as self-renewal potential that turn them into cancer stem cells can in some cases be explained by mutational transformation of either normal stem cells or differentiated cells (Takahashi and Yamanaka 2006). Another theory suggests that hypoxia, through activation of HIF-1α and HIF-2α, contributes by activating pathways that induce dedifferentiation of cancer cells, maintenance of stem cell identity, and increased metastatic potential (Barnhart and Simon 2007). For example, HIF-1α stabilizes Notch1, which maintains the undifferentiated state, and induces lysyl oxidase (LOX) and matrix metalloproteases (MMP) that are important for invasive and metastatic phenotypes. HIF-2α, on the other hand, induces the expression of OCT-4, one of the most important stem cell maintenance factors, and enhances the activity of c-Myc which increases proliferation. Thus, despite being mostly speculative at this stage, the idea that hypoxia, through HIF-1/2α, may impact specific pathways supporting stem cell maintenance is highly intriguing and holds promise for future novel therapies.

3.6 HIF-1 as a Cancer Drug Target

HIF-1 provides a major defense against hypoxic stress in the growing tumor by increasing the expression of survival genes. However, the fact that HIF-1 also increases the expression of proapoptotic genes such as BNIP3, BNIP3L (NIX) (Bruick 2000; Sowter et al. 2001), RTP801(DDIT4) (Shoshani et al. 2002) and Noxa (Kim et al. 2004) has raised the question of whether HIF-1α is a good target for chemotherapy because inhibition of the proapoptotic effects of hypoxia could conceivably lead to increased tumor growth (Patiar and Harris 2006). It is well known that anoxia or severe and prolonged hypoxia induces apoptotic death in cells (Brown and Giaccia 1998). This is likely to occur in areas of the tumor where blood vessels are compressed or obstructed by tumor cells. However, the type of hypoxia that has been observed within tumors appears to be less severe due to the abnormal architecture and blood-flow dynamics of tumor vasculature that leads to cycles of vasoconstriction and dilation, and periods of poor perfusion (Nordsmark et al. 1996; Thomlinson and Gray 1955). Thus, under the levels of hypoxia found within tumors, HIF-1-induced proapoptotic genes may play little role in inducing apoptotic cell death. Indeed, the overwhelming evidence is that the antiapototic effects of HIF-1 outweigh any proapoptotic effects and that HIF-1 expression increases tumor growth. Studies with HIF-1α null knockout immortalized murine embryonic fibroblasts (MEFs) (Ryan et al. 2000; Unruh et al. 2003), CHO cells with mutagen-induced loss of HIF-1α (Williams et al. 2002) and human colon tumor cells with deleted HIF-1α (Dang et al. 2006) have all shown decreased tumor growth with increased apoptosis when injected into mice. The ability of antisense RNA (Chang et al. 2006; Sun et al. 2001; Sun et al. 2003), RNAi (Li et al. 2005), and dominant negative HIF-1α (Chen et al. 2003) to inhibit tumor growth in animal models also suggest that the cell survival effects of HIF-1 outweigh its apoptotic effects. There are, however, a few reports that HIF-1α inhibition may stimulate tumor growth. Murine embryonic stem (ES) cells with deleted HIF-1α injected into mice were reported to form tumors and after several weeks delay, shown to grow faster and show decreased apoptosis compared to tumors from wild type cells (Carmeliet et al. 1998). However, this could not be confirmed in another study where ES HIF-1α null cells formed tumors that grew more slowly and had increased apoptosis (Ryan et al. 1998). Human HIF-1α deficient transformed astrocytes injected subcutaneously into mice have been reported to form tumors with poor vascularization and slower growth than wild type astrocytomas. However, when the same cells were injected intracranially, the HIF-1α deficient astrocytomas were highly vascularized and grew faster than wild type astrocytomas (Blouw et al. 2003), although apoptosis was similar in both HIF-1α and wild type tumors. A study with A549 human non small cell lung cancer cells overexpressing HIF-1α also reported slower growth together with increased apoptosis compared to empty vector transfected control tumors, although this occurred despite increased angiogenesis in the HIF-1α transfected tumors (Savai et al. 2005). It is noteworthy that A549 tumors have only low levels of HIF-1α and VEGF, and their growth does not respond to HIF-1α inhibition, suggesting that A-549 is a tumor where HIF-1α is not critical for angiogenesis and tumor growth (Jordan et al. 2005). Thus, except for the limited examples given here, there is overwhelming evidence that HIF-1α is a rational and an exciting target for anticancer drug discovery.

3.7 HIF-1 Inhibitors

The relative ease of cell-based screening for inhibitors of HIF-1 transcriptional activity typically using an HRE-fluorescent or chemiluminescent reporter under conditions where HIF-1α is elevated, such as by hypoxia or artificially with a chemical inhibitor of HIF-1α degradation such as cobalt chloride or desferrioxamine, has led to the identification of a number of HIF-1 inhibitors (reviewed in (Melillo 2007; Patiar and Harris 2006; Powis and Kirkpatrick

2004; Semenza 2007)). Although such screens provide little information on the mechanism of HIF-1 inhibition, follow-up studies have identified potential mechanisms for the inhibition of transcription by the CDK inhibitor flavopiridol (Newcomb et al. 2005), inhibition of translation by temsirolimus, an inhibitor of mTOR (Del Bufalo et al. 2006), increased HIF-1α degradation by Hsp90 inhibitors (Hur et al. 2002; Isaacs et al. 2002; Kurebayashi et al. 2001), and by SCH6636, a farnesyl transferase inhibitor (Han et al. 2005), inhibition of growth factor-induced HIF-1 signaling by imatinib, a BCR-ABL, c-Kit inhibitor (Mayerhofer et al. 2002), by the EGF receptor small molecule inhibitors imatinib and erlotinib (Pore et al. 2006) and the EGF receptor monoclonal antibody cetuximab (Luwor et al. 2005). Specific screens have also identified agents that inhibit the interaction of HIF-1α with p300 (Kung et al. 2004). However, for most of the agents, the ability to inhibit tumor HIF-1 transcriptional activity in an in vivo setting has not been demonstrated. Agents that have been shown to inhibit tumor HIF-1α are listed in Table 3.2, and those that have antitumor activity in animal models are described below.

YC-1 [3-(5′-hydroxymethyl-2-furyl)-1-benzyl indazole] was developed as an activator of soluble guanyl cyclase for treating circulatory disorders caused by platelet aggregation and vascular contraction. It was also found to decrease HIF-1α levels in vitro (Chun et al. 2001) and in tumors (Yeo et al. 2003). YC-1 has been reported to accelerate HIF-1α degradation (Kim et al. 2006), to inhibit PI-3K/AKT/mTor mediated HIF-1α synthesis (Sun et al. 2007) and most recently, to stimulate the FIH-dependent dissociation of p300 from HIF-1α (Li et al. 2008). Although used experimentally, a clinical application for YC-1 as an antitumor agent remains in doubt because of its potential for increasing bleeding time, to cause hypotension and to act as an erectogenic (Chun et al. 2004).

Topotecan, a cytotoxic agent that causes DNA replication-mediated DNA damage through its action as a topoisomerase poison and approved for clinical use in lung and ovarian cancer, was identified as an inhibitor of HIF-1 activity in a cell-based screen (Rapisarda et al. 2002). It was subsequently shown to be an inhibitor of HIF-1α translation through a topoisomerase dependent mechanism (Rapisarda et al. 2004a). When administered on a daily schedule to mice with human glioma tumor xenografts, topotecan inhibited tumor growth, accompanied by decreased tumor HIF-1α expression and angiogenesis (Rapisarda et al. 2004b). Based on these results, topotecan is being tested in a pilot study in patients with advanced malignancies to determine if it inhibits HIF-1α in patients with tumor over-expressing HIF-1α (Melillo et al. 2007). If HIF-1α inhibition can be confirmed, it will still have to be demonstrated that this contributes to the antitumor activity of topotecan.

It is worth noting that a number of histone deacetylase (HDAC) inhibitors, particularly those targeting Class I and II HDACs, decrease HIF-1α levels in cells (Liang et al. 2006). It is generally accepted that a major function of HDAC inhibitors is to decrease tumor angiogenesis by inhibiting the formation of proangiogenic factors such as VEGF (Kim et al. 2001; Mie Lee et al. 2003). This has led to the assumption that it is inhibition of HIF-1 that is responsible for this effect (Liang et al. 2006). The mechanism responsible for this activity is a subject of debate, but may involve pVHL and p53 independent HIF-1α destabilization and proteasomal degradation. This could be due to either direct HIF-1α acetylation (Kim et al. 2001) or a mechanism involving Hsp90 acetylation (Liang et al. 2006). HDAC inhibitors could also repress HIF-1 transactivating activity by targeting the HIF-1α/p300 complex (Fath et al. 2006). However, what is lacking is the clear demonstration that HDAC inhibitors at doses that inhibit tumor growth also lower tumor HIF-1α levels or decrease HIF-1 transactivating activity. In two early studies of the HDAC inhibitors trichostatin A (Kim et al. 2001) and FK228 (Mie Lee et al. 2003), HIF-1α levels appear to be increased or unchanged in tumors on drug treatment.

3

Table 3.2 Compounds reported to inhibit HIF-1α

Compound	Mechanism of HIF inhibition	Reference
Hsp90 inhibitors		
17AAG	Degradation	(Isaacs et al. 2002)
Radicicol	DNA binding	(Hur et al. 2002)
KF58333 (radicicol analog)	Degradation	(Kurebayashi et al. 2001)
Topoisomerase inhibitors		
Topotecan (topoisomerase 1)	Translation	(Rapisarda et al. 2002; Rapisarda et al. 2004a)
GL331 (toposiomerase 2)	Transcription	(Chang et al. 2003)
Antimicrotubule		
Taxol	Translation	(Mabjeesh et al. 2003)
Vincristine	Translation	(Mabjeesh et al. 2003)
2ME2	Translation	(Mabjeesh et al. 2003)
HDAC inhibitors		
Trichostatin A	Degradation/transactivation	(Fath et al. 2006; Kong et al. 2006)
FK228	Transcription	(Mie Lee et al. 2003)
mTOR inhibitors		
Temsirolimus (CCI779)	Translation	(Del Bufalo et al. 2006; Wan et al. 2006)
Everolimus (RAD001)	Translation	(Majumder et al. 2004)
Thioredoxin inhibitors		
PX-12	Unknown	(Welsh and Powis 2003)
Pleurotin	Unknown	(Welsh and Powis 2003)
PX-916 (TXN reductase I)	Unknown	(Powis et al. 2006)
Soluble guanyl cyclase stimulator		
YC-1	Degradation/transactivation	(Yeo et al. 2003)
Farnesyl transferase inhibitor		
SCH66336	Degradation	(Han et al. 2005)
Growth factor signaling inhibitors		
Imatinib (BCR-ABL, c-Kit)	Translation/ Other	(Litz and Krystal 2006)
Erlotinib, gefitinib (EGFR)	Translation	(Pore et al. 2006)
Cetuximab (EGFR)	Translation	(Luwor et al. 2005)
Other		
Chetomin	Transactivation	(Kung et al. 2004)
PX-478	Translation/other	(Koh et al. 2008b; Welsh et al. 2004)

A more exhaustive list of compounds has been provided elsewhere (Melillo 2007; Powis and Kirkpatrick 2004)

2-Methoxyestradiol (2ME2) is an antiproliferative and antiangiogenic estrogen metabolite with weak estrogen receptor-binding activity (Sutherland et al. 2007). 2ME2 has been reported to have a number of effects which could account for its biological activity, including oxidative stress associated with inhibition of superoxide dismutase and increased production of nitric oxide and binding to tubulin to cause microtubule disruption and mitotic arrest (reviewed in (Sutherland et al. 2007)). 2ME2 has also been identified as an inhibitor of HIF-1α translation and nuclear translocation (Mabjeesh et al. 2003). It is noteworthy that other microtubule agents destabilizing agents such as *Vinca* alkaloids and colchicine-like compounds, as well as microtubule stabilizing agents such as taxanes and epothilones, have also been reported to inhibit HIF-1α expression (Escuin et al. 2005). 2ME2 has been reported to lower HIF-1α protein in an animal human orthotopic human glioblastoma model (Kang et al. 2006) and is currently in Phase II clinical trials. It may be difficult to separate HIF-1α inhibitory activity from 2ME2's other effects in relation to its antitumor activity.

Chetomin, a dithiodiketopiperazine fungal metabolite, was identified in a high-throughput screen of over half a million natural and synthetic compounds for inhibitors of the interaction of HIF-1α with p300 that regulates HIF-1 transcriptional activity (Kung et al. 2004). Chetomin also disrupts the binding of other proteins to p300, including HIF-2α and STAT2, indicating that it is a nonspecific inhibitor of transcription. When administered intravenously to mice with tumor xenografts, chetomin was shown to inhibit the interaction of HIF-1α and p300, and to block HIF-1 transcriptional activity and downstream gene expression. Significant antitumor activity was also seen against HCT-116 colon and PC-3 prostate tumor xenografts. Unfortunately, local toxicity at the site of intravenous injection limited the amount of chetomin that could be administered and whether it will be pursued as an antitumor agent is in doubt.

The small redox protein thioredoxin, which is found in high levels in many human tumors, has been reported to increase HIF-1α protein levels in hypoxic cells by an unknown mechanism (Welsh et al. 2002). The thioredioxin inhibitor PX-12 (1-methylpropyl-2-imidazoly disulfide) has been found to decrease HIF-1α protein levels, HIF-1 transactivating activity and downstream gene expression, including *VEGF* in cells and in tumor xenografts in mice (Jordan et al. 2005; Welsh et al. 2004). PX-12 is currently in Phase I/II clinical trial as an antitumor agent, but whether HIF-1α inhibition contributes to its activity remains to be determined. An inhibitor of thioredoxin reductase, PX-916, a water-soluble prodrug of the naphthoquinone spiroketal fungal metabolite palmarumycin CP1, has also shown the ability to decrease HIF-1α and VEGF protein levels,in tumor xenografts in mice, and to cause growth inhibition in a number of tumor xenografts (Powis et al. 2006).

PX-478 (S-2-amino-3-[4'-*N,N*,-bis(chloroethyl)amino]-phenyl propionic acid *N*-oxide dihydrochloride) was identified through a screen for compounds that lowered cellular HIF-1α levels, HIF-1 transactivating activity and downstream gene expression through a process that is independent of oxygen, pVHL, or p53. The primary mechanism for lowering of HIF-1α protein by PX-478 appears to be inhibition of HIF-1α translation since HIF-1α translation is maintained in hypoxia, whereas translation of most proteins is inhibited. However, PX478 also decreases levels of HIF-1α mRNA and causes inhibition of HIF-1α deubiquitination (Koh et al. 2008b). PX-478 administered intravenously or per orem to mice lowered HIF-1α levels in tumor xenografts and inhibited the expression of HIF-1 target genes *VEGF* and *GLUT-1*. PX-478 showed antitumor activity against a variety of established tumors with marked tumor regression accompanied by massive apoptosis, and in some cases cures (Jordan et al. 2005; Welsh et al. 2004). The antitumor response to PX-478 positively correlated with tumor HIF-1α levels. PX-478 is currently in Phase I clinical trial as an antitumor agent and HIF-1 inhibitor.

3.8 Conclusions

While a number of agents have been found to inhibit HIF-1α levels in cells, only a few agents have been demonstrated to inhibit HIF-1α or

HIF-1 activity in tumors in vivo. This has, however, been accompanied by antitumor activity that in some cases, is quite marked. In most cases the exact molecular target of the agent is not known. Some agents have properties or biological activities that preclude their use in humans. Of agents that are currently being tested in humans, some have other mechanisms of action that could more rationally account for their activity. For these agents it will be difficult, if not impossible, to determine whether HIF-1 inhibition contributes in any way to antitumor activity. In this regard, PX-478 is one agent that appears to show selective inhibition of HIF-1α. Thus, HIF-1 presents a novel target for cancer drug discovery and development and, while it is still early days, agents are being tested in the clinic that will show whether its preclinical potential as a target will be realized.

Aknowledgments Supported by NIH grants CA-0179094, CA095060, CA0179094 and CA109552.

References

Adhikary S, Eilers M (2005) Transcriptional regulation and transformation by Myc proteins. Nat Rev Mol Cell Biol 6:635–645

An WG, Kanekal M, Simon MC, Maltepe E, Blagosklonny MV, Neckers LM (1998) Stabilization of wild-type p53 by hypoxia-inducible factor 1alpha. Nature 392:405–408

Arany Z, Huang LE, Eckner R, Bhattacharya S, Jiang C, Goldberg MA, Bunn HF, Livingston DM (1996) An essential role for p300/CBP in the cellular response to hypoxia. Proc Natl Acad Sci U S A 93:12969–12973

Barnhart BC, Simon MC (2007) Metastasis and stem cell pathways. Cancer Metastasis Rev 26:261–271

Berchner-Pfannschmidt U, Petrat F, Doege K, Trinidad B, Freitag P, Metzen E, de Groot H, Fandrey J (2004) Chelation of cellular calcium modulates hypoxia-inducible gene expression through activation of hypoxia-inducible factor-1alpha. J Biol Chem 279:44976–44986

Bergers G, Benjamin LE (2003) Tumorigenesis and the angiogenic switch. Nat Rev Cancer 3:401–410

Bernardi R, Guernah I, Jin D, Grisendi S, Alimonti A, Teruya-Feldstein J, Cordon-Cardo C, Simon MC, Rafii S, Pandolfi PP (2006) PML inhibits HIF-1alpha translation and neoangiogenesis through repression of mTOR. Nature 442:779–785

Berra E, Milanini J, Richard DE, Le Gall M, Vinals F, Gothie E, Roux D, Pages G, Pouyssegur J (2000) Signaling angiogenesis via p42/p44 MAP kinase and hypoxia. Biochem Pharmacol 60:1171–1178

Bert AG, Grepin R, Vadas MA, Goodall GJ (2006) Assessing IRES activity in the HIF-1alpha and other cellular 5' UTRs. Rna 12:1074–1083

Blouw B, Song H, Tihan T, Bosze J, Ferrara N, Gerber HP, Johnson RS, Bergers G (2003) The hypoxic response of tumors is dependent on their microenvironment. Cancer Cell 4:133–146

Braunstein S, Karpisheva K, Pola C, Goldberg J, Hochman T, Yee H, Cangiarella J, Arju R, Formenti SC, Schneider RJ (2007) A hypoxia-controlled cap-dependent to cap-independent translation switch in breast cancer. Mol Cell 28:501–512

Bristow RG, Hill RP (2008) Hypoxia and metabolism. Hypoxia, DNA repair and genetic instability. Nat Rev Cancer 8:180–192

Brown JM, Giaccia AJ (1998) The unique physiology of solid tumors: opportunities (and problems) for cancer therapy. Cancer Res 58:1408–1416

Brugarolas J, Lei K, Hurley RL, Manning BD, Reiling JH, Hafen E, Witters LA, Ellisen LW, Kaelin WG Jr (2004) Regulation of mTOR function in response to hypoxia by REDD1 and the TSC1/TSC2 tumor suppressor complex. Genes Dev 18:2893–2904

Bruick RK (2000) Expression of the gene encoding the proapoptotic Nip3 protein is induced by hypoxia. Proc Natl Acad Sci U S A 97:9082–9087

Carmeliet P, Dor Y, Herbert JM, Fukumura D, Brusselmans K, Dewerchin M, Neeman M, Bono F, Abramovitch R, Maxwell P, Koch CJ, Ratcliffe P, Moons L, Jain RK, Collen D, Keshert E, Keshet E (1998) Role of HIF-1alpha in hypoxia-mediated apoptosis, cell proliferation and tumour angiogenesis. Nature 394:485–490

Carrero P, Okamoto K, Coumailleau P, O'Brien S, Tanaka H, Poellinger L (2000) Redox-regulated recruitment of the transcriptional coactivators CREB-binding protein and SRC-1 to hypoxia-inducible factor 1alpha. Mol Cell Biol 20: 402–415

Chang H, Shyu KG, Lee CC, Tsai SC, Wang BW, Hsien Lee Y, Lin S (2003) GL331 inhibits

HIF-1alpha expression in a lung cancer model. Biochem Biophys Res Commun 302:95–100

Chang Q, Qin R, Huang T, Gao J, Feng Y (2006) Effect of antisense hypoxia-inducible factor 1alpha on progression, metastasis, and chemosensitivity of pancreatic cancer. Pancreas 32:297–305

Chen J, Zhao S, Nakada K, Kuge Y, Tamaki N, Okada F, Wang J, Shindo M, Higashino F, Takeda K, Asaka M, Katoh H, Sugiyama T, Hosokawa M, Kobayashi M (2003) Dominant-negative hypoxia-inducible factor-1 alpha reduces tumorigenicity of pancreatic cancer cells through the suppression of glucose metabolism. Am J Pathol 162:1283–1291

Chun YS, Yeo EJ, Choi E, Teng CM, Bae JM, Kim MS, Park JW (2001) Inhibitory effect of YC-1 on the hypoxic induction of erythropoietin and vascular endothelial growth factor in Hep3B cells. Biochem Pharmacol 61:947–954

Chun YS, Yeo EJ, Park JW (2004) Versatile pharmacological actions of YC-1: anti-platelet to anticancer. Cancer Lett 207:1–7

Corn PG, Ricci MS, Scata KA, Arsham AM, Simon MC, Dicker DT, El-Deiry WS (2005) Mxi1 is induced by hypoxia in a HIF-1-dependent manner and protects cells from c-Myc-induced apoptosis. Cancer Biol Ther 4:1285–1294

Dang CV, Kim JW, Gao P, Yustein J (2008) The interplay between MYC and HIF in cancer. Nat Rev Cancer 8:51–56

Dang DT, Chen F, Gardner LB, Cummins JM, Rago C, Bunz F, Kantsevoy SV, Dang LH (2006) Hypoxia-inducible factor-1alpha promotes non-hypoxia-mediated proliferation in colon cancer cells and xenografts. Cancer Res 66:1684–1936

Del Bufalo D, Ciuffreda L, Trisciuoglio D, Desideri M, Cognetti F, Zupi G, Milella M (2006) Antiangiogenic potential of the Mammalian target of rapamycin inhibitor temsirolimus. Cancer Res 66:5549–5554

Escuin D, Kline ER, Giannakakou P (2005) Both microtubule-stabilizing and microtubule-destabilizing drugs inhibit hypoxia-inducible factor-1alpha accumulation and activity by disrupting microtubule function. Cancer Res 65: 9021–9028

Fath DM, Kong X, Liang D, Lin Z, Chou A, Jiang Y, Fang J, Caro J, Sang N (2006) Histone deacetylase inhibitors repress the transactivation potential of hypoxia-inducible factors independently of direct acetylation of HIF-alpha. J Biol Chem 281:13612–13619

Galban S, Kuwano Y, Pullmann R Jr, Martindale JL, Kim HH, Lal A, Abdelmohsen K, Yang X, Dang Y, Liu JO, Lewis SM, Holcik M, Gorospe M (2008) RNA-binding proteins HuR and PTB promote the translation of hypoxia-inducible factor 1alpha. Mol Cell Biol 28:93–107

Giaccia AJ, Kastan MB (1998) The complexity of p53 modulation: emerging patterns from divergent signals. Genes Dev 12:2973–2983

Giordano FJ, Johnson RS (2001) Angiogenesis: the role of the microenvironment in flipping the switch. Curr Opin Genet Dev 11:35–40

Gordan JD, Bertout JA, Hu CJ, Diehl JA, Simon MC (2007) HIF-2alpha promotes hypoxic cell proliferation by enhancing c-myc transcriptional activity. Cancer Cell 11:335–347

Graeber TG, Peterson JF, Tsai M, Monica K, Fornace AJ Jr, Giaccia AJ (1994) Hypoxia induces accumulation of p53 protein, but activation of a G1-phase checkpoint by low-oxygen conditions is independent of p53 status. Mol Cell Biol 14:6264–6277

Gray MJ, Zhang J, Ellis LM, Semenza GL, Evans DB, Watowich SS, Gallick GE (2005) HIF-1alpha, STAT3, CBP/p300 and Ref-1/APE are components of a transcriptional complex that regulates Src-dependent hypoxia-induced expression of VEGF in pancreatic and prostate carcinomas. Oncogene 24:3110–3120

Gu W, Shi XL, Roeder RG (1997) Synergistic activation of transcription by CBP and p53. Nature 387:819–823

Gu YZ, Moran SM, Hogenesch JB, Wartman L, Bradfield CA (1998) Molecular characterization and chromosomal localization of a third alpha-class hypoxia inducible factor subunit, HIF3alpha. Gene Expr 7:205–213

Hagen T, Taylor CT, Lam F, Moncada S (2003) Redistribution of intracellular oxygen in hypoxia by nitric oxide: effect on HIF1alpha. Science 302:1975–1978

Han JY, Oh SH, Morgillo F, Myers JN, Kim E, Hong WK, Lee HY (2005) Hypoxia-inducible factor 1alpha and antiangiogenic activity of farnesyltransferase inhibitor SCH66336 in human aerodigestive tract cancer. J Natl Cancer Inst 97:1272–1286

Harding HP, Novoa I, Zhang Y, Zeng H, Wek R, Schapira M, Ron D (2000) Regulated translation initiation controls stress-induced gene expression in mammalian cells. Mol Cell 6:1099–1108

Holmquist-Mengelbier L, Fredlund E, Lofstedt T, Noguera R, Navarro S, Nilsson H, Pietras A,

3

Vallon-Christersson J, Borg A, Gradin K, Poellinger L, Pahlman S (2006) Recruitment of HIF-1alpha and HIF-2alpha to common target genes is differentially regulated in neuroblastoma: HIF-2alpha promotes an aggressive phenotype. Cancer Cell 10:413–423

Hu CJ, Wang LY, Chodosh LA, Keith B, Simon MC (2003) Differential roles of hypoxia-inducible factor 1alpha (HIF-1alpha) and HIF-2alpha in hypoxic gene regulation. Mol Cell Biol 23:9361–9374

Huang LE (2008) Carrot and stick: HIF-alpha engages c-Myc in hypoxic adaptation. Cell Death Differ 15:672–677

Hudson CC, Liu M, Chiang GG, Otterness DM, Loomis DC, Kaper F, Giaccia AJ, Abraham RT (2002) Regulation of hypoxia-inducible factor 1alpha expression and function by the mammalian target of rapamycin. Mol Cell Biol 22:7004–7014

Hui AS, Bauer AL, Striet JB, Schnell PO, Czyzyk-Krzeska MF (2006) Calcium signaling stimulates translation of HIF-alpha during hypoxia. Faseb J 20:466–475

Hur E, Kim HH, Choi SM, Kim JH, Yim S, Kwon HJ, Choi Y, Kim DK, Lee MO, Park H (2002) Reduction of hypoxia-induced transcription through the repression of hypoxia-inducible factor-1alpha/aryl hydrocarbon receptor nuclear translocator DNA binding by the 90-kDa heat-shock protein inhibitor radicicol. Mol Pharmacol 62:975–982

Isaacs JS, Jung YJ, Mimnaugh EG, Martinez A, Cuttitta F, Neckers LM (2002) Hsp90 regulates a von Hippel Lindau-independent hypoxia-inducible factor-1 alpha-degradative pathway. J Biol Chem 277:29936–29944

Jaakkola P, Mole DR, Tian YM, Wilson MI, Gielbert J, Gaskell SJ, Kriegsheim A, Hebestreit HF, Mukherji M, Schofield CJ, Maxwell PH, Pugh CW, Ratcliffe PJ (2001) Targeting of HIF-alpha to the von Hippel-Lindau ubiquitylation complex by O2-regulated prolyl hydroxylation. Science 292:468–472

Jiang BH, Liu LZ (2008) PI3K/PTEN signaling in tumorigenesis and angiogenesis. Biochim Biophys Acta 1784:150–158

Jiang BH, Rue E, Wang GL, Roe R, Semenza GL (1996) Dimerization, DNA binding, and transactivation properties of hypoxia-inducible factor 1. J Biol Chem 271:17771–17778

Jordan BF, Runquist M, Raghunand N, Baker A, Williams R, Kirkpatrick L, Powis G, Gillies RJ (2005) Dynamic contrast-enhanced and diffusion MRI show rapid and dramatic changes in tumor microenvironment in response to inhibition of HIF-1alpha using PX-478. Neoplasia 7:475–485

Kaelin WG (2007) Von hippel-lindau disease. Annu Rev Pathol 2:145–173

Kang SH, Cho HT, Devi S, Zhang Z, Escuin D, Liang Z, Mao H, Brat DJ, Olson JJ, Simons JW, Lavallee TM, Giannakakou P, Van Meir EG, Shim H (2006) Antitumor effect of 2-methoxyestradiol in a rat orthotopic brain tumor model. Cancer Res 66:11991–11997

Kim HL, Yeo EJ, Chun YS, Park JW (2006) A domain responsible for HIF-1alpha degradation by YC-1, a novel anticancer agent. Int J Oncol 29:255–260

Kim JW, Gao P, Liu YC, Semenza GL, Dang CV (2007) Hypoxia-inducible factor 1 and dysregulated c-Myc cooperatively induce vascular endothelial growth factor and metabolic switches hexokinase 2 and pyruvate dehydrogenase kinase 1. Mol Cell Biol 27:7381–7393

Kim JY, Ahn HJ, Ryu JH, Suk K, Park JH (2004) BH3-only protein Noxa is a mediator of hypoxic cell death induced by hypoxia-inducible factor 1alpha. J Exp Med 199:113–124

Kim MS, Kwon HJ, Lee YM, Baek JH, Jang JE, Lee SW, Moon EJ, Kim HS, Lee SK, Chung HY, Kim CW, Kim KW (2001) Histone deacetylases induce angiogenesis by negative regulation of tumor suppressor genes. Nat Med 7:437–443

Koh MY, Darnay BG, Powis G (2008a) Hypoxia-associated factor, a novel E3-ubiquitin ligase, binds and ubiquitinates hypoxia-inducible factor 1alpha, leading to its oxygen-independent degradation. Mol Cell Biol 28:7081–7095

Koh MY, Spivak-Kroizman T, Venturini S, Welsh S, Williams RR, Kirkpatrick DL, Powis G (2008b) Molecular mechanisms for the activity of PX-478, an antitumor inhibitor of the hypoxia-inducible factor-1alpha. Mol Cancer Ther 7:90–100

Koh MY, Spivak-Kroizman TR, Powis G (2008c) HIF-1 regulation: not so easy come, easy go. Trends Biochem Sci 33(11):526–534

Koivunen P, Tiainen P, Hyvarinen J, Williams KE, Sormunen R, Klaus SJ, Kivirikko KI, Myllyharju J (2007) An endoplasmic reticulum transmembrane prolyl 4-hydroxylase is induced by hypoxia and acts on hypoxia-inducible factor alpha. J Biol Chem 282:30544–30552

Kong X, Lin Z, Liang D, Fath D, Sang N, Caro J (2006) Histone deacetylase inhibitors induce VHL and ubiquitin-independent proteasomal degradation of hypoxia-inducible factor 1alpha. Mol Cell Biol 26:2019–2028

Koshiji M, Kageyama Y, Pete EA, Horikawa I, Barrett JC, Huang LE (2004) HIF-1alpha induces cell cycle arrest by functionally counteracting Myc. Embo J 23:1949–1956
Kung AL, Zabludoff SD, France DS, Freedman SJ, Tanner EA, Vieira A, Cornell-Kennon S, Lee J, Wang B, Wang J, Memmert K, Naegeli HU, Petersen F, Eck MJ, Bair KW, Wood AW, Livingston DM (2004) Small molecule blockade of transcriptional coactivation of the hypoxia-inducible factor pathway. Cancer Cell 6:33–43
Kurebayashi J, Otsuki T, Kurosumi M, Soga S, Akinaga S, Sonoo H (2001) A radicicol derivative, KF58333, inhibits expression of hypoxia-inducible factor-1alpha and vascular endothelial growth factor, angiogenesis and growth of human breast cancer xenografts. Jpn J Cancer Res 92:1342–1351
Lando D, Peet DJ, Whelan DA, Gorman JJ, Whitelaw ML (2002) Asparagine hydroxylation of the HIF transactivation domain a hypoxic switch. Science 295:858–861
Lang KJD, Kappel A, Goodall GJ (2002) Hypoxia-inducible factor-1 contains an interna ribosome entry site that allows efficient translation during normoxia and hypoxia. Mol Biol Cell 13:1792–1801
Levine AJ (1997) p53, the cellular gatekeeper for growth and division. Cell 88:323–331
Li L, Lin X, Staver M, Shoemaker A, Semizarov D, Fesik SW, Shen Y (2005) Evaluating hypoxia-inducible factor-1alpha as a cancer therapeutic target via inducible RNA interference in vivo. Cancer Res 65:7249–7258
Li SH, Shin DH, Chun YS, Lee MK, Kim MS, Park JW (2008) A novel mode of action of YC-1 in HIF inhibition: stimulation of FIH-dependent p300 dissociation from HIF-1{alpha}. Mol Cancer Ther 7:3729–3738
Liang D, Kong X, Sang N (2006) Effects of histone deacetylase inhibitors on HIF-1. Cell Cycle 5:2430–2435
Litz J, Krystal GW (2006) Imatinib inhibits c-Kit-induced hypoxia-inducible factor-1alpha activity and vascular endothelial growth factor expression in small cell lung cancer cells. Mol Cancer Ther 5:1415–1422
Liu Q, Moller U, Flugel D, Kietzmann T (2004) Induction of plasminogen activator inhibitor I gene expression by intracellular calcium via hypoxia-inducible factor-1. Blood 104:3993–4001
Liu YV, Baek JH, Zhang H, Diez R, Cole RN, Semenza GL (2007a) RACK1 competes with HSP90 for binding to HIF-1alpha and is required for O(2)-independent and HSP90 inhibitor-induced degradation of HIF-1alpha. Mol Cell 25:207–217
Liu YV, Hubbi ME, Pan F, McDonald KR, Mansharamani M, Cole RN, Liu JO, Semenza GL (2007b) Calcineurin promotes hypoxia-inducible factor 1alpha expression by dephosphorylating RACK1 and blocking RACK1 dimerization. J Biol Chem 282:37064–37073
Luwor RB, Lu Y, Li X, Mendelsohn J, Fan Z (2005) The antiepidermal growth factor receptor monoclonal antibody cetuximab/C225 reduces hypoxia-inducible factor-1 alpha, leading to transcriptional inhibition of vascular endothelial growth factor expression. Oncogene 24:4433–4441
Mabjeesh NJ, Escuin D, LaVallee TM, Pribluda VS, Swartz GM, Johnson MS, Willard MT, Zhong H, Simons JW, Giannakakou P (2003) 2ME2 inhibits tumor growth and angiogenesis by disrupting microtubules and dysregulating HIF. Cancer Cell 3:363–375
Mahon PC, Hirota K, Semenza GL (2001) FIH-1: a novel protein that interacts with HIF-1alpha and VHL to mediate repression of HIF-1 transcriptional activity. Genes Dev 15:2675–2686
Majumder PK, Febbo PG, Bikoff R, Berger R, Xue Q, McMahon LM, Manola J, Brugarolas J, McDonnell TJ, Golub TR, Loda M, Lane HA, Sellers WR (2004) mTOR inhibition reverses Akt-dependent prostate intraepithelial neoplasia through regulation of apoptotic and HIF-1-dependent pathways. Nat Med 10:594–601
Makino Y, Kanopka A, Wilson WJ, Tanaka H, Poellinger L (2002) Inhibitory PAS domain protein (IPAS) is a hypoxia-inducible splicing variant of the hypoxia-inducible factor-3alpha locus. J Biol Chem 277:32405–32408
Maxwell PH, Pugh CW, Ratcliffe PJ (2001) Activation of the HIF pathway in cancer. Curr Opin Genet Dev 11:293–299
Mayerhofer M, Valent P, Sperr WR, Griffin JD, Sillaber C (2002) BCR/ABL induces expression of vascular endothelial growth factor and its transcriptional activator, hypoxia inducible factor-1alpha, through a pathway involving phosphoinositide 3-kinase and the mammalian target of rapamycin. Blood 100:3767–3775
Melillo G (2007) Targeting hypoxia cell signaling for cancer therapy. Cancer Metastasis Rev 26:341–352
Melillo G, Gutierrez M, Holkova B, Rapisarda A, Raffeld M, Horneffer Y, Chang R, Murgo AJ, Doroshow JH, Kummar S (2007) A pilot trial of topotecan administered orally in patients with

3

advanced solid tumors expressing hypoxia inducible factor (HIF)- 1alpha. J Clin Oncol 25:14103

Metzen E, Fandrey J, Jelkmann W (1999) Evidence against a major role for Ca2+ in hypoxia-induced gene expression in human hepatoma cells (Hep3B). J Physiol 517(Pt 3):651–657

Mie Lee Y, Kim SH, Kim HS, Jin Son M, Nakajima H, Jeong Kwon H, Kim KW (2003) Inhibition of hypoxia-induced angiogenesis by FK228, a specific histone deacetylase inhibitor, via suppression of HIF-1alpha activity. Biochem Biophys Res Commun 300:241–246

Mottet D, Michel G, Renard P, Ninane N, Raes M, Michiels C (2002) ERK and calcium in activation of HIF-1. Ann N Y Acad Sci 973:448–453

Nakayama K, Ronai Z (2004) Siah: new players in the cellular response to hypoxia. Cell Cycle 3:1345–1347

Newcomb EW, Ali MA, Schnee T, Lan L, Lukyanov Y, Fowkes M, Miller DC, Zagzag D (2005) Flavopiridol downregulates hypoxia-mediated hypoxia-inducible factor-1alpha expression in human glioma cells by a proteasome independent pathway: implications for in vivo therapy. Neuro Oncol 7:225–235

Nordsmark M, Hoyer M, Keller J, Nielsen OS, Jensen OM, Overgaard J (1996) The relationship between tumor oxygenation and cell proliferation in human soft tissue sarcomas. Int J Radiat Oncol Biol Phys 35:701–708

Ohh M, Park CW, Ivan M, Hoffman MA, Kim TY, Huang LE, Pavletich N, Chau V, Kaelin WG (2000) Ubiquitination of hypoxia-inducible factor requires direct binding to the beta-domain of the von Hippel-Lindau protein. Nat Cell Biol 2:423–427

Pan Y, Oprysko PR, Asham AM, Koch CJ, Simon MC (2004) p53 cannot be induced by hypoxia alone but responds to the hypoxic microenvironment. Oncogene 23:4975–4983

Pardal R, Clarke MF, Morrison SJ (2003) Applying the principles of stem-cell biology to cancer. Nat Rev Cancer 3:895–902

Patiar S, Harris AL (2006) Role of hypoxia-inducible factor-1alpha as a cancer therapy target. Endocr Relat Cancer 13(Suppl 1):S61–S75

Pore N, Jiang Z, Gupta A, Cerniglia G, Kao GD, Maity A (2006) EGFR tyrosine kinase inhibitors decrease VEGF expression by both hypoxia-inducible factor (HIF)-1-independent and HIF-1-dependent mechanisms. Cancer Res 66:3197–3204

Powis G, Kirkpatrick L (2004) Hypoxia inducible factor-1alpha as a cancer drug target. Mol Cancer Ther 3:647–654

Powis G, Wipf P, Lynch SM, Birmingham A, Kirkpatrick DL (2006) Molecular pharmacology and antitumor activity of palmarumycin-based inhibitors of thioredoxin reductase. Mol Cancer Ther 5:630–636

Rapisarda A, Uranchimeg B, Scudiero DA, Selby M, Sausville EA, Shoemaker RH, Melillo G (2002) Identification of small molecule inhibitors of hypoxia-inducible factor 1 transcriptional activation pathway. Cancer Res 62:4316–4324

Rapisarda A, Uranchimeg B, Sordet O, Pommier Y, Shoemaker RH, Melillo G (2004a) Topoisomerase I-mediated inhibition of hypoxia-inducible factor 1: mechanism and therapeutic implications. Cancer Res 64:1475–1482

Rapisarda A, Zalek J, Hollingshead M, Braunschweig T, Uranchimeg B, Bonomi CA, Borgel SD, Carter JP, Hewitt SM, Shoemaker RH, Melillo G (2004b) Schedule-dependent inhibition of hypoxia-inducible factor-1alpha protein accumulation, angiogenesis, and tumor growth by topotecan in U251-HRE glioblastoma xenografts. Cancer Res 64:6845–6848

Ravi R, Mookerjee B, Bhujwalla ZM, Sutter CH, Artemov D, Zeng Q, Dillehay LE, Madan A, Semenza GL, Bedi A (2000) Regulation of tumor angiogenesis by p53-induced degradation of hypoxia-inducible factor 1alpha. Genes Dev 14:34–44

Richard DE, Berra E, Gothie E, Roux D, Pouyssegur J (1999) p42/p44 mitogen-activated protein kinases phosphorylate hypoxia-inducible factor 1alpha (HIF-1alpha) and enhance the transcriptional activity of HIF-1. J Biol Chem 274:32631–32637

Roe JS, Kim H, Lee SM, Kim ST, Cho EJ, Youn HD (2006) p53 stabilization and transactivation by a von Hippel-Lindau protein. Mol Cell 22:395–405

Ron D, Walter P (2007) Signal integration in the endoplasmic reticulum unfolded protein response. Nat Rev Mol Cell Biol 8:519–529

Ryan HE, Lo J, Johnson RS (1998) HIF-1 alpha is required for solid tumor formation and embryonic vascularization. Embo J 17:3005–3015

Ryan HE, Poloni M, McNulty W, Elson D, Gassmann M, Arbeit JM, Johnson RS (2000) Hypoxia-inducible factor-1alpha is a positive factor in solid tumor growth. Cancer Res 60:4010–4015

Salnikow K, Kluz T, Costa M, Piquemal D, Demidenko ZN, Xie K, Blagosklonny MV (2002) The regulation of hypoxic genes by calcium involves c-Jun/AP-1, which cooperates with hypoxia-inducible factor 1 in response to hypoxia. Mol Cell Biol 22:1734–1741

Savai R, Schermuly RT, Voswinckel R, Renigunta A, Reichmann B, Eul B, Grimminger F, Seeger W, Rose F, Hanze J (2005) HIF-1alpha attenuates tumor growth in spite of augmented vascularization in an A549 adenocarcinoma mouse model. Int J Oncol 27:393–400

Schepens B, Tinton SA, Bruynooghe Y, Beyaert R, Cornelis S (2005) The polypyrimidine tract-binding protein stimulates HIF-1alpha IRES-mediated translation during hypoxia. Nucleic Acids Res 33:6884–6894

Semenza G (2002) Signal transduction to hypoxia-inducible factor 1. Biochem Pharmacol 64: 993–998

Semenza GL (2007) Evaluation of HIF-1 inhibitors as anticancer agents. Drug Discov Today 12: 853–859

Semenza GL (2004) Intratumoral hypoxia, radiation resistance, and HIF-1. Cancer Cell 5:405–406

Semenza GL (1999) Regulation of mammalian O_2 homeostasis by hypoxia-inducible factor 1. Annu Rev Cell Dev Biol 15:551–578

Semenza GL (2003) Targeting HIF-1 for cancer therapy. Nat Rev Cancer 3:721–732

Semenza GL, Wang GL (1992) A nuclear factor induced by hypoxia via de novo protein synthesis binds to the human erythropoietin gene enhancer at a site required for transcriptional activation. Mol Cell Biol 12:5447–5454

Seta KA, Yuan Y, Spicer Z, Lu G, Bedard J, Ferguson TK, Pathrose P, Cole-Strauss A, Kaufhold A, Millhorn DE (2004) The role of calcium in hypoxia-induced signal transduction and gene expression. Cell Calcium 36:331–340

Shchors K, Evan G (2007) Tumor angiogenesis: cause or consequence of cancer? Cancer Res 67:7059–7061

Shoshani T, Faerman A, Mett I, Zelin E, Tenne T, Gorodin S, Moshel Y, Elbaz S, Budanov A, Chajut A, Kalinski H, Kamer I, Rozen A, Mor O, Keshet E, Leshkowitz D, Einat P, Skaliter R, Feinstein E (2002) Identification of a novel hypoxia-inducible factor 1-responsive gene, RTP801, involved in apoptosis. Mol Cell Biol 22:2283–2293

Simon MC (2006) Mitochondrial reactive oxygen species are required for hypoxic HIF alpha stabilization. Adv Exp Med Biol 588:165–170

Sowter HM, Ratcliffe PJ, Watson P, Greenberg AH, Harris AL (2001) HIF-1-dependent regulation of hypoxic induction of the cell death factors BNIP3 and NIX in human tumors. Cancer Res 61:6669–6673

Sun HC, Qiu ZJ, Liu J, Sun J, Jiang T, Huang KJ, Yao M, Huang C (2007) Expression of hypoxia-inducible factor-1 alpha and associated proteins in pancreatic ductal adenocarcinoma and their impact on prognosis. Int J Oncol 30:1359–1367

Sun X, Kanwar JR, Leung E, Lehnert K, Wang D, Krissansen GW (2001) Gene transfer of antisense hypoxia inducible factor-1 alpha enhances the therapeutic efficacy of cancer immunotherapy. Gene Ther 8:638–645

Sun X, Kanwar JR, Leung E, Vale M, Krissansen GW (2003) Regression of solid tumors by engineered overexpression of von Hippel-Lindau tumor suppressor protein and antisense hypoxia-inducible factor-1alpha. Gene Ther 10:2081–2089

Sutherland TE, Anderson RL, Hughes RA, Altmann E, Schuliga M, Ziogas J, Stewart AG (2007) 2-Methoxyestradiol–a unique blend of activities generating a new class of anti-tumour/anti-inflammatory agents. Drug Discov Today 12:577–584

Takahashi K, Yamanaka S (2006) Induction of pluripotent stem cells from mouse embryonic and adult fibroblast cultures by defined factors. Cell 126:663–676

Thomas GV, Tran C, Mellinghoff IK, Welsbie DS, Chan E, Fueger B, Czernin J, Sawyers CL (2006) Hypoxia-inducible factor determines sensitivity to inhibitors of mTOR in kidney cancer. Nat Med 12:122–127

Thomlinson RH, Gray LH (1955) The histological structure of some human lung cancers and the possible implications for radiotherapy. Br J Cancer 9:539–549

Unruh A, Ressel A, Mohamed HG, Johnson RS, Nadrowitz R, Richter E, Katschinski DM, Wenger RH (2003) The hypoxia-inducible factor-1 alpha is a negative factor for tumor therapy. Oncogene 22:3213–3220

Vaupel P, Mayer A (2007) Hypoxia in cancer: significance and impact on clinical outcome. Cancer Metastasis Rev 26:225–239

Wan X, Shen N, Mendoza A, Khanna C, Helman LJ (2006) CCI-779 inhibits rhabdomyosarcoma xenograft growth by an antiangiogenic mechanism linked to the targeting of mTOR/Hif-1alpha/VEGF signaling. Neoplasia 8:394–401

Wang GL, Jiang BH, Rue EA, Semenza GL (1995) Hypoxia-inducible factor 1 is a basic-helix-loop-helix-PAS heterodimer regulated by cellular O2 tension. Proc Natl Acad Sci U S A 92:5510–5514

Welsh S, Williams R, Kirkpatrick L, Paine-Murrieta G, Powis G (2004) Antitumor activity and pharmacodynamic properties of PX-478, an inhibitor of

3

hypoxia-inducible factor-1alpha. Mol Cancer Ther 3:233–244
Welsh SJ, Bellamy WT, Briehl MM, Powis G (2002) The redox protein thioredoxin-1 (Trx-1) increases hypoxia-inducible factor 1alpha protein expression: Trx-1 overexpression results in increased vascular endothelial growth factor production and enhanced tumor angiogenesis. Cancer Res 62:5089–5095
Welsh SJ, Koh MY, Powis G (2006) The hypoxic inducible stress response as a target for cancer drug discovery. Semin Oncol 33:486–497
Welsh SJ, Powis G (2003) Hypoxia inducible factor as a cancer drug target. Curr Cancer Drug Targets 3:391–405
Wenger RH, Camenisch G, Desbaillets I, Chilov D, Gassmann M (1998) Up-regulation of hypoxia-inducible factor-1alpha is not sufficient for hypoxic/anoxic p53 induction. Cancer Res 58:5678–5680
Werno C, Zhou J, Brune B (2008) A23187, ionomycin and thapsigargin upregulate mRNA of HIF-1alpha via endoplasmic reticulum stress rather than a rise in intracellular calcium. J Cell Physiol 215:708–714
Wiesener MS, Jurgensen JS, Rosenberger C, Scholze CK, Horstrup JH, Warnecke C, Mandriota S, Bechmann I, Frei UA, Pugh CW, Ratcliffe PJ, Bachmann S, Maxwell PH, Eckardt KU (2003) Widespread hypoxia-inducible expression of HIF-2alpha in distinct cell populations of different organs. Faseb J 17:271–273
Williams KJ, Telfer BA, Airley RE, Peters HP, Sheridan MR, van der Kogel AJ, Harris AL, Stratford IJ (2002) A protective role for HIF-1 in response to redox manipulation and glucose deprivation: implications for tumorigenesis. Oncogene 21:282–290
Yeo EJ, Chun YS, Cho YS, Kim J, Lee JC, Kim MS, Park JW (2003) YC-1: a potential anticancer drug targeting hypoxia-inducible factor 1. J Natl Cancer Inst 95:516–525
Young RM, Wang SJ, Gordan JD, Ji X, Liebhaber SA, Simon MC (2008) Hypoxia-mediated selective mRNA translation by an internal ribosome entry site-independent mechanism. J Biol Chem 283: 16309–16319
Zhang H, Gao P, Fukuda R, Kumar G, Krishnamachary B, Zeller KI, Dang CV, Semenza GL (2007) HIF-1 inhibits mitochondrial biogenesis and cellular respiration in VHL-deficient renal cell carcinoma by repression of C-MYC activity. Cancer Cell 11:407–420
Zhong H, Chiles K, Feldser D, Laughner E, Hanrahan C, Georgescu MM, Simons JW, Semenza GL (2000) Modulation of hypoxia-inducible factor 1alpha expression by the epidermal growth factor/phosphatidylinositol 3-kinase/PTEN/AKT/FRAP pathway in human prostate cancer cells: implications for tumor angiogenesis and therapeutics. Cancer Res 60:1541–1545
Zhong H, De Marzo AM, Laughner E, Lim M, Hilton DA, Zagzag D, Buechler P, Isaacs WB, Semenza GL, Simons JW (1999) Overexpression of hypoxia-inducible factor 1alpha in common human cancers and their metastases. Cancer Res 59:5830–5835
Zhou J, Callapina M, Goodall GJ, Brune B (2004) Functional integrity of nuclear factor kappaB, phosphatidylinositol 3'-kinase, and mitogen-activated protein kinase signaling allows tumor necrosis factor alpha-evoked Bcl-2 expression to provoke internal ribosome entry site-dependent translation of hypoxia-inducible factor 1alpha. Cancer Res 64:9041–9048
Zhou J, Kohl R, Herr B, Frank R, Brune B (2006) Calpain mediates a von Hippel-Lindau protein-independent destruction of hypoxia-inducible factor-1alpha. Mol Biol Cell 17:1549–1558
Zimmer M, Ebert BL, Neil C, Brenner K, Papaioannou I, Melas A, Tolliday N, Lamb J, Pantopoulos K, Golub T, Iliopoulos O (2008) Small-molecule inhibitors of HIF-2a translation link its 5'UTR iron-responsive element to oxygen sensing. Mol Cell 32:838–848
Zundel W, Schindler C, Haas-Kogan D, Koong A, Kaper F, Chen E, Gottschalk AR, Ryan HE, Johnson RS, Jefferson AB, Stokoe D, Giaccia AJ (2000) Loss of PTEN facilitates HIF-1-mediated gene expression. Genes Dev 14:391–396

Chemokines

4

Andreas Hippe, Bernhard Homey, and Anja Mueller-Homey

Abstract Tumor growth is restricted to approximately 2 μm diameters by simple dissociation of nutrients and oxygen. Hence, tumors require the formation of new blood vessels for further growth progression. This process is referred to as tumor neo-angiogenesis. The process of tumor neo-angiogenesis is directed by complex bidirectional interactions between the tumor and the vessels, and creates a favorable microenvironment for angiogenesis. The tumor vessel system not only facilitates tumor growth by providing nutrients and oxygen but also functions as a convenient route for metastasis.

A group of small cytokine-like molecules called chemokines have been shown to participate in angiogenesis under homeostatic and neoplastic conditions. This review summarizes their role in tumor-associated angiogenesis.

B. Homey (✉)
Department of Dermatology,
Heinrich-Heine-University, Moorenstrasse 5,
40225, Düsseldorf, Germany
e-mail: Bernhard.Homey@uni-duesseldorf.de

4.1 Angiogenesis

The physiological process of blood vessel formation from preexisting microvasculature is referred to as angiogenesis. The process of angiogenesis has been reported to play an important role in both health and disease (Auerbach et al. 1976; Folkman 1995; Folkman and Shing 1992; Polverini 1995). The regulation of angiogenesis is dependent on the balance of angiogenic and angiostatic factors present in the microenvironment. Under homeostatic conditions, turnover of endothelial cells forming the vasculature is measured in months or years (Engerman et al. 1967; Tannock and Hayashi 1972). However, under conditions requiring rapid neo-vascularization such as wound healing, the balance between angiogenic and angiostatic factors in the microenvironment is rapidly shifted in favor of angiogenic factors, enabling the development of new vessels efficiently within days (Leibovich and Wiseman 1988). Such a predominance of angiogenic factors is transient and is followed by an equally rapid decline of these factors to achieve a steady state. Thus, under healthy conditions, the process of angiogenesis is controlled, fast, and transient, regressing back to a steady-state level (Strieter et al. 1995a). The termination of angiogenesis after wound healing is accomplished at

R. Liersch et al. (eds.), *Angiogenesis Inhibition,* Recent Results in Cancer Research,
DOI: 10.1007/978-3-540-78281-0_4, © Springer Verlag Berlin Heidelberg 2010

4

Table 4.1 Known chemokines, their synonyms, as well as their corresponding receptors are shown on the table

Name	Synonyms	Chemokine receptor	ELR-motif	Role in angiogenesis
CXC family				
CXCL1	Groα	CXCR2>CXCR1	+	Angiogenic
CXCL2	Groβ	CXCR2	+	Angiogenic
CXCL3	Groγ	CXCR2	+	Angiogenic
CXCL4	PF4	CXCR3B	–	Angiostatic
CXCL5	ENA-78	CXCR2	+	Angiogenic
CXCL6	GCP-2	CXCR1, CXCR2	+	Angiogenic
CXCL7	NAP-2	Unknown	+	Angiogenic
CXCL8	IL-8	CXCR1, CXCR2	+	Angiogenic
CXCL9	MIG	CXCR3, CXCR3B	–	Angiostatic
CXCL10	IP-10	CXCR3, CXCR3B	–	Angiostatic
CXCL11	I-TAC	CXCR3, CXCR3B	–	Angiostatic
CXCL12	SDF-1α/β	CXCR4, CXCR7	–	Angiogenic
CXCL13	BLC, BCA-1	Unknown	–	Angiostatic
CXCL14	BRAK, Bolekine	Unknown	–	
CXCL15	Unknown	Unknown	+	
CXCL16		CXCR6	–	
CXCL17	DMC	Unknown	–	
CC family				
CCL1	I-309	CCR8	–	Angiogenic
CCL2	MCP-1	CCR2	–	Angiogenic
CCL3	Mip-1α, LD78α	CCR1, CCR5	–	
CCL3L1	LD78β		–	
CCL3L3	LD78β		–	
CCL4	MIP-1β	CCR5	–	
CCL4L1	AT744.2		–	
CCL4L2			–	
CCL5	RANTES	CCR1, CCR3, CCR5	–	Angiogenic
CCL7	MCP-3	CCR1, CCR2, CCR3	–	
CCL8	MCP-2	CCR1, CCR2, CCR3, CCR5	–	
CCL11	Eotaxin	CCR3	–	Angiogenic
CCL13	MCP-4	CCR1, CCR2, CCR3	–	
CCL14	HCC-1	CCR1	–	
CCL15	HCC-2	CCR1, CCR3	–	Angiogenic
CCL16	HCC-4	CCR1, CCR2, CCR5	–	Angiogenic
CCL17	TARC	CCR4	–	
CCL18	DC-CK1, PARC	Unknown	–	
CCL19	MIP-3β, ELC	CCR7	–	
CCL20	MIP-3α, LARC	CCR6	–	
CCL21	SLC, 6Ckine	CCR7	–	Angiostatic
CCL22	MDC, STCP-1	CCR4	–	

Table 4.1 (continued)

Name	Synonyms	Chemokine receptor	ELR-motif	Role in angiogenesis
CCL23	MPIF-1	CCR1	–	Angiogenic
CCL24	Eotaxin-2	CCR3	–	
CCL25	TECK	CCR9	–	
CCL26	Eotaxin-3	CCR3	–	
CCL27	CTACK/ILC	CCR10	–	
CCL28	MEC	CCR10S	–	
C family			–	
XCL1	Lymphotactin, SCM-1α	XCR1	–	
XCL2	SCM-1β		–	
CX3C family			–	
CX3CL1	Fractalkine	CX3CR1	–	Angiogenic

The occurrence of the ELR-motif in CXC chemokines is listed, as well as any known angiogenic or angiostatic properties. If the entry under role in angiogenesis is left blank, the chemokine in question either has no or no known role in angiogenesis

two levels: (a) a reduction of angiogenic factors, and (b) an increase in expression of angiostatic molecules (Bouck 1990).

If this tightly controlled mechanism is defective, pathological conditions occur, as exemplified by aberrant angiogenesis during tumor progression or rheumatoid arthritis (Harris 1976).

4.2 Chemokines in Angiogenesis

Chemokines are a family of small (8–14 kDa) cytokine-like, mostly basic, structurally related molecules that are known to regulate leukocyte trafficking through interactions with G-protein-coupled receptors with seven transmembrane-spanning domains (Zlotnik and Yoshie 2000). Chemokines can be subdivided into four classes based on the alignment of the first two cysteine residues in their amino acid sequence. If the cysteines follow each other, the respective chemokine is part of the CC subgroup, whereas if the two cysteines are separated by one amino acid in between, then the respective chemokine is part of the CXC subgroup. In addition, there are two subgroups consisting of chemokines with only one residue (XC) or with three residues between the cysteines (CX3C) (Zlotnik and Yoshie 2000). A comprehensive listing of known chemokines, their receptors, and known roles in angiogenesis is summarized in Table 4.1.

4.2.1 CXC Chemokine Subfamily

First, the angiogenic potential of members of the CXC subfamily was identified. The CXC chemokines can be further subdivided based on the presence or absence of a three-amino-acid motif (Glu-Leu-Arg) present at the NH_2-terminus, namely the ELR-motif (Strieter et al. 1995b). Initially, CXC chemokines lacking an ELR-motif such as CXCL4 (PF4), CXCL9 (MIG), and CXCL10 (IP-10) were considered as angiostatic chemokines, whereas those CXC chemokines endowed with the ELR-motif such as CXCL1-3 (GRO-α-γ), CXCL5 (ENA-78), CXCL6 (GCP-2), CXCL7 (NAP-2), and CXCL8 (IL-8) were considered as angiogenic chemokines

(Belperio et al. 2000). The role of the motif as a structural domain for angiogenic activity was first demonstrated by a site-directed mutagenesis substitution of the motif. A switch of the ELR motif from CXCL8 to CXCL9 caused a shift in the angiogenic properties of these molecules both *in vitro* and *in vivo* (Strieter et al. 1995b). In addition, angiostatic interferons upregulated ELR-motif lacking angiostatic chemokines (Cole et al. 1998; Miller and Krangel 1992) and downregulated the expression of ELR-motif containing angiogenic chemokines (Strieter et al. 1995a). Analysis of chemokine–chemokine receptor interactions demonstrated that angiogenic ELR-motif containing chemokines bound to CXCR2. The angiostatic non-ELR-motif chemokines bound to CXCR3 instead, suggesting receptor-specificity to be responsible for effects on angiogenesis. Indeed, Martins-Green and Hanafusa demonstrated that CXCL12 (SDF-1), a chemokine lacking the motif, had angiogenic properties (Martins-Green and Hanafusa 1997). CXCL12 binds to CXCR4; therefore the more important factor contributing to the angiogenic property of a chemokine is receptor specificity. A typical example is the non-ELR-motif angiostatic chemokine CXCL4. Recently, Lasagni et al. demonstrated that CXCL4 along with CXCL9, 10, 11 bound to CXCR3-B (a splice variant of CXCR3) where as CXCL 9, 10, 11 bound to an another variant (CXCR3-A) (Lasagni et al. 2003). CXCR3-B and not CXCR3-A was specifically expressed by primary cultures of human microvascular endothelial cells (HMEC) and a treatment with CXCL4, 9, 10, 11 resulted in inhibition of growth, thus implicating not only CXCR3-B to be the angiostatic receptor but consequently CXCL4 to be an angiostatic chemokine by virtue of its receptor specificity (Lasagni et al. 2003).

The chemokine CXCL14 (BRAK) was first reported in 1999 by Hromas et al. It is a non-ELR-motif chemokine (Hromas et al. 1999) reported to induce chemotaxis in prostaglandin E_2-treated monocytes (Kurth et al. 2001), neutrophils, and dendritic cells (Cao et al. 2000), as well as cell lines from B-cell and monocytic cell lineages (Sleeman et al. 2000). In one report by Shellenberger et al., CXCL14 potently inhibited angiogenesis in vivo in a rat corneal micropocket assay (Shellenberger et al. 2004). The corresponding receptor for CXCL14 is still unknown and might present itself as another putative angiostatic CXC receptor.

4.2.2 CC Chemokine Subfamily

Recent findings indicate that CC chemokines, in addition to the CXC chemokine sub-family members, also modulate angiogenesis. (Yan et al. 2006). Out of the CC chemokine subfamily CCL1, 2, 11, 15, 16, 21, and 23 are involved under homeostatic, inflammatory, and neoplastic conditions (Bernardini et al. 2000; Goede et al. 1999; Hwang et al. 2004; Salcedo et al. 2001; Soto et al. 1998; Strasly et al. 2004). CCL2 induced migration of human endothelial cells (Salcedo et al. 2000) and exhibited an angiogenic potency similar to vascular endothelial growth factor (VEGF)-A (Goede et al. 1999). However, unlike angiogenesis induced by angiogenic factors such as VEGF, CCL2-mediated angiogenesis was also accompanied by macrophage recruitment (Goede et al. 1999). Hence, indirect effects might be involved as well.

CCL11, a ligand for the receptor CCR3, has been demonstrated to induce angiogenesis in vivo. In a study by Salcedo et al. HMEC migrated toward CCL11 (Salcedo et al. 2001). In rat aortic assays, matrigel plug assays, as well as chicken chorian allantois membrane (CAM) assays, CCL11 was able to induce vascularization (Salcedo et al. 2001). Additionally, CCL15, which also binds to CCR3, induced angiogenic effects (Hwang et al. 2004). This effect was stronger when using a truncated form of CCL15, which consisted of the amino acids 25–92 of full-length CCL15 (Hwang et al. 2004). It promoted sprouting from rat aortic rings, as well as induced neovascularization in a chicken CAM assay (Hwang et al. 2004). Therefore, CCR3 is considered to be an angiogenic receptor.

An interesting case is presented by the CC chemokine CCL21. CCL21 differs from other CC chemokines, having six cysteines in its amino acid sequence rather than the four cysteines characterizing most of the CC chemokine family members (Hedrick and Zlotnik 1997). It is known for the recruitment of activated, matured dendritic cells and naive T cells to T cell zones of lymph nodes (Arenberg et al. 2001). Interestingly, it has been demonstrated that murine CCL21 is able to bind to CCR7 and CXCR3 (Soto et al. 1998), whereas human CCL21 can only bind to CCR7 (Jenh et al. 1999). Hence, murine CCL21 is able to act as an angiostatic chemokine, as demonstrated in a rat corneal micropocket assay in vivo (Soto et al. 1998). Contrary to mCCL21, human CCL21 was not able to bind to either human CXCR3 or murine CXCR3, as well as showing no effect on tumor growth, demonstrating that the angiostatic effect of CCL21 is caused by CXCR3 binding and is specific to the mouse model (Arenberg et al. 2001).

4.2.3 CX3C Chemokine Subfamily

CX3CL1 (Fractalkine) presents itself as a unique chemokine not only by being the sole member of the CX3C chemokine family, but also by its presence as a membrane-bound form as well as a cleaved soluble one (Fong et al. 2000). Inflammatory cytokines induce CX3CL1 expression on endothelial cells, and in the membrane-bound form, it is able to promote a robust adhesion of CX3CR1-expressing monocytes and T-lymphocytes (Imaizumi et al. 2004). By proteolytic cleavage, CX3CL1 enters a soluble state, acting as a chemotatic agent for monocytes and lymphocytes (Imaizumi et al. 2004). Recently, CX3CL1 has also been implicated to play a role in angiogenesis. It was found to be an angiogenic mediator in rheumatoid arthritis (Volin et al. 2001), as well as in ocular angiogenesis (You et al. 2007). CX3CL1/CX3CR1 interaction on endothelial cells activates the Raf-1/MEK/ERK- and PI3K/Akt/eNOS-dependent signal pathways (Lee et al. 2006). This induces hypoxia inducible factor 1α (HIF-1α), which in turn induces VEGF-A production, inducing angiogenesis via VEGF receptor 2 (Ryu et al. 2007).

4.3 Chemokine Receptor Repertoire of Endothelial Cells

For modulation of angiogenesis by chemokines, chemokine–chemokine receptor interaction is necessary. This necessity implicates the study of receptor repertoires of cells involved in angiogenesis. The typical vessel is comprised of an inner lining of endothelial cells and an outer layer of mural cells, which can be smooth muscle cells in larger vessels and pericytes in the microvasculature, divided by a basal membrane (Alberts et al. 2007). Both cell types play a role in angiogenesis. Since the mid-1990s, several studies were published investigating the presence of chemokine receptors on endothelial cells. These studies were reviewed in Bernardini et al. 2003, and demonstrated that HMEC expressed CXCR2, CXCR3, CXCR4, and CX3CR1 (Bernardini et al. 2003). HMECs of a dermal lineage were reported to additionally express CCR2 (Salcedo et al. 2000). There are two isoforms of CCR2, namely CCR2A and B, encoded in a single gene, created by alternative splicing (Charo et al. 1994). De Paepe and De Bleecker studied the expression of these two isoforms, demonstrating CCR2A as the most prominent endothelial CCR2 variant (De Paepe and De Bleecker 2005). Human umbilical vein endothelial cells (HUVEC) expressed only low levels of CXCR2 and CXCR3, while abundantly expressing CXCR4. Additionally, HUVECs expressed CXCR5, CCR2, CCR3, CCR4, and CCR8, which were not expressed on HMEC, but they lacked the HMEC receptor CX3CR1

(Bernardini 2003). Aortic endothelial cells were shown to express CXCR4, CCR2, CCR4, and CCR5 (Bernardini 2003).

Knockout of CXCR4 in mice demonstrated a prenatal lethal phenotype due to defects in development of arteries of the gastrointestinal tract as well as defects in vascular development and cardiogenesis (Tachibana et al. 1998). Similarly, CXCR2-deficient mice demonstrated impaired angiogenesis in the cornea in response to CXCR2-ligand-induced angiogenic activity (Addison et al. 2000). These observations emphasize the importance of both CXCR2 and CXCR4 in angiogenesis and organogenesis in vivo.

Despite this progress, there are several challenges and limitations in the identification of endothelial cell receptor repertoires. Three major concerns being, (a) differential expression of the aforesaid receptors in different endothelial cells of different origin in vitro, (b) faithfulness of model systems, and (c) expression in vivo. For instance, HUVEC (derived from umbilical vessels) are part of the macrocirculation, as described by Garlanda and Dejana (Garlanda and Dejana 1997), and hence may not be an ideal representative for cells involved in angiogenic processes. Similarly, most microvascular endothelial cells in culture are derived from both blood and lymphatic vessels, raising the issue of differences between these lineages of endothelial cells. These differences were observed by Kriehuber et al. after separation of podoplanin-positive lymphatic endothelial cells and podoplanin-negative blood endothelial cells from dermal cell suspensions. Besides podoplanin, LYVE-1 and VEGF-C receptor, among others, were found to be differentially expressed (Kriehuber et al. 2001). Currently, no data for the differential expression of chemokine receptors between lymphatic and blood endothelial cells have been reported. The expression data acquired to date mostly concentrates on cell line receptor expression. The few data on in vivo tissue expression showed that CXCR3 was on middle and large endothelial cells in vivo (Garcia-Lopez et al. 2001), while CXCR4 was expressed on aortic endothelium as well as on coronary vessels of the heart (Berger et al. 1999; Volin et al. 1998). Of the CC chemokine receptors, high CCR2a expression could be demonstrated on coronary vessels, while only low expression of CCR3 and 5 could be demonstrated on these cells (Berger et al. 1999).

Mural cells associated with the endothelial cell, for example, pericytes, have not yet been extensively studied for their chemokine receptor repertoire. Some studies reported chemokine receptor expression of pericytes, for example, CXCR3 was demonstrated to be functionally expressed (Bonacchi et al. 2001). Additionally, CXCR4 (Pablos et al. 1999) and CCR2 (Carulli et al. 2005) expression on pericytes was demonstrated.

4.4 Angiogenesis, Chemokines, and Cancer

Tumor-associated angiogenesis is dependent on several key factors to accomplish neovascularization. Microvascular endothelial and mural cells need to proliferate and sprout from preexisting microvasculature in a directional migration toward the tumor. Tumors therefore need to establish a favorable microenvironment (consisting of extracellular matrix and stromal cells, e.g., fibroblasts, endothelial cells, and leukocytes), which in turn influences the preexisting nearby microvasculature to change from a homeostatic condition to a migratory one. Tumor-associated chemokine production is an important event in forming the tumor microenvironment as it plays a key role in facilitating angiogenesis and attracting endothelial cells and leukocytes to the tumor (Belperio et al. 2000; Ben-Baruch 2003; Bernardini et al. 2003). The neo-vasculature of the tumor then (a) feeds the tumor mass and allows tumor growth and (b) presents an accessible route for metastasizing cells from the primary site to distant locations. Here we focus on three cancer types, namely breast cancer, malignant melanoma, and lung cancer, and summarize the current knowledge on chemokine-associated angiogenesis in these malignancies.

4.4.1 Breast Cancer

Breast cancer represents the leading cause of cancer-related deaths among women in developed countries (Parkin et al. 2005). Lack of estrogen receptor (ER) has been associated with a poor prognosis of the disease (Skoog et al. 1987). Interestingly, ER-negative breast cancer cells express CCL2 abundantly (Chavey et al. 2007). In xenomodels, immunodeficient mice infected with human MDA-MB 231 tumor cells show significantly inhibited formation of lung metastases following neutralization of CCL2. This decrease of metastatic dissemination was associated with decreased tumor angiogenesis in vivo (Salcedo et al. 2000). Interestingly, CCL2 expression of breast cancer cells was accompanied by the recruitment of tumor-associated macrophages (Chavey et al. 2007). These macrophages secreted TNF-α and in turn were able to stimulate breast cancer cells to express more CCL2 and 5, forming a vicious circle (Yaal-Hahoshen et al. 2006). Tumor-secreted CCL2 is therefore able to both stimulate angiogenesis and draw macrophages into the tumor. These tumor-associated macrophages are then able to modulate the microenvironment via their cytokine and growth factor expression to a tumor-favorable state. Similarly, CXCL8 expression was inversely correlated with the expression of ER in breast cancers (Freund et al. 2003). The CXCL8-expressing tumor cells not only demonstrated increased invasiveness into matrigel, but also when media-conditioned by CXCL8-expressing tumor cells matrigel was able to facilitate angiogenesis when injected subcutaneously into nude mice (Lin et al. 2004). Therefore, apart from CCL2, CXCL8 might also increase angiogenesis in breast tumors. Interestingly, CCL2 and CXCL8 expression was inversely correlated to ER expression (Chavey et al. 2007; Lin et al. 2004). Loss of ER in breast cancer cells is accompanied by poor prognosis and high risk of locoregional recurrence and distant metastases (Kyndi et al. 2008), giving evidence that an increase in angiogenic chemokine expression might increase the probability of metastasis formation.

4.4.2 Malignant Melanoma

Melanoma, a malignant tumor of melanocytes, is the main cause for skin-cancer-related deaths. The large variety of different chemokines expressed by melanoma cells is evidence for tumor-associated angiogenesis in this malignancy. Hs294T melanoma cell culture supernatants contained CXCL1, which induced autocrine growth stimulatory activity (Balentien et al. 1991; Richmond and Thomas 1986). CXCL1 mRNA was also reported to be constitutively expressed in cultured nevocytes and melanoma cells, but was undetectable in primary melanocytes (Bordoni et al. 1990). This change in expression from melanocytes to premalignant and malignant forms was identified to be dependent on NF-κB activation (Shattuck-Brandt and Richmond 1997). CXCL8 has been demonstrated to be constitutively expressed by melanoma cell lines in vitro, too. CXCL8 exhibited an autocrine effect on melanoma cells as inferred from the decrease of melanoma cell proliferation either by neutralizing CXCL8 by antibodies or by decreasing CXCL8 expression in melanoma cells by transfection of antisense oligonucleotides (Schadendorf et al. 1993). As expected, CXCR1 and CXCR2 expression (the chemokine receptors of CXCL8) could be identified on melanoma cells in tissue sections by immunohistochemistry

(Varney et al. 2006). Interestingly, CXCR2 expression was more abundant in Clark level III to V specimens, than in Clark level I–II specimens. In contrast, CXCR1 expression was ubiquitously detected in the majority of analyzed specimens (Varney et al. 2006). Therefore, autocrine stimulation of melanoma cells by CXCL8, which enhances proliferation, might be dependent on CXCR2 signaling, as more advanced stages of melanoma express more CXCR2. In addition, CXCL8 expression by melanoma cells enhanced angiogenesis. Increased proliferation of endothelial cells was observed during both in vitro and in vivo vessel formation assays using matrigel plugs containing conditioned media of M14 melanoma cells, which was enriched with CXCL8 (Giorgini et al. 2007). Furthermore, the importance of the tumor microenvironment for tumor progression and angiogenesis could be observed in melanoma. Metastatic human melanoma cells harvested from subcuteanous areas expressed CXCL8 much more abundantly than metastases from liver. Subcutaneous metastases lost their abundant CXCL8 expression when reinjected and reharvested from liver lesions. This could be reproduced in coculture experiments of melanoma cells with either keratinocytes or hepatocytes. Paracrine induction of CXCL8 in melanoma cells by keratinocyte-derived IL-1 was observed to be the reason for high levels of CXCL8, while hepatocyte-derived TGF-β was responsible for a negative regulation of CXCL8 in melanoma, demonstrating the vital importance of the microenvironment for tumors (Gutman et al. 1995). Furthermore, CCL2 is expressed in melanoma and blocking of CCL2 function was able to prevent tumor angiogenesis and tumor growth (Koga et al. 2008). The role of CCL2 might therefore be similar to its role in breast cancers. Additionally, a more aggressive behaviour of melanoma in nude mice was observed after CCL5 induction in melanoma cells by TNF-α (Mrowietz et al. 1999). This is compelling evidence that tumor infiltrating macrophages might, through enhancement of CCL2 and CCL5 production, transform the microenvironment to one favorable for angiogenesis and tumor progression, which in turn leads to a tumor in a more aggressive stage.

4.4.3 Lung Cancer

The role of chemokines in lung cancer angiogenesis has been well established by Strieter et al. CXCL8 expression was elevated in non-small cell lung cancer (NSCLC) and significantly contributed to tumor-derived angiogenesis (Smith et al. 1994). Neutralizing antibodies to CXCL8 were able to significantly reduce endothelial cell chemotactic activity in response to NSCLC tissue (Smith et al. 1994). Furthermore, in a human NSCLC/SCID mouse chimera model, the cell line A549 (adenocarcinoma) and the cell line Calu 1 (squamous cell carcinoma) were studied. In A549-bearing animals, a progressive increase of tumor size was observed, while Calu 1-bearing mice demonstrated little tumor growth (Arenberg et al. 1996a). Correspondingly, A549 tumors produced greater levels of CXCL8 than Calu 1 tumors and were up to 50-fold larger in size than Calu 1 tumors (Arenberg et al. 1996a). When A549 tumors were treated with neutralizing antibodies to CXCL8, a marked reduction of tumor growth compared to control tumors followed (Arenberg et al. 1996a). Furthermore, in corneal micropocket assays and assessments of vessel density in tumors, inhibition of CXCL8 by antibody treatment resulted in lower vessel density as well as reduced angiogenesis, demonstrating that tumor-associated CXCL8 mediated tumor angiogenesis in A549 (Arenberg et al. 1996a). It is important to note that, although CXCL8 is unknown in mice (Zlotnik and Yoshie 2000), both corresponding receptors,

CXCR1 and CXCR2, have been identified in mice and being responsive to human CXCL8 (Fan et al. 2007). Interestingly, an inversely correlated phenomenon was observed after assessing expression of CXCL10 in adenocarcinomas compared to squamous cell carcinomas. In squamous cell carcinomas elevated levels of CXCL10 were observed (Arenberg et al. 1996b). Corresponding to the CXCL8 experiments, CXCL10 expression was studied in the same NSCLC/SCID mouse chimera model. Not surprisingly, CXCL10 expression was inversely correlated to tumor growth showing high levels in Calu 1 tumors and low levels in A549 tumors, and the antibody neutralization of CXCL10 caused an increase in growth of Calu 1 tumors (Arenberg et al. 1996b). Furthermore, neutralization of CXCL10 by antibodies increased neovascularization of squamous cell carcinomas in the cornea as well as showing an increased endothelial cell chemotactic activity (Arenberg et al. 1996b). The balance of CXCL8 vs. CXCL10 expression of adenocarcinomas and squamous cell carcinomas of the lung corresponded to the prognosis of patients. Patient survival is poorer and metastatic potential is greater in patients with adenocarcinomas when compared to patients with squamous cell carcinomas (Carney 1988; Minna 1991). Therefore, the difference of behavior observed in these two tumor entities might be dependent on the balance of angiogenic CXCL8 and angiostatic CXCL10, demonstrating an opposing system of angiogenic and angiostatic factors in the microenvironment controlling tumorangiogenesis. Furthermore, tumor-infiltrating macrophages were able to induce CXCL8 expression in lung cancer cells, as demonstrated by a significant increase in CXCL8 mRNA in lung cancer cells cocultured with phorbol myristate acetate-treated THP-1 cells and human primary lung macrophages (Yao et al. 2005), demonstrating the vital importance of crosstalk between tumor-associated macrophages and tumor cells in modulating the microenvironment.

In contrast, abundant CXCL8 expression could not be observed in small cell lung cancer (SCLC) (Zhu et al. 2004). Instead, SCLC cell lines H711, H69, H345, Lu165, and GLC19 expressed CXCL6 abundantly, where as in tested NSCLC cell lines CXCL6 expression could not be observed (Zhu et al. 2006). Additionally, IL-1β as well as hypoxic conditions induced the production of CXCL6 in SCLC cell lines. Furthermore, CXCL6 is able to promote cell proliferation by autocrine stimulation, as evidenced by inhibition of proliferation when SCLC cells were treated with neutralizing anti-CXCL6 antibodies (Zhu et al. 2006). Interestingly, the receptor for CXCL6 is the same as for CXCL8, namely CXCR2 (Zlotnik and Yoshie 2000). It might be possible that CXCL6 is the agent modulating angiogenesis in a SCLC scenario, instead of CXCL8, although this still needs to be further elucidated.

4.5 Inhibition of Chemokine-Induced Angiogenesis as a Therapeutic Strategy

Today, cancer therapeutic strategies targeting angiogenesis are in clinical use. The most prominent of antiangiogenic drugs for cancer therapy is bevacizumab, an antibody targeting VEGF (John et al. 2008). Use of bevacizumab in addition to standard chemotherapy shows some promising results in prolonging the survival of treated patients (John et al. 2008). There are several other drugs in preclinical and clinical evaluation which target the receptors of VEGF, matrix-metallo proteinases, and cyclooxygenase-2 (COX-2) (John et al. 2008). COX-2 is an inducible enzyme, which catalyzes the conversion of arachidonic acid to prostaglandin H_2 (PGH_2) (Williams et al. 1999). PGH_2 serves as a subtrate for a number of prostaglandin synthetases (Williams et al. 1999). One prostaglandin endproduct, prostaglandin E_2 (PGE_2), has been implicated in acting as an inducer of angiogenesis regulators like VEGF, endothelin-1 and others (Chiarugi et al. 1998). Not surprisingly, COX-2 is upregulated in many cancer types and represents a valuable target for antitumor therapy (Harris 2007).

The role of chemokines in angiogenesis presents an opportunity for novel approaches in cancer therapy. It might be worthwhile to pursue a therapeutic role for angiostatic chemokines like CXCL4, CXCL9, CXCL10, and CXCL11. These chemokines could be introduced into a tumor either by direct application or by gene therapy approaches to shift the balance of the tumor microenvironment towards angiostasis, thereby inhibiting tumor growth. One prominent example of a tumor therapy strategy utilizing an inhibiting drug is exemplified by Interferon-α (INFα). A tumor-limiting effect of INFα was demonstrated more than 25 years ago in B16 melanoma (Bart et al. 1980). Today, it has found clinical application as a treatment of several malignancies, including non-Hodgkin's lymphoma, Kaposi sarcoma, melanoma, and renal cell carcinoma (Parmar and Platanias 2003). INFα not only acts through activation of immune cells, but it was demonstrated to also directly act on tumor cells by induction of apoptosis (Parmar and Platanias 2003).

One risk involved in such an approach could be that the loss of vasculature inside the tumor could result in hypoxic conditions. Hypoxia in the tumor might drive the tumor cells toward different ways to escape hypoxic-related cell death. In fact, antiangiogenic therapies might select resistant subclones and boost tumor progression and growth, giving rise to the paradox, that in antiangiogenic therapy, the induced hypoxic condition of the tumor needs to be fought, too (Abbadessa et al. 2007). For example, hypoxia induced CXCR4 expression in mononuclear phagocytes, HUVEC, and the ovarian cancer cell line CAOV3 (Schioppa et al. 2003). Furthermore, in mouse embryonic fibroblasts hypoxia-induced CXCR4 induction was alleviated in HIF-1α-deficient cells, implicating that CXCR4 is under regulation by HIF-1α (Schioppa et al. 2003). CXCR4 expression on cancer cells plays a role in invasion and targeted metastasis to distant sites (Muller et al. 2001). Therefore, chemokine receptor expression induced by hypoxia might represent the danger involved in therapy targeting angiogensis.

Another approach might be the inhibition of angiogenic chemokines present in the tumor microenvironment. Drugs which inhibit the corresponding chemokine receptor or using chemokine-specific antibodies to neutralize the angiogenic effect would realize this approach. This strategy is already in use with VEGF or VEGFR-targeting drugs mentioned at the beginning of this chapter. The goal of both general strategies (a) supplementing the tumor microenvironment with agents inhibiting angiogenesis directly or (b) agents targeting angiogenic modulators, thereby inhibiting angiogenesis indirectly, are to shift the microenvironment from an angiogenesis favoring to an angiogenesis limiting state.

The research for chemokine-based cancer therapy has mostly been directed toward stimulating immune response (immunotherapy) to tumors or to inhibit metastasis. One prominent example is the use of antagonists against CXCR4. The focus on research of CXCR4 antagonists is founded on its role as a coreceptor for viral infection in HIV (Feng et al. 1996), as well as its role in cancer metastasis (Geminder et al. 2001; Muller et al. 2001; Payne and Cornelius 2002; Taichman et al. 2002; Zeelenberg et al. 2001). Several small molecule antagonists to CXCR4 are in development, among them BKT140 and its analogs (Takenaga et al. 2004; Tamamura et al. 2003), CTCE-9908 by Chemokine Therapeutics (Vancouver, Canada) (Kim et al. 2005), as well as AMD3100 by AnorMED Inc. (Langley, Canada) (De Clercq 2003). AMD3100, now renamed Mozobil™, completed Phase II studies (Devine et al. 2004) for stem cell transplantaion treatment of multiple myeloma and non-Hodgkin's lymphoma patients in 2004. Recently, GenzymeCorporation (Cambridge,MA,USA),developingMozobil(TM) after its acquisition of AnorMED Inc., announced after successful Phase III trials the FDA approval for Mozobil(TM) at the end of 2008 for the mobilization of stem cells from the bone marrow for collection and autologous transplantation. Incidentally, CXCR4 antagonists might not only present a way to inhibit metastasis, but also due to its role in angiogenesis (see Chap. 2), be a viable antiangiogenesis therapeutic.

The research focusing on finding chemokine-derived agents which inhibit angiogenesis is much smaller. Abgenix (Thousand Oaks, CA, USA) has developed an anti-CXCL8 antibody, ABX-IL8 (Yang et al. 1999). ABX-IL8 inhibited angiogenesis, tumor growth, and metastasis in human melanoma both in vitro and in vivo (Huang et al. 2002) in preclinical trials and inhibited tumor growth and matrix metalloproteinase activity in orthotopic bladder cancer xenografts as well (Mian et al. 2003). A Phase II study of ABX-IL8 in patients with malignant melanoma was planned in 2002, but this study never commenced due to failure to meet its endpoint in a seperate psoriasis trial (Yan et al. 2006).

About 25% of human malignancies contain activated forms of the *Ras* protooncogene (Bos 1989). Interestingly, CXCL8, a chemokine with a prominent role in angiogenesis, is induced by activation of the epidermal growth factor receptor (EGFR)/Ras signal transduction pathway (Sparmann and Bar-Sagi 2004). Moreover, activation of EGFR/Ras signal transduction in skin malignancies facilitates escape of immune surveillance via downregulation of homeostatic CCL27 by the tumor (Pivarcsi et al. 2007). Targeting the EGFR/Ras signal transduction pathway therefore might not only inhibit angiogenesis but also establish an immune response to the tumor. EGFR inhibitors like erlotinib, geftinib, and cetuximab (John et al. 2008) are either already in clinical use or in clinical study phases and present a promising antiproliferative, immunomodulating, apoptosis-enhancing, and antiangiogenetic therapeutic approach in cancer therapy.

The possibility of inhibiting tumor angiogenesis by (a) antibodies to angiogenic chemokines or anatgonists against angiogenic receptors, (b) raising the angiostatic chemokine level in the tumor microenvironment or (c) targeting signal transduction pathways modulating chemokine expression, presents a promising strategy for novel anticancer therapeutics. Further investigations and screening for new antagonists to chemokine receptors or chemokines might provide physicians with further tools to inhibit tumor growth and to combat progression of tumors.

References

Abbadessa G, Vogiatzi P, Rimassa L, Claudio PP (2007) Antiangiogenic drugs currently used for colorectal cancer: what other pathways can we target to prolong responses? Drug News Perspect 20:307–313

Addison CL, Daniel TO, Burdick MD, Liu H, Ehlert JE, Xue YY, Buechi L, Walz A, Richmond A, Strieter RM (2000) The CXC chemokine receptor 2, CXCR2, is the putative receptor for ELR+ CXC chemokine-induced angiogenic activity. J Immunol 165:5269–5277

Arenberg DA, Kunkel SL, Polverini PJ, Glass M, Burdick MD, Strieter RM (1996a) Inhibition of interleukin-8 reduces tumorigenesis of human non-small cell lung cancer in SCID mice. J Clin Invest 97:2792–2802

Arenberg DA, Kunkel SL, Polverini PJ, Morris SB, Burdick MD, Glass MC, Taub DT, Iannettoni MD, Whyte RI, Strieter RM (1996b) Interferon-gamma-inducible protein 10 (IP-10) is an angiostatic factor that inhibits human non-small cell lung cancer (NSCLC) tumorigenesis and spontaneous metastases. J Exp Med 184:981–992

Arenberg DA, Zlotnick A, Strom SR, Burdick MD, Strieter RM (2001) The murine CC chemokine, 6C-kine, inhibits tumor growth and angiogenesis in a human lung cancer SCID mouse model. Cancer Immunol Immunother 49:587–592

Auerbach R, Kubai L, Sidky Y (1976) Angiogenesis induction by tumors, embryonic tissues, and lymphocytes. Cancer Res 36:3435–3440

Alberts B, Johnson A, Lewis J, Raff M, Roberts K, Walter P (2007) Molecular biology of the cell. Garland Science, London

4

Balentien E, Mufson BE, Shattuck RL, Derynck R, Richmond A (1991) Effects of MGSA/GRO alpha on melanocyte transformation. Oncogene 6:1115–1124

Bart RS, Porzio NR, Kopf AW, Vilcek JT, Cheng EH, Farcet Y (1980) Inhibition of growth of B16 murine malignant melanoma by exogenous interferon. Cancer Res 40:614–619

Belperio JA, Keane MP, Arenberg DA, Addison CL, Ehlert JE, Burdick MD, Strieter RM (2000) CXC chemokines in angiogenesis. J Leukoc Biol 68:1–8

Ben-Baruch A (2003) Host microenvironment in breast cancer development: inflammatory cells, cytokines and chemokines in breast cancer progression: reciprocal tumor-microenvironment interactions. Breast Cancer Res 5:31–36

Berger O, Gan X, Gujuluva C, Burns AR, Sulur G, Stins M, Way D, Witte M, Weinand M, Said J, Kim KS, Taub D, Graves MC, Fiala M (1999) CXC and CC chemokine receptors on coronary and brain endothelia. Mol Med 5:795–805

Bernardini G, Ribatti D, Spinetti G, Morbidelli L, Ziche M, Santoni A, Capogrossi MC, Napolitano M (2003) Analysis of the role of chemokines in angiogenesis. J Immunol Methods 273: 83–101

Bernardini G, Spinetti G, Ribatti D, Camarda G, Morbidelli L, Ziche M, Santoni A, Capogrossi MC, Napolitano M (2000) I-309 binds to and activates endothelial cell functions and acts as an angiogenic molecule in vivo. Blood 96: 4039–4045

Bonacchi A, Romagnani P, Romanelli RG, Efsen E, Annunziato F, Lasagni L, Francalanci M, Serio M, Laffi G, Pinzani M, Gentilini P, Marra F (2001) Signal transduction by the chemokine receptor CXCR3: activation of Ras/ERK, Src, and phosphatidylinositol 3-kinase/Akt controls cell migration and proliferation in human vascular pericytes. J Biol Chem 276:9945–9954

Bordoni R, Fine R, Murray D, Richmond A (1990) Characterization of the role of melanoma growth stimulatory activity (MGSA) in the growth of normal melanocytes, nevocytes, and malignant melanocytes. J Cell Biochem 44:207–219

Bos JL (1989) ras oncogenes in human cancer: a review. Cancer Res 49:4682–4689

Bouck N (1990) Tumor angiogenesis: the role of oncogenes and tumor suppressor genes. Cancer Cells 2:179–185

Cao X, Zhang W, Wan T, He L, Chen T, Yuan Z, Ma S, Yu Y, Chen G (2000) Molecular cloning and characterization of a novel CXC chemokine macrophage inflammatory protein-2 gamma chemoattractant for human neutrophils and dendritic cells. J Immunol 165:2588–2595

Carney DN (1988) Cancers of the lungs. In: Fishman AP (ed) Pulmonary diseases and disorders. McGraw-Hill, New York, pp 1885–2068

Carulli MT, Ong VH, Ponticos M, Shiwen X, Abraham DJ, Black CM, Denton CP (2005) Chemokine receptor CCR2 expression by systemic sclerosis fibroblasts: evidence for autocrine regulation of myofibroblast differentiation. Arthritis Rheum 52:3772–3782

Charo IF, Myers SJ, Herman A, Franci C, Connolly AJ, Coughlin SR (1994) Molecular cloning and functional expression of two monocyte chemoattractant protein 1 receptors reveals alternative splicing of the carboxyl-terminal tails. Proc Natl Acad Sci U S A 91:2752–2756

Chavey C, Bibeau F, Gourgou-Bourgade S, Burlinchon S, Boissiere F, Laune D, Roques S, Lazennec G (2007) Oestrogen receptor negative breast cancers exhibit high cytokine content. Breast Cancer Res 9:R15

Chiarugi V, Magnelli L, Gallo O (1998) Cox 2, iNOS and p53 as play-makers of tumor angiogenesis (review). Int J Mol Med 2:715–719

Cole KE, Strick CA, Paradis TJ, Ogborne KT, Loetscher M, Gladue RP, Lin W, Boyd JG, Moser B, Wood DE, Sahagan BG, Neote K (1998) Interferon-inducible T cell alpha chemoattractant (I-TAC): a novel non-ELR CXC chemokine with potent activity on activated T cells through selective high affinity binding to CXCR3. J Exp Med 187:2009–2021

De Clercq E (2003) The bicyclam AMD3100 story. Nat Rev Drug Discov 2:581–587

De Paepe B, De Bleecker JL (2005) Beta-chemokine receptor expression in idiopathic inflammatory myopathies. Muscle Nerve 31:621–627

Devine SM, Flomenberg N, Vesole DH, Liesveld J, Weisdorf D, Badel K, Calandra G, DiPersio JF (2004) Rapid mobilization of CD34+ cells following administration of the CXCR4 antagonist AMD3100 to patients with multiple myeloma and non-Hodgkin's lymphoma. J Clin Oncol 22:1095–1102

Engerman RL, Pfaffenbach D, Davis MD (1967) Cell turnover of capillaries. Lab Invest 17:738–743

Fan X, Patera AC, Pong-Kennedy A, Deno G, Gonsiorek W, Manfra DJ, Vassileva G, Zeng M, Jackson C, Sullivan L, Sharif-Rodriguez W,

Opdenakker G, Van Damme J, Hedrick JA, Lundell D, Lira SA, Hipkin RW (2007) Murine CXCR1 is a functional receptor for GCP-2/CXCL6 and interleukin-8/CXCL8. J Biol Chem 282:11658–11666

Feng Y, Broder CC, Kennedy PE, Berger EA (1996) HIV-1 entry cofactor: functional cDNA cloning of a seven-transmembrane, G protein-coupled receptor. Science 272:872–877

Folkman J (1995) Angiogenesis in cancer, vascular, rheumatoid and other disease. Nat Med 1:27–31

Folkman J, Shing Y (1992) Angiogenesis. J Biol Chem 267:10931–10934

Fong AM, Erickson HP, Zachariah JP, Poon S, Schamberg NJ, Imai T, Patel DD (2000) Ultrastructure and function of the fractalkine mucin domain in CX(3)C chemokine domain presentation. J Biol Chem 275:3781–3786

Freund A, Chauveau C, Brouillet JP, Lucas A, Lacroix M, Licznar A, Vignon F, Lazennec G (2003) IL-8 expression and its possible relationship with estrogen-receptor-negative status of breast cancer cells. Oncogene 22:256–265

Garcia-Lopez MA, Sanchez-Madrid F, Rodriguez-Frade JM, Mellado M, Acevedo A, Garcia MI, Albar JP, Martinez C, Marazuela M (2001) CXCR3 chemokine receptor distribution in normal and inflamed tissues: expression on activated lymphocytes, endothelial cells, and dendritic cells. Lab Invest 81:409–418

Garlanda C, Dejana E (1997) Heterogeneity of endothelial cells. Specific markers. Arterioscler Thromb Vasc Biol 17:1193–1202

Geminder H, Sagi-Assif O, Goldberg L, Meshel T, Rechavi G, Witz IP, Ben-Baruch A (2001) A possible role for CXCR4 and its ligand, the CXC chemokine stromal cell-derived factor-1, in the development of bone marrow metastases in neuroblastoma. J Immunol 167:4747–4757

Giorgini S, Trisciuoglio D, Gabellini C, Desideri M, Castellini L, Colarossi C, Zangemeister-Wittke U, Zupi G, Del Bufalo D (2007) Modulation of bcl-xL in tumor cells regulates angiogenesis through CXCL8 expression. Mol Cancer Res 5:761–771

Goede V, Brogelli L, Ziche M, Augustin HG (1999) Induction of inflammatory angiogenesis by monocyte chemoattractant protein-1. Int J Cancer 82:765–770

Gutman M, Singh RK, Xie K, Bucana CD, Fidler IJ (1995) Regulation of interleukin-8 expression in human melanoma cells by the organ environment. Cancer Res 55:2470–2475

Harris ED Jr (1976) Recent insights into the pathogenesis of the proliferative lesion in rheumatoid arthritis. Arthritis Rheum 19:68–72

Harris RE (2007) Cyclooxygenase-2 (cox-2) and the inflammogenesis of cancer. Subcell Biochem 42:93–126

Hedrick JA, Zlotnik A (1997) Identification and characterization of a novel beta chemokine containing six conserved cysteines. J Immunol 159:1589–1593

Hromas R, Broxmeyer HE, Kim C, Nakshatri H, Christopherson K 2nd, Azam M, Hou YH (1999) Cloning of BRAK, a novel divergent CXC chemokine preferentially expressed in normal versus malignant cells. Biochem Biophys Res Commun 255:703–706

Huang S, Mills L, Mian B, Tellez C, McCarty M, Yang XD, Gudas JM, Bar-Eli M (2002) Fully humanized neutralizing antibodies to interleukin-8 (ABX-IL8) inhibit angiogenesis, tumor growth, and metastasis of human melanoma. Am J Pathol 161:125–134

Hwang J, Kim CW, Son KN, Han KY, Lee KH, Kleinman HK, Ko J, Na DS, Kwon BS, Gho YS, Kim J (2004) Angiogenic activity of human CC chemokine CCL15 in vitro and in vivo. FEBS Lett 570:47–51

Imaizumi T, Yoshida H, Satoh K (2004) Regulation of CX3CL1/fractalkine expression in endothelial cells. J Atheroscler Thromb 11:15–21

Jenh CH, Cox MA, Kaminski H, Zhang M, Byrnes H, Fine J, Lundell D, Chou CC, Narula SK, Zavodny PJ (1999) Cutting edge: species specificity of the CC chemokine 6Ckine signaling through the CXC chemokine receptor CXCR3: human 6Ckine is not a ligand for the human or mouse CXCR3 receptors. J Immunol 162:3765–3769

John AR, Bramhall SR, Eggo MC (2008) Antiangiogenic therapy and surgical practice. Br J Surg 95:281–293

Kim S, Mendoza A, Midura B et al (2005) Inhibition of murine osteosarcoma lung metastases using the CXCR4 antagonist, CTCE-9908. In Proceedings of the 96th AACR annual meeting. Anaheim, CA.

Koga M, Kai H, Egami K, Murohara T, Ikeda A, Yasuoka S, Egashira K, Matsuishi T, Kai M, Kataoka Y, Kuwano M, Imaizumi T (2008) Mutant MCP-1 therapy inhibits tumor angiogenesis and growth of malignant melanoma in mice. Biochem Biophys Res Commun 365:279–284

4

Kriehuber E, Breiteneder-Geleff S, Groeger M, Soleiman A, Schoppmann SF, Stingl G, Kerjaschki D, Maurer D (2001) Isolation and characterization of dermal lymphatic and blood endothelial cells reveal stable and functionally specialized cell lineages. J Exp Med 194: 797–808

Kurth I, Willimann K, Schaerli P, Hunziker T, Clark-Lewis I, Moser B (2001) Monocyte selectivity and tissue localization suggests a role for breast and kidney-expressed chemokine (BRAK) in macrophage development. J Exp Med 194:855–861

Kyndi M, Sorensen FB, Knudsen H, Overgaard M, Nielsen HM, Overgaard J (2008) Estrogen receptor, progesterone receptor, HER-2, and response to postmastectomy radiotherapy in high-risk breast cancer: the Danish Breast Cancer Cooperative Group. J Clin Oncol 26(9):1419–1426

Lasagni L, Francalanci M, Annunziato F, Lazzeri E, Giannini S, Cosmi L, Sagrinati C, Mazzinghi B, Orlando C, Maggi E, Marra F, Romagnani S, Serio M, Romagnani P (2003) An alternatively spliced variant of CXCR3 mediates the inhibition of endothelial cell growth induced by IP-10, Mig, and I-TAC, and acts as functional receptor for platelet factor 4. J Exp Med 197:1537–1549

Lee SJ, Namkoong S, Kim YM, Kim CK, Lee H, Ha KS, Chung HT, Kwon YG (2006) Fractalkine stimulates angiogenesis by activating the Raf-1/MEK/ERK- and PI3K/Akt/eNOS-dependent signal pathways. Am J Physiol Heart Circ Physiol 291:H2836–H2846

Leibovich SJ, Wiseman DM (1988) Macrophages, wound repair and angiogenesis. Prog Clin Biol Res 266:131–145

Lin Y, Huang R, Chen L, Li S, Shi Q, Jordan C, Huang RP (2004) Identification of interleukin-8 as estrogen receptor-regulated factor involved in breast cancer invasion and angiogenesis by protein arrays. Int J Cancer 109:507–515

Martins-Green M, Hanafusa H (1997) The 9E3/CEF4 gene and its product the chicken chemotactic and angiogenic factor (cCAF): potential roles in wound healing and tumor development. Cytokine Growth Factor Rev 8:221–232

Mian BM, Dinney CP, Bermejo CE, Sweeney P, Tellez C, Yang XD, Gudas JM, McConkey DJ, Bar-Eli M (2003) Fully human anti-interleukin 8 antibody inhibits tumor growth in orthotopic bladder cancer xenografts via down-regulation of matrix metalloproteases and nuclear factor-kappaB. Clin Cancer Res 9:3167–3175

Miller MD, Krangel MS (1992) Biology and biochemistry of the chemokines: a family of chemotactic and inflammatory cytokines. Crit Rev Immunol 12:17–46

Minna JD (1991) Neoplasms of the lung. In: Isselbacher KJ (ed) Principles of internal medicine. McGraw-Hill, New York, pp 1102–1110

Mrowietz U, Schwenk U, Maune S, Bartels J, Kupper M, Fichtner I, Schroder JM, Schadendorf D (1999) The chemokine RANTES is secreted by human melanoma cells and is associated with enhanced tumour formation in nude mice. Br J Cancer 79:1025–1031

Muller A, Homey B, Soto H, Ge N, Catron D, Buchanan ME, McClanahan T, Murphy E, Yuan W, Wagner SN, Barrera JL, Mohar A, Verastegui E, Zlotnik A (2001) Involvement of chemokine receptors in breast cancer metastasis. Nature 410:50–56

Pablos JL, Amara A, Bouloc A, Santiago B, Caruz A, Galindo M, Delaunay T, Virelizier JL, Arenzana-Seisdedos F (1999) Stromal-cell derived factor is expressed by dendritic cells and endothelium in human skin. Am J Pathol 155: 1577–1586

Parkin DM, Bray F, Ferlay J, Pisani P (2005) Global cancer statistics, 2002. CA Cancer J Clin 55: 74–108

Parmar S, Platanias LC (2003) Interferons: mechanisms of action and clinical applications. Curr Opin Oncol 15:431–439

Payne AS, Cornelius LA (2002) The role of chemokines in melanoma tumor growth and metastasis. J Invest Dermatol 118:915–922

Pivarcsi A, Muller A, Hippe A, Rieker J, van Lierop A, Steinhoff M, Seeliger S, Kubitza R, Pippirs U, Meller S, Gerber PA, Liersch R, Buenemann E, Sonkoly E, Wiesner U, Hoffmann TK, Schneider L, Piekorz R, Enderlein E, Reifenberger J, Rohr UP, Haas R, Boukamp P, Haase I, Nurnberg B, Ruzicka T, Zlotnik A, Homey B (2007) Tumor immune escape by the loss of homeostatic chemokine expression. Proc Natl Acad Sci U S A 104:19055–19060

Polverini PJ (1995) The pathophysiology of angiogenesis. Crit Rev Oral Biol Med 6:230–247

Richmond A, Thomas HG (1986) Purification of melanoma growth stimulatory activity. J Cell Physiol 129:375–384

Ryu J, Lee CW, Hong KH, Shin JA, Lim SH, Park CS, Shim J, Nam KB, Choi KJ, Kim YH, Han KH (2007) Activation of Fractalkine/CX3CR1 by

Vascular Endothelial Cells Induces Angiogenesis through VEGF-A/KDR and Reverses Hindlimb Ischemia. Cardiovasc Res 78(2):333–340

Salcedo R, Ponce ML, Young HA, Wasserman K, Ward JM, Kleinman HK, Oppenheim JJ, Murphy WJ (2000) Human endothelial cells express CCR2 and respond to MCP-1: direct role of MCP-1 in angiogenesis and tumor progression. Blood 96:34–40

Salcedo R, Young HA, Ponce ML, Ward JM, Kleinman HK, Murphy WJ, Oppenheim JJ (2001) Eotaxin (CCL11) induces in vivo angiogenic responses by human CCR3+ endothelial cells. J Immunol 166:7571–7578

Schadendorf D, Moller A, Algermissen B, Worm M, Sticherling M, Czarnetzki BM (1993) IL-8 produced by human malignant melanoma cells in vitro is an essential autocrine growth factor. J Immunol 151:2667–2675

Schioppa T, Uranchimeg B, Saccani A, Biswas SK, Doni A, Rapisarda A, Bernasconi S, Saccani S, Nebuloni M, Vago L, Mantovani A, Melillo G, Sica A (2003) Regulation of the chemokine receptor CXCR4 by hypoxia. J Exp Med 198: 1391–1402

Shattuck-Brandt RL, Richmond A (1997) Enhanced degradation of I-kappaB alpha contributes to endogenous activation of NF-kappaB in Hs294T melanoma cells. Cancer Res 57:3032–3039

Shellenberger TD, Wang M, Gujrati M, Jayakumar A, Strieter RM, Burdick MD, Ioannides CG, Efferson CL, El-Naggar AK, Roberts D, Clayman GL, Frederick MJ (2004) BRAK/CXCL14 is a potent inhibitor of angiogenesis and a chemotactic factor for immature dendritic cells. Cancer Res 64:8262–8270

Skoog L, Humla S, Axelsson M, Frost M, Norman A, Nordenskjold B, Wallgren A (1987) Estrogen receptor levels and survival of breast cancer patients. A study on patients participating in randomized trials of adjuvant therapy. Acta Oncol 26:95–100

Sleeman MA, Fraser JK, Murison JG, Kelly SL, Prestidge RL, Palmer DJ, Watson JD, Kumble KD (2000) B cell- and monocyte-activating chemokine (BMAC), a novel non-ELR alpha-chemokine. Int Immunol 12:677–689

Smith DR, Polverini PJ, Kunkel SL, Orringer MB, Whyte RI, Burdick MD, Wilke CA, Strieter RM (1994) Inhibition of interleukin 8 attenuates angiogenesis in bronchogenic carcinoma. J Exp Med 179:1409–1415

Soto H, Wang W, Strieter RM, Copeland NG, Gilbert DJ, Jenkins NA, Hedrick J, Zlotnik A (1998) The CC chemokine 6Ckine binds the CXC chemokine receptor CXCR3. Proc Natl Acad Sci U S A 95:8205–8210

Sparmann A, Bar-Sagi D (2004) Ras-induced interleukin-8 expression plays a critical role in tumor growth and angiogenesis. Cancer Cell 6:447–458

Strasly M, Doronzo G, Capello P, Valdembri D, Arese M, Mitola S, Moore P, Alessandri G, Giovarelli M, Bussolino F (2004) CCL16 activates an angiogenic program in vascular endothelial cells. Blood 103:40–49

Strieter RM, Polverini PJ, Arenberg DA, Kunkel SL (1995a) The role of CXC chemokines as regulators of angiogenesis. Shock 4:155–160

Strieter RM, Polverini PJ, Kunkel SL, Arenberg DA, Burdick MD, Kasper J, Dzuiba J, Van Damme J, Walz A, Marriott D et al (1995b) The functional role of the ELR motif in CXC chemokine-mediated angiogenesis. J Biol Chem 270:27348–27357

Tachibana K, Hirota S, Iizasa H, Yoshida H, Kawabata K, Kataoka Y, Kitamura Y, Matsushima K, Yoshida N, Nishikawa S, Kishimoto T, Nagasawa T (1998) The chemokine receptor CXCR4 is essential for vascularization of the gastrointestinal tract. Nature 393:591–594

Taichman RS, Cooper C, Keller ET, Pienta KJ, Taichman NS, McCauley LK (2002) Use of the stromal cell-derived factor-1/CXCR4 pathway in prostate cancer metastasis to bone. Cancer Res 62:1832–1837

Takenaga M, Tamamura H, Hiramatsu K, Nakamura N, Yamaguchi Y, Kitagawa A, Kawai S, Nakashima H, Fujii N, Igarashi R (2004) A single treatment with microcapsules containing a CXCR4 antagonist suppresses pulmonary metastasis of murine melanoma. Biochem Biophys Res Commun 320:226–232

Tamamura H, Hori A, Kanzaki N, Hiramatsu K, Mizumoto M, Nakashima H, Yamamoto N, Otaka A, Fujii N (2003) T140 analogs as CXCR4 antagonists identified as anti-metastatic agents in the treatment of breast cancer. FEBS Lett 550:79–83

Tannock IF, Hayashi S (1972) The proliferation of capillary endothelial cells. Cancer Res 32:77–82

Varney ML, Johansson SL, Singh RK (2006) Distinct expression of CXCL8 and its receptors CXCR1 and CXCR2 and their association with vessel density and aggressiveness in malignant melanoma. Am J Clin Pathol 125:209–216

Volin MV, Joseph L, Shockley MS, Davies PF (1998) Chemokine receptor CXCR4 expression

4

in endothelium. Biochem Biophys Res Commun 242:46–53

Volin MV, Woods JM, Amin MA, Connors MA, Harlow LA, Koch AE (2001) Fractalkine: a novel angiogenic chemokine in rheumatoid arthritis. Am J Pathol 159:1521–1530

Williams CS, Mann M, DuBois RN (1999) The role of cyclooxygenases in inflammation, cancer, and development. Oncogene 18:7908–7916

Yaal-Hahoshen N, Shina S, Leider-Trejo L, Barnea I, Shabtai EL, Azenshtein E, Greenberg I, Keydar I, Ben-Baruch A (2006) The chemokine CCL5 as a potential prognostic factor predicting disease progression in stage II breast cancer patients. Clin Cancer Res 12:4474–4480

Yan L, Anderson GM, DeWitte M, Nakada MT (2006) Therapeutic potential of cytokine and chemokine antagonists in cancer therapy. Eur J Cancer 42:793–802

Yang XD, Corvalan JR, Wang P, Roy CM, Davis CG (1999) Fully human anti-interleukin-8 monoclonal antibodies: potential therapeutics for the treatment of inflammatory disease states. J Leukoc Biol 66:401–410

Yao PL, Lin YC, Wang CH, Huang YC, Liao WY, Wang SS, Chen JJ, Yang PC (2005) Autocrine and paracrine regulation of interleukin-8 expression in lung cancer cells. Am J Respir Cell Mol Biol 32:540–547

You JJ, Yang CH, Huang JS, Chen MS, Yang CM (2007) Fractalkine, a CX3C chemokine, as a mediator of ocular angiogenesis. Invest Ophthalmol Vis Sci 48:5290–5298

Zeelenberg IS, Ruuls-Van Stalle L, Roos E (2001) Retention of CXCR4 in the endoplasmic reticulum blocks dissemination of a T cell hybridoma. J Clin Invest 108:269–277

Zhu YM, Bagstaff SM, Woll PJ (2006) Production and upregulation of granulocyte chemotactic protein-2/CXCL6 by IL-1beta and hypoxia in small cell lung cancer. Br J Cancer 94: 1936–1941

Zhu YM, Webster SJ, Flower D, Woll PJ (2004) Interleukin-8/CXCL8 is a growth factor for human lung cancer cells. Br J Cancer 91: 1970–1976

Zlotnik A, Yoshie O (2000) Chemokines: a new classification system and their role in immunity. Immunity 12:121–127

Angiogenesis Inhibition in Cancer Therapy

5

Platelet-Derived Growth Factor (PDGF) and Vascular Endothelial Growth Factor (VEGF) and their Receptors: Biological Functions and Role in Malignancy

Iris Appelmann, Rüdiger Liersch, Torsten Kessler, Rolf M. Mesters, and Wolfgang E. Berdel

Abstract Vascular endothelial growth factor (VEGF) is an endothelial cell-specific mitogen in vitro and an angiogenic inducer in a variety of in vivo models. VEGF gene transcription is induced in particular in hypoxic cells. In developmental angiogenesis, the role of VEGF is demonstrated by the finding that the loss of a single VEGF allele results in defective vascularization and early embryonic lethality. Substantial evidence also implicates VEGF as a mediator of pathological angiogenesis. In situ hybridization studies demonstrate expression of VEGF mRNA in the majority of human tumors. Platelet-derived growth factor (PDGF) is mainly believed to be an important mitogen for connective tissue, and also has important roles during embryonal development. Its overexpression has been linked to different types of malignancies. Thus, it is important to understand the physiology of VEGF and PDGF and their receptors as well as their roles in malignancies in order to develop antiangiogenic strategies for the treatment of malignant disease.

I. Appelmann (✉)
Department of Medicine/Hematology and Oncology, University of Münster, Albert-Schweitzer-Strasse 33, 48129 Münster, Germany
e-mail: Iris.Appelmann@ukmuenster.de

5.1 Introduction

In vertebrates, virtually all tissues depend on oxygen and nutrition supply provided by the blood-vessel system (Risau 1997). The diffusion limit for oxygen is between 100 and 200 µm; thus nearly all cells need to reside in proximity of a capillary (Carmeliet 2003). In addition, the progression of major diseases and of malignancies in particular is related to an abnormally increased formation of vascular networks (Hanahan and Folkman 1996), whereas other important diseases such as cardiac or brain infarction are caused by poor blood supply. Thus, in order to overcome diseases related to the vascular system, an understanding of the molecular basis of angiogenesis is of major importance. Several factors have been identified to play relevant roles in angiogenesis, for example, VEGF, PDGF, and angiopoietin. Among them, VEGF and its receptors are involved in mammalian blood and lymph vessel formation from earliest stages in embryogenesis (Alitalo and Carmeliet 2002; Ferrara and Davis-Smyth 1997), and also play pivotal roles in pathologic angiogenesis (Cornali et al. 1996; Ferrara et al. 1998; Ferrara and Gerber 2001; Plate et al. 1992; Shweiki et al. 1992). PDGF is mainly believed to be an important mitogen for connective

R. Liersch et al. (eds.), *Angiogenesis Inhibition,* Recent Results in Cancer Research,
DOI: 10.1007/978-3-540-78281-0_5,

tissue, especially for fibroblasts that serve in wound healing. However, PDGF also has important roles during embryonal development, and its overexpression has been linked to different types of fibrotic disorders and malignancies. Thus, it is important to understand the physiology of VEGF and PDGF and their receptors as well as their roles in malignancies. This chapter summarizes the biosynthesis and physiologic activity of VEGF and PDGF, and the role of VEGF and PDGF expression in malignant disease. For detailed information on particular aspects of VEGF and PDGF biology (e.g., signal transduction) the reader is kindly referred to other reviews and original literature, some of which are cited later in the chapter.

5.2 VEGF

5.2.1 VEGF Isoforms and Their Expression

In 1983, VEGF was first described as having an important impact on vessel formation (Senger et al. 1983). It was observed that this factor induced vascular leakage, and thus it was first called vascular permeability factor (VPF). Sequencing and purification of VPF took place in 1990 (Connolly et al. 1989a). Independently, the term "vascular endothelial growth factor" was used by Ferrara and Henzel for a specific endothelial mitogen isolated from conditioned medium. Finally, Connolly was able to prove in 1989 that VPF and VEGF were the same molecule (Connolly et al. 1989a, b).

VEGF is now recognized to play an essential role in physiological as well as pathological angiogenesis (Cornali et al. 1996; Ferrara et al. 1998; Ferrara and Gerber 2001; Plate et al. 1992; Shweiki et al. 1992). Different structurally related dimeric glycoproteins which are highly homologous to PDGF have been identified (Keck et al. 1989; Leung et al. 1989), and constitute the VEGF family. This VEGF family includes VEGF-A, VEGF-B (Olofsson et al. 1996), VEGF-C (Joukov et al. 1996), VEGF-D (Achen et al. 1998), VEGF-E, and placenta-derived growth factor (PlGF) (Maglione et al. 1991; Maglione et al. 1993). Homodimers or heterodimers of the VEGF family form the active VEGF molecule. VEGF-A as the predominant form is a heparin-binding homodimeric glycoprotein of 45 kDa and is generated by alternative exon splicing in four different isoforms (VEGF121, VEGF165, VEGF189, VEGF205) (Houck et al. 1992; Keyt et al. 1996; Tischer et al. 1991) which are generated concomitantly (Fig. 5.1). In humans, the VEGF gene consists of eight exons with seven introns

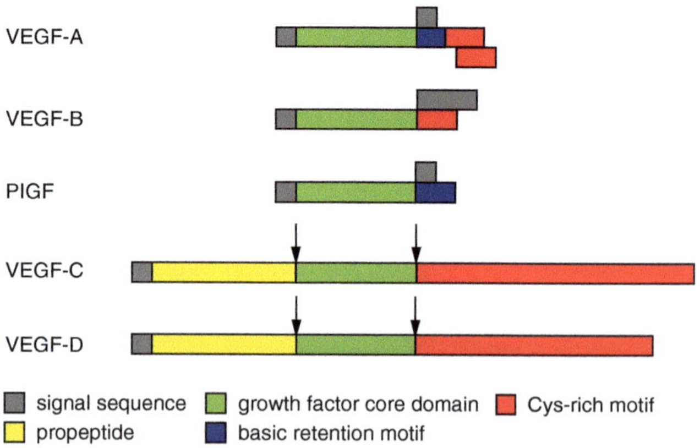

Fig. 5.1 Mammalian VEGFs. *Arrows* indicates proteolytic cleavage sites

and is localized on chromosome 6p21.3 (Vincenti et al. 1996). The two shorter isoforms show mitogenic activity as well as permeability-inducing activity. The longer isoforms are only capable of inducing vascular permeability (Keyt et al. 1996). VEGF 121 lacks the parts encoded by Exon 6 and 7 so that it loses its heparin-binding capability. This lack of heparin-binding capacity causes a significant reduction of the mitogenic potential of VEGF (Keyt et al. 1996). A complete recovery of a tumorigenic phenotype in VEGF −/− mice is only caused by the murine isoform VEGF164 (which is shorter by one amino acid compared to the human isoform) (Grunstein et al. 2000). Furthermore, mice which exclusively express VEGF120 die as newborns or within the first two weeks (Carmeliet et al. 1999). Thus, for the initiation of vascular branch formation, the heparin-binding capacity seems to play a pivotal role (Carmeliet 1999). An increase in VEGF levels has been observed in several different human malignancies, for example, breast, lung, pancreatic, ovarian, kidney, and bladder carcinomas (Boocock et al. 1995; Brown et al. 1993a; Ellis et al. 1998; Hatva et al. 1995; Volm et al. 1997a; Yoshiji et al. 1996). Since low oxygen tension serves as major stimulus for VEGF expression, the highest expression is found in proximity to necrotic areas (Ferrara et al. 1998; Shweiki et al. 1992). There is a close relationship between the hypoxic mechanism leading to VEGF expression and the regulative mechanism of erythropoietin (Epo) expression (Goldberg and Schneider 1994). The VEGF gene, as well as the Epo gene, contains a highly homologous promoter region with similar affinity to hypoxia-inducible factor 1 (HIF-1) (Levy et al. 1995; Liu et al. 1995), which is one of the essential mediators for a response to low oxygen tension (Madan and Curtin 1993). Other important mediators linked to the HIF-1 pathway include products of tumor suppressor genes like the von-Hippel-Lindau (VHL) protein (Iliopoulos et al. 1996) and the tumor suppressor gene PTEN. PTEN is a negative regulator to the PI3-kinase pathway and is constitutively mutated in glioblastomas (Li et al. 1997; Zundel et al. 2000). Furthermore, a stimulus for increased VEGF expression is the amplification of the oncogene ras (Grugel et al. 1995; Rak et al. 1995), which directly links an upregulation of VEGF to oncogenic transformation in malignant cells. This strongly suggests a role for VEGF as autocrine growth factor not only for endothelial cells. In addition, the expression of VEGF is upregulated by other growth factors, cytokines, and hormones such as PDGF, fibroblast growth factor (FGF), insulin-like growth factor 1 (IGF-1), tumor necrosis factor α (TNF-α), and estradiol (Cohen et al. 1996; Frank et al. 1995; Mueller et al. 2000; Mueller et al. 2003; Pertovaara et al. 1994; Warren et al. 1996).

5.2.2 VEGF Receptors

There is evidence that mammalian VEGF receptors (VEGFRs) are derived from the tyrosine kinase receptor D-VEGFR/PVR found in Drosophila, where it is mainly needed to mediate cell migration (e.g., migration of border cells, hematopoietic cells, and epithelial cells for thorax closure) (Cho et al. 2002; Duchek et al. 2001; Ishimaru et al. 2004). Only one VEGFR-related gene has been identified in nonvertebrates like Drosophila; thus it is believed that the variety of VEGFR family genes and structurally similar PDGFR genes in vertebrates have been generated by gene duplication or triplication during early stages of evolution of vertebrates. The phylogenetical developments of VEGFRs and PDGFRs in vertebrates seem to have occured in a step-wise manner due to which a gain of function has developed. It explains that vertebrate VEGFRs do not only transduce signals for cell migration, but also generate mitotic signals for vascular/lymphatic endothelial cells. In close relationship, PDGFRs even generate signals

5

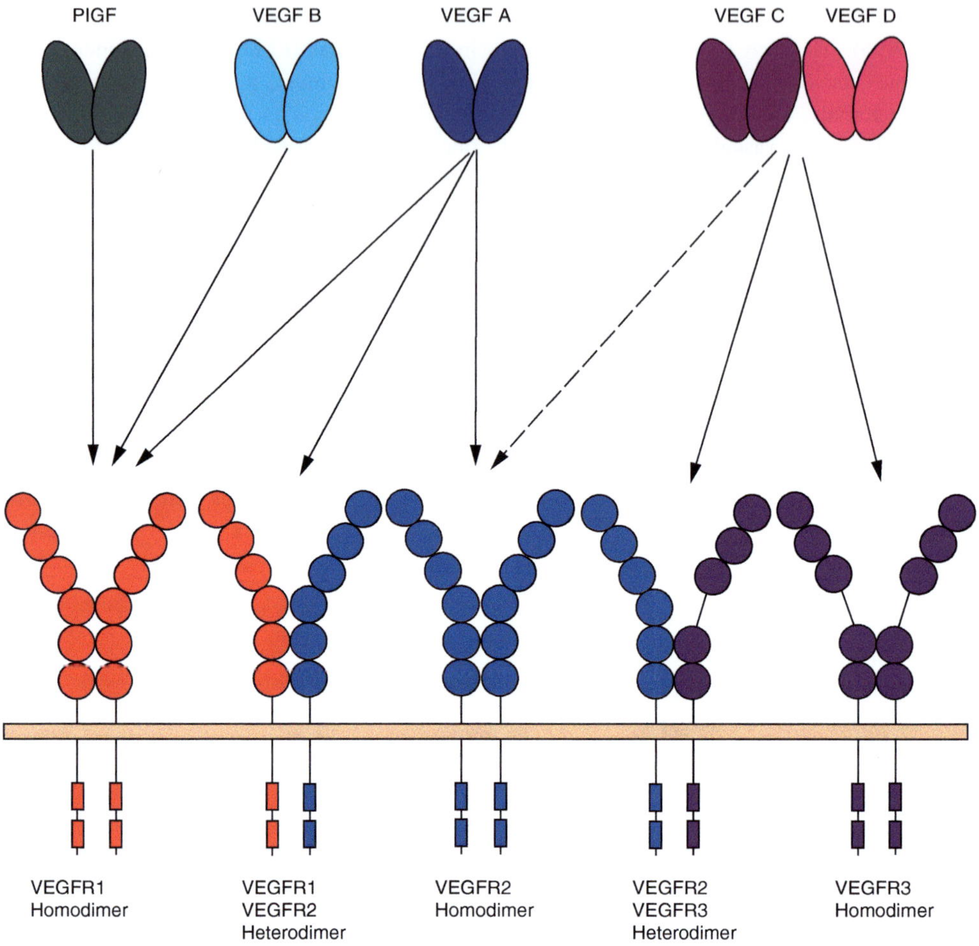

Fig. 5.2 VEGF receptor-binding properties and signaling complexes

for the activation of the PI3-kinase and ras pathways for cell growth and transformation (Shibuya 2002; Shibuya and Claesson-Welsh 2006) (Fig 5.2).

5.2.3 Structure of VEGFR1 and VEGFR2

In humans the VEGFR1 consists of 1338 amino acids and VEGFR2 contains 1356 amino acids. Both receptors can be separated into four regions: an extracellular ligand-binding domain, a transmembrane domain, a tyrosine kinase domain, and a downstream carboxy terminal region (Matthews et al. 1991; Millauer et al. 1993; Shibuya et al. 1990; Terman et al. 1991). There is a homology in the overall structure of VEGFR1 (Flt1), VEGFR2 (KDR/Flk-1), and VEGFR3 (Flt-4) (Alitalo and Carmeliet 2002; Shibuya et al. 1990). The VEGF receptors are closely related to the PDGF receptor family, for example, PDGFR, CSF-1 receptor (c-Fms), SCF receptor (c-Kit), and Flt-3. There is, however, a difference between the two receptor families in the number of Ig-like domains: the VEGFRs contain 7 Ig-like domains, whereas the PDGFRs contain only 5 Ig-like domains.

The binding sites for VEGF-A are located on the second Ig-like domain in the VEGFR1 and on the second/third Ig-like domain in VEGFR2. Several authors observed that the downstream structure of the fourth to seventh Ig-like domains plays an important role for receptor dimerization and thus activation (Fuh et al. 1998; Keyt et al. 1996; Shinkai et al. 1998; Tanaka et al. 1997). In both VEGFR and PDGFR, a tyronsine residue can be found in position 801, which in PDGFR is phosphorylated and binds to c-Src, thereby provoking a negative signaling (Heldin and Westermark 1999). In contrast to PDGFR, this tyrosine residue is not well autophosphorylated in VEGFR2. Even an exchange of this tyrosine residue in a phenylalanine mutant did not elicit a significant difference in MAP-kinase activation and DNA synthesis (Takahashi et al. 2001).

In the tyrosine kinase domain of VEGFR1 and R2 and PDGFR, similarities can again be found: the length of the kinase insert shows a high grade of homology (two inserts of 70 amino acids), whereas the structure differs between VEGFRs and PDGFRs. (Shibuya 1995; Terman et al. 1991). Two Tyr-x-x-Met motifs for autophosphorylation can be found in the PDGFR insert sequence. These are critical activating sites for the PI3-kinase/Akt pathway to activate Ras as survival signal. In the entire sequence of VEGFR1 and R2, these motifs are not present. The lack of these critical motifs suggests only a weak cross-talk between VEGFR1/R2 and the PI3K/Akt pathway (Gerber et al. 1998).

The neuropilins (NRP-1 and NRP-2) act as coreceptors for the VEGFs and increase the binding affinity of VEGF to VEGFRs. There is evidence that NRP-1 and NRP-2 can also induce signal transduction independent from their coreceptor function. The effects of NRP-mediated VEGF activation have not yet been completely understood. However, recent studies have shown that dual targeting of the vasculature with antibodies to VEGF and NRP is more effective than single-agent therapy (Pan et al. 2007).

5.2.4 Signaling and Biological Functions of VEGFR1

On the one hand, different authors observed that the affinity of VEGF-A to VEGFR1 is very high with a kDa of 2–10 pM (de Vries et al. 1992; Sawano et al. 1997). On the other hand, the tyrosine kinase activity of VEGFR1 is relatively weak and it does not stimulate the proliferation of NIH3T3 cells overexpressing VEGFR1. Furthermore, the proliferation of VEGFR1 and R2-expressing endothelial cells is not stimulated by VEGFR1-specific ligands (PlGF, VEGF-B) (Waltenberger et al. 1994).

The VEGFR1 gene encodes not only the mRNA for a full-length receptor, but also a short mRNA for a soluble form of the VEGFR1 protein, which carries only the extracellular ligand-binding domain (Kendall and Thomas 1993; Shibuya et al. 1990). The soluble ligand-binding domain could serve as a natural inhibitor of VEGF-A. Thus, VEGFR1 seems to function as a positive regulator via its tyrosine kinase domain and also as a negative regulator via its ligand-binding domain.

The relatively weak biological activity of VEGFR1 makes it difficult to assess the downstream signaling of VEGFR1. It is autophosphorylated in five positions: Tyr-1169, 1213, 1242, 1327, and 1333 (Cunningham et al. 1995; Ito et al. 2001; Sawano et al. 1997). The major binding site for the MAP-kinase pathway leading toward angiogenesis in VEGFR2 is Tyr-1175. In VEGFR1, Tyr-1169 corresponds to this binding site, but the phosphorylation here is again relatively weak, and in conclusion the aforementioned pathway is only mildly activated (Sawano et al. 1997). 1213-Tyr is highly autophosphorylated on VEGFR1 but its downstream pathway remains unclear.

It was observed by Fong et al. that VEGFR1-null mutant mice die at embryonic stage E-8.5–9.0 due to the overgrowth and disorganization of blood vessels (Fong et al. 1995). This strongly suggests a negative role for VEGFR1 by suppressing proangiogenic signals in the early embryo in order to establish a balance essential for physiological angiogenesis. Hiratsuka et al. tested if the negative role of VEGFR1 involves the ligand-binding domain or not. Knock-out mice lacking the tyrosine kinase domain of VEGFR1 were basically healthy with nearly normal blood vessels but showed a defect in the migration of macrophages toward VEGF-A (Hiratsuka et al. 2001; Hiratsuka et al. 1998). These results indicate that ligand-binding domain and transmembrane domain of VEGFR1 together are sufficient for a suppressive effect on angiogenesis in embryogenesis.

In contrast to the negative role in embryogenesis, a positive role of VEGFR1 has been described concerning tumor growth, metastasis, and inflammation. The rate of tumor growth in VEGFR1 TK (–/–) mice is slower than in wildtype mice. In particular, the tumor cells grow faster in VEGFR1 TK (–/–) mice if PlGF. a VEGFR1-specific ligand, is overexpressed at the same time (Hiratsuka et al. 2001). The mechanisms underlying this phenomenon remain unclear.

In lung carcinomas, the rate of growth in VEGFR TK (–/–) mice was similar to the rate of growth in wildtype mice, but the VEGFR TK (–/–) mice showed a significant reduction in the rate of lung-orientated metastasis (Hiratsuka et al. 2002). Hiratsuka et al. reported furthermore that there was a significant infiltration of monocytes/macrophages in the pulmonary tissue before the occurrence of metastasis in tumor-bearing wildtype mice. This infiltration also occurs in VEGFR TK (–/–) mice, but to a considerably lower degree. It was also observed that the expression of matrix metalloproteinase 9 (MMP9) was induced in both tumor-bearing wildtype mice and VEGFR TK (–/–) mice, but the extent was again different: the expression of MMP9 was threefold higher in VEGFR TK (–/–) mice than in tumor-bearing wildtype mice. In tumor-bearing MMP9-knockout mice, macrophage-lineage cells also infiltrate the lung but metastasis is significantly decreased. These results support the theory that signaling of VEGFR1 tyrosine kinase promotes lung metastasis by premetastatic induction of MMP9 expression. Similar results have been reported by Kaplan et al. in 2005 when bone-marrow derived cells (e.g., macrophage lineage cells) infiltrate the lung before the occurrence of metastasis and thus provide a pre-metastatic niche for the original tumor (Kaplan et al. 2005). This implies the importance of VEGFR signaling as target for the suppression of tumor metastasis.

5.2.5 Expression and Signaling of VEGFR2

The expression of VEGFR2 is first perceived at E7.5 in murine development in mesodermal cells of the tail (Kaipainen et al. 1993; Shalaby et al. 1995). Differentiation into primitive endothelial cells then takes place in E 7.5–8.0 when VEGFR2-positive cells migrate into the head region and yolk sac (Hiratsuka et al. 2005; Shalaby et al. 1995). In the yolk sac, these cells begin to form blood islands and initiate hematopoiesis (Eichmann et al. 1997; Shalaby et al. 1995). Postnatally, there is still an expression of VEGFR2 on hematopoietic cells found, but to a much lower extent compared to its expression on vascular endothelial cells. The role of these relatively low expression levels of VEGFR2 on hematopoietic cells remains to be determined as well as its role in nonendothelial cells (lower levels are also described on neuronal cells, osteoblasts, pancreatic duct cells, retinal progenitor cells, and megakaryocytes) (Matsumoto and Claesson-Welsh 2001).

Plate et al. reported a 3–5-fold higher expression of VEGFR2 on tumor vessels compared to normal vasculature, and VEGF-A is a stimulus for VEGFR2 expression via a positive feedback loop (Ferrara and Davis-Smyth 1997; Plate et al. 1992). Within the tumor tissue, in contrast to tumor vasculature, only little VEGFR2 is expressed, whereas expression levels of VEGF-A are high. Hence this implies a paracrine regulation loop of VEGF-A and VEGFR2 between tumor cells and vascular endothelial cells to stimulate pathological angiogenesis (Alitalo and Carmeliet 2002; Ferrara and Davis-Smyth 1997; Shibuya 1995).

VEGFR2 has a pivotal role for signal transduction in both physiological and pathological angiogenesis: VEGFR2 knockout mice die at E 8.0–8.5 with a lack of vasculogenesis. This shows the importance of VEGFR2 signaling for the differentiation of VEGFR2-positive endothelial precursor cells into vascular endothelial cells and for their proliferation (Shalaby et al. 1995). Carmeliet et al. and other groups reported a lethal effect of reduced VEGFR2 signaling due to VEGF-A (+/−) heterozygosity and neuropilin 1 (−/−) gene homozygosity. Death in this case was caused by a critical abnormality of the vascular system, in particular by an impaired aortic heart connection and vascular remodeling in the yolk sac, although the blood vessel formation itself was carried out normally (Carmeliet et al. 1996; Ferrara et al. 1996; Kawasaki et al. 1999; Maes et al. 2002). These results signify that vasculogenesis may sufficiently be promoted with reduced VEGFR2 TK activation, but in this condition, however, critical steps such as morphogenesis of the aorta and the heart are carried out insufficiently.

Several tyrosine inserts are phosphorylated in the carboxy tail and kinase insert region when stimulation of VEGFR2 by VEGF-A takes place, whereas only one of them, Tyr-1175, is the only binding site for the SH2 domain of phospholipase Cγ (PLCγ). The PKC-c-Raf-MEK-MAP pathway is activated by tyrosine phosphorylation of PLCγ (Takahashi et al. 2001). Despite this, DURING VEGFR2 pathway activation the active Ras (GTP-form of Ras) is only rarely found. Furthermore, dominant negative Ras mutants were not able to inhibit PKC-dependent MAP-kinase activation via VEGFR2 (Takahashi et al. 1999). This is unique since other growth-promoting receptor tyrosine kinases such as EGFR utilize the activation of Ras for various downstream signaling events. In addition, Sakurai et al. detected a death at embryonic stage 9.0 which was again due to a lack of vasculogenesis in knock-in mutant carrying a Tyr-to-Ph substitution at position 1173 (in analogy to human 1175-Tyr) (Sakurai et al. 2005). These results suggest that the VEGFR2-1175PY-PLCγ-PKC pathway has an important role in vivo, although its exact biological meaning remains unclear. There is evidence that signaling via VEGFR2 might be critical for the maintenance of the tubular structure of blood vessels during angiogenesis as well as vascular remodeling. Interactions of VEGFR2 and VE-cadherin and integrins have been observed (Shay-Salit et al. 2002; Stupack and Cheresh 2004). The exact mechanism and the interacting residues involved have not yet been detected. VEGFR2 is also expressed on lymph vessels, and thus might be involved in lymphangiogenesis (Hirakawa et al. 2005; Veikkola et al. 2001).

5.2.6 VEGF and Malignancy

Neovascularization in the proximity of tumors was first described a century ago, (Goldmann 1907; Ide et al. 1939) and was named angiogenesis in contrast to the term vasculogenesis referring to the development of the vascular system in embryogenesis. In 1971, the paradigm-shifting work of Folkman (Folkman 1971; Folkman et al. 1971) proposed a new strategy against malignant tumor: blocking angiogenesis. In the concerted play of growth factors (e.g., FGF, PDGF, VEGF, angiopoietins), which at least partly causes the angiogenic switch in malignant tumors, VEGF is believed to be one of the key molecules as it stimulates permeability, endothelial cell activation, survival and proliferation, proliferation of tumor cells, and facilitates invasion and migration. In situ hybridization studies have demonstrated the expression of VEGF mRNA in the majority of human tumors, including carcinoma of the lung (Volm et al. 1997a, b), breast (Brown et al. 1995; Yoshiji et al. 1996), gastrointestinal tract (Brown et al. 1993b; Ellis et al. 1998; Suzuki et al. 1996; Uchida et al. 1998), kidney (Nicol et al. 1997; Tomisawa et al. 1999), bladder (Brown et al. 1993a), ovary (Olson et al. 1994; Sowter et al. 1997; Yamamoto et al. 1997), endometrium (Guidi et al. 1996), and several intracranial tumors, for example, glioblastoma multiforme (Plate et al. 1992; Shweiki et al. 1992). Sporadic expression has also been observed in capillary hemangioblastoma (Wizigmann-Voos et al. 1995). In a variety of pituitary tumors, VEGF expression has also been described (Lloyd et al. 1999). VEGF is expressed in various cell lines derived from different hematological malignancies, including T-cell lymphoma, acute lymphoblastic leukemia, Burkitt's lymphoma, acute lymphocytic leukemia, histiocytic lymphoma, promyelocytic leukemia, etc. (for review see (Gerber and Ferrara 2003)). Expression of both VEGFRs has been detected in some, but not all, leukemia cell lines, and VEGFR-1 was found to be more frequently expressed than VEGFR-2. These observations suggest that the production of VEGF by malignant myeloid precursors might serve both as an autocrine growth stimulus and a diffusible, paracrine, signal-mediating angiogenesis within the bone marrow.

Although tumor cells usually represent the major source of VEGF, tumor-associated stroma is also an important site of VEGF production (Fukumura et al. 1998; Gerber et al. 2000). Chemotactic signals from tumor cells cause recruitment of stromal cells, which also produce VEGF and other angiogenic factors. The growth of several human tumor cell lines transplanted in nude mice is substantially reduced, but not completely suppressed, by antihuman VEGF monoclonal antibodies (Kim et al. 1993). Administration of mFlt (1–3)-IgG, a chimeric receptor containing the first three Ig-like domains of VEGFR-1, that binds both human and mouse VEGF, results in a nearly complete suppression of tumor growth and tumor cells necrosis in a nude mouse model of human rhabdomyosarcoma (Gerber et al. 2000). Similar observations were made using a chimeric soluble receptor consisting of domain 2 of VEGFR-1 fused with domain 3 of VEGFR-2, referred to as "VEGF-trap" (Holash et al. 2002). Thus, the use of VEGF inhibitors that only target human VEGF in human xenograft models might result in an underestimation of the role of VEGF in the process of tumor angiogenesis.

The overexpression of VEGF has been observed to be a bad prognostic parameter in carcinomas of the lung (Imoto et al. 1998; O'Byrne et al. 2000; Volm et al. 1997a), breast (Gasparini et al. 1997; Toi et al. 1995), gastrointestinal tract (Amaya et al. 1997; Ishigami et al. 1998; Maeda et al. 2000; Ogata et al. 2003; Shih et al. 2000), kidney (Jacobsen et al. 2004), and ovary (Paley et al. 1997; Yamamoto et al. 1997). Klein et al. (2001) have shown that VEGF expression detected by immunohistochemistry is a negative prognostic marker in papillary thyroid carcinoma. In prostate carcinoma, VEGF expression is regulated by androgens, and recent studies suggest a correlation between angiogenesis and biological aggressiveness of the disease. In hematologic malignancies, the overexpression of VEGF also led to an unfavorable outcome (Aguayo et al. 2002).

A potent inhibitory effect on the growth of several tumor cell lines in nude mice is exerted by anti-VEGF monoclonal antibodies (Kim et al. 1993), but this antibody had no effect on the tumor cells in vitro. As a consequence, various other tumor cell lines were found to be inhibited in vivo by anti-VEGF monoclonal antibodies (Asano et al. 1995; Borgstrom et al. 1996, 1998,

1999; Melnyk et al. 1996; Mesiano et al. 1998; Warren et al. 1995). Tumor growth inhibition was demonstrated also with other anti-VEGF treatments, including a retrovirus-delivered dominant negative Flk-1 mutant (Millauer et al. 1994), small molecule inhibitors of VEGFR-2 signaling (Fiedler et al. 2003; Strawn et al. 1996; Wedge et al. 2000; Wood et al. 2000), antisense oligonucleotides (Oku et al. 1998; Saleh et al. 1996), anti-VEGFR-2 antibodies (334), and soluble VEGF receptors (Gerber et al. 2000; Goldman et al. 1998; Kong et al. 1998; Prewett et al. 1999). The inhibitory effects of small molecule inhibitors targeting VEGFR-1 and VEGFR-2 on the growth of human myeloid leukemia cell lines have been documented (Smolich et al. 2001). Further evidence for a functional role of VEGFR-2 in leukemic cell growth was provided by experiments showing that an anti-VEGFR-2 antibody inhibits proliferation of xenotransplanted human leukemia cells and significantly increased survival of nude mice (Dias et al. 2000). Clinical results with anti-VEGF strategies are detailed in Chap. 9 in this volume.

5.3 PDGF

PDGFs and their receptors are known to play important roles in animal development, for example, in gastrulation, the development of cranial and cardiac neural crest, gonads, lung, intestine, skin, CNS, and skeleton, and thus have been intensively studied over the past two decades. Similarly, models for PDGFR-β signaling have been developed in angiogenesis and early hematopoiesis and are widely accepted. Furthermore, PDGF signaling is observed in various pathological conditions and diseases. Autocrine activation of PDGF signaling pathways is observed in gliomas, sarcomas, and leukemias, whereas paracrine PDGF signaling pathways are important for the development of epithelial cancers. Here PDGF triggers the recruitment of stromal cells and seems to be involved in epithelial–mesenchymal transition. This has an influence on tumor growth by affecting angiogenesis, invasion, and metastasis. Besides, PDGF is not only important in malignancy, but also drives the development of various other pathological conditions such as vascular disorders (e.g., atherosclerosis, pulmonary hypertension, retinopathies) and fibrotic diseases (e.g., pulmonary or hepatic fibrosis, scleroderma, and glomerulosclerosis). In the following paragraphs, current knowledge on PDGF functions in health and disease are summarized and a background to PDGF biochemistry and cell biology is discussed. The regulation of bioavailability and tissue distribution of the PDGFs by certain different mechanisms are shown.

5.3.1 Platelet-Derived Growth Factor and Its Isoforms

PDGF was identified more than three decades ago for the first time as a serum growth factor for fibroblasts, smooth muscle cells (SMCs), and glia cells (Kohler and Lipton 1974; Ross et al. 1974; Wasteson et al. 1976), and was shown to be a cationic disulfide-linked homo- or heterodimer of two different polypeptide chains, A and B, separable by using reversed phase chromatography (Johnsson et al. 1982).

For almost two decades, the theory existed that the PDGF family consists of three proteins—PDGF-AA, PDGF-AB, and PDGF-BB—encoded by two genes, PDGF-A and PDGF-B.

Between the B-chain of PDGF (PDGF-B) and the product of the retroviral oncogene v-sis of simian sarcoma virus (SSV) (Doolittle et al. 1983; Waterfield et al. 1983) some homology was characterized by amino acid sequencing. Subsequently, it was confirmed by different studies that the human cellular counterpart to v-sis was identical to PDGF-B, and that autocrine PDGF activity was sufficient for SSV transformation in vitro. For the relationship between neoplastic cell transformation and normal growth control, this was a staggering discovery because the importance of autocrine growth stimulation in neoplastic transformation was demonstrated for the first time. It is now a well-established model that autocrine PDGF stimulation is also of significance in some human cancers.

PDGF-A was characterized by cDNA cloning (Betsholtz et al. 1986) and most cell lines express PDGF-A and secrete PDGF-AA homodimers (Heldin et al. 1986), whereas PDGF-BB homodimers are produced by SSV-transformed or PDGF-B-expressing cells. The view of two encoding genes for PDGF dimers was corrected 20 years after the first description of PDGF when two additional PDGF genes were identified by Li et al. and Bergsten et al. (PDGF-C and PDGF-D) (Bergsten et al. 2001; Li et al. 2000). To current knowledge, the PDGF genes and polypeptides belong to a family of growth factors that also includes the VEGFs (see earlier) (Fredriksson et al. 2004).

Although the PDGFs play crucial roles during development, there is only limited evidence for, and knowledge about, their physiological functions in the adult. However, increased PDGF activity is important in several diseases and pathological conditions, and even causal pathogenic roles of the PDGFs have been established for some diseases. This might provide prospects for therapy, using PDGF antagonists. Intensive testing of PDGF receptor-inhibiting substances on the one hand and recombinant human PDGF-BB on the other hand is now taking place in preclinical models as well as in human clinical trials.

Nine different genes encode four different PDGF chains (PDGF-A, PDGF-B, PDGF-C, and PDGF-D) and five different VEGF chains (VEGF-A, VEGF-B, VEGF-C, VEGF-D, and placenta growth factor, PlGF) in mammals (Ferrara et al. 2003; Fredriksson et al. 2004) (Fig. 5.3). All PDGFs and VEGFs are dimers of disulfide-linked polypeptide chains (Heldin and Westermark 1999).

One heterodimer (PDGF-AB) has been demonstrated specifically in human platelets whose physiological importance remains unclear although its signaling properties have been shown to be different from those of the homodimers (Ekman et al. 1999; Stroobant and Waterfield 1984).

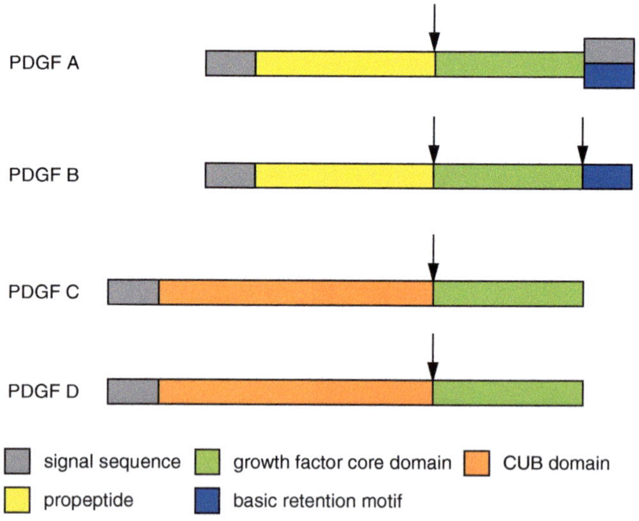

Fig. 5.3 Mammalian PDGFs. *Arrows* indicate proteolytic cleavage sites

The nonoverlapping endogenous expression patterns of PDGF-A and PDGF-B (Hoch and Soriano 2003) suggest that heterodimers are infrequent in vivo. Also, there is no evidence for genetic interactions between PDGF-A and PDGF-B (Li et al. 2000). Thus, homodimers appear to dominate, at least during development. Mammalian PDGFs and VEGFs separate into four distinguishable classes of proteins (VEGF structure and isoforms shown earlier). All members have a growth factor core domain containing a set of cysteine residues. The core domain is necessary and sufficient for receptor binding and activation. The classification into PDGFs or VEGFs is based on receptor binding. The model that PDGFs and VEGFs are selective for their own receptors had been generally accepted until recently this was challenged by the demonstration that VEGF-A may bind to and activate PDGF receptors in bone-marrow-derived mesenchymal stem cells (Ball et al. 2007). The view that VEGFs target mainly endothelial cells, whereas mesenchymal cells are targeted by PDGFs is also called into question by the study mentioned earlier and by findings that VEGF-C and PDGF-A both regulate oligodendrocyte development, however, through distinct receptors. Both VEGFs and PDGFs also appear to be of importance in hematopoietic development, neurogenesis, and neuroprotection (Andrae et al. 2008).

5.3.2 PDGF Receptors

PDGFs act via two RTKs that share structures with c-Kit, c-Fms, and Flt3. The domain structures include five extracellular immunoglobulin loops and an intracellular tyrosine kinase (TK) domain (Fig. 5.4).

Receptor dimerization is promoted by ligand binding. The dimerization then initiates signaling. Depending on ligand configuration and the pattern of receptor expression, different receptor dimers may form (Heldin and Westermark 1999). Only a few interactions between PDGF and the PDGF receptors have been shown in vivo, whereas in cell culture experiments, the interactions seem to be multiple and complex. An overview of PDGF receptor signal transduction mechanisms is provided in further reviews on this topic (Heldin and Westermark 1999; Ronnstrand and Heldin 2001; Tallquist and Kazlauskas 2004).

5.3.3 PDGF Ligand and Receptor Expression Patterns

Although there is evidence for paracrine as well as autocrine functions of PDGF, autocrine roles, similar to those recently described for VEGF-A in endothelial cells (Lee et al. 2007), have not been demonstrated for the PDGFs. Their function as paracrine growth factors seems to be of greater importance; they act locally to drive different cellular responses (Betsholtz 2004; Hoch and Soriano 2003). The expression patterns of PDGF and PDGFR are spatio-temporally regulated in vivo during development and in some physiological hypertrophic responses. Expression of PDGF in cultured cells is dynamic and responds to certain stimuli, for example, low oxygen tension, thrombin, cytokines, and growth factors including PDGF itself (Heldin and Westermark 1999). Expression of PDGF-A also increases in human uterine SMCs during pregnancy (physiological hypertrophy). Similarly, the expression of PDGFR is dynamic. In physiological conditions, the expression of PDGFR on mesenchymal cells is low in vivo but increases in conditions of inflammation. Several factors induce PDGFR expression, including TGF-β, estrogen, interleukin-1 (IL-1), fibroblast growth factor-2 (FGF-2), tumor necrosis factor-α, and lipopolysaccharide (Heldin and Westermark 1999). Although the detailed expression patterns of the individual PDGF ligands and receptors are complex and have been reviewed elsewhere

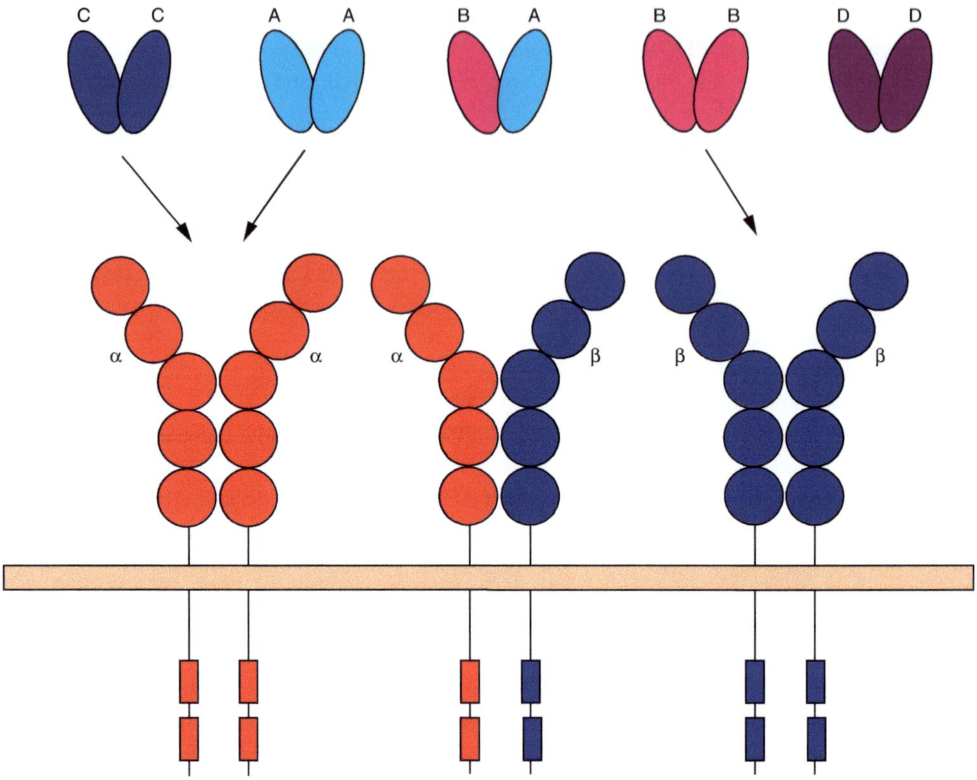

Fig. 5.4 PDGF and PDGF receptor interactions. Each part of the PDGF dimer interacts with the PDGFR and thus influences receptor configuration and activity. *Arrows* show interactions which have been observed to be of importance in mammalian development

(Heldin and Westermark 1999; Hoch and Soriano 2003), there are some general patterns of expression: PDGF-B is mainly expressed in vascular endothelial cells, megakaryocytes, and neurons. PDGF-A and PDGF-C are expressed in epithelial cells, muscle, and neuronal progenitors. PDGF-D expression has been described in fibroblasts and SMCs at certain locations but is less well-characterized. PDGFR-α is expressed in mesenchymal cells as well as in subtypes of mesenchymal progenitors in lung, skin, and intestine and in pericytes of the vessel wall. In mesenchymal progenitors, a particularly strong expression of PDGFR-α has been described. The PDGF and PDGFR genes are located on different chromosomes. Their transcriptional regulation seems mostly independent. The transcriptional regulation of the PDGF-A and PDGF-B genes has been extensively studied and is reviewed elsewhere (Heldin and Westermark 1999; Kaetzel 2003). The transcriptional regulation of PDGF-C and PDGF-D and the PDGFRs has not been widely studied to date.

5.3.4 PDGF Biosynthesis, Secretion, and Distribution

There are control mechanisms of PDGF biosynthesis and processing at multiple levels. Biosynthesis and processing vary for the different PDGFs. There is currently no evidence for regulated secretion of the PDGFs. PDGFs instead appear to be constitutively released (Fruttiger et al. 2000). PDGF-A and PDGF-B become disulfide-linked into dimers already as propeptides. PDGF-C and PDGF-D have been less studied in this regard. Intracellularly, the N-terminal prodomains of PDGF-A and PDGF-B are removed by furin or related proprotein convertases (for review, see (Fredriksson et al. 2004)). N-terminal processing is necessary for PDGF-A to acquire receptor-binding ability (for review, see (Fredriksson et al. 2004; Heldin and Westermark 1999)). Likewise, PDGF-B also requires N-terminal propeptide removal to become active. PDGF-C and PDGF-D are not processed intracellularly but are instead secreted as conditionally inactive ligands (Fredriksson et al. 2004; Reigstad et al. 2005). Dissociation of the growth factor domain from the CUB domain leads to activation in the extra-cellular space. Plasmin and tissue plasminogen activator (tPA) have been shown to remove the CUB domain in PDGF-C proteolytically, leading to biological activity (Fredriksson et al. 2004). Although the endogenous protease responsible for PDGF-C activation in vivo remains to be identified, tPA endogenously expressed in cultured fibroblasts activates PDGF-CC expressed by the same cells. Activation of PDGF-D can also take place by plasmin cleavage, but not tPA cleavage (Fredriksson et al. 2004). The tPA needs to interact with both the CUB domain and the core domain in order to cleave and activate PDGF-C, which likely explains its specificity. Biological activity and action range of growth factors, cytokines, and morphogens is explained by their uneven distribution with gradients and depots. Binding to extracellular matrix components plays an important role for the diffusion of PDGF in the tissue interstitium. The binding is attained partly by the positively charged C-terminal motifs (referred to as retention motifs) for PDGF-A and PDGF-B. The C-terminal motifs contain a high proportion of basic amino acid residues. PDGF-C and PDGF-D lack basic retention motifs. Still, the existence of CUB domains results in protein–protein and protein–carbohydrate interactions in other contexts. This may be a regulatory factor for extracellular distribution of constitutively inactive PDGF-C and PDGF-D. Proteolytic processing determines the retention motifs in PDGF-B, whereas alternative splicing is the major determinant for the retention motif in PDGF-A. Alternative splicing of the PDGF-A transcript is specific for different cell types and also differs among tumor cell lines (Afrakhte et al. 1996) and in different organs during development. The C-terminal proteolytic processing of PDGF-B may take place intracellularly or extracellularly. There are hints that thrombin is the endogenous protease for extracellular proteolysis, and thus might release endogenously expressed PDGF-B adherent to the cell surface and the extracellular matrix (Kelly et al. 1993; Soyombo and DiCorleto 1994).

PDGF interacts with heparin and heparan sulfate proteoglycans (HSPGs) like many other growth factor and morphogens as well, and the roles of these interactions remained unclear until phenotypic analysis of PDGF-B retention motif knockout mice were carried out by different groups (Abramsson et al. 2007; Feyzi et al. 1997; Hacker et al. 2005; Lin et al. 2004; Lustig et al. 1999). Targeted deletion of the retention motif led to detachment of pericytes from the microvessel wall (Abramsson et al. 2003; Lindblom et al. 2003). Reduced heparan sulfate (HS) *N*-sulfation (caused by lack of the responsible enzyme *N*-deacetylase/*N*- sulfotransferase-1) similarly led to pericyte detachment and delayed pericyte migration in vivo (Abramsson et al. 2007). This might be caused by reduced PDGF-BB binding to HS. PDGF-BB/HS interaction appears to depend on overall *N*- and *O*-sulfation of HS. Considering these observations, a model in which PDGF-BB secreted from endothelial cells interacts with HS at the endothelial surface or in the periendothelial matrix can be developed. Consecutively, this would lead to local deposits of PDGF-BB that are critical for the correct investment of pericytes in the vessel wall. HS binding is also necessary for proper localization and function of VEGF-A (Ruhrberg et al. 2002).

PDGF also binds to certain non-HSPG extracellular proteins. The physiological significance of these interactions remains unclear. Binding of PDGF-B to α-2-macroglobulin (Bonner et al. 1995; Bonner and Osornio-Vargas 1995) has been observed. In this context, α-2-macroglobulin is potentially acting as a scavenger for PDGF-B through low-density lipoprotein (LDL) receptor-related protein (LRP) receptors on macrophages and other cells (Bonner et al. 1995). PDGF-B also binds to SPARC and adiponectin, which may keep the growth factor in the extracellular space (Arita et al. 2002; Raines et al. 1992; Raines and Ross 1992).

5.3.5 PDGFR Signal Transduction

Dimerization is crucial in PDGF receptor activation as it causes receptor autophosphorylation on tyrosine residues in the intracellular domain (Kelly et al. 1991). By autophosphorylation the receptor kinase is activated and docking sites for downstream signaling molecules are allocated (Kazlauskas and Cooper 1989). Docking of receptor substrates and further signal transmission involves protein–protein interactions. For these interactions specific domains are essential; for example, Src homology 2 (SH2) and phosphotyrosine-binding (PTB) domains recognizing phosphorylated tyrosines, SH3 domains recognizing proline-rich regions, pleckstrin homology (PH) domains recognizing membrane phospholipids, and PDZ domains recognizing C-terminal-specific sequences (for review, see (Heldin et al. 1998)). Binding to specific sites on the phosphorylated receptors is mostly affected by the SH2 domains of the PDGFR effectors. PDGFR-α and PDGFR-β signaling involves several well-described signaling pathways, for example, Ras-MAPK, PI3K, and PLC. These signaling pathways are involved in various cellular and developmental responses (Fig. 5.5).

PDGFRs connect to Ras-MAPK through the adaptor proteins Grb2 and Shc. Grb2 binds the activated PDGFR through its SH2 domain and complexes Sos1 through its SH3 domains. Sos1 then activates Ras, followed by downstream activation of Raf-1 and the MAPK cascade. Gene transcription is activated by MAPK signaling, leading to stimulation of cell growth, differentiation, and migration (Bar-Sagi and Feramisco 1986; Campbell et al. 1995). PI3K is a family of enzymes phosphorylating phosphoinositides, and effectors of PI3K signaling include serine/threonine kinases such as Akt/PKB (Burgering and Coffer 1995; Franke et al. 1995), some members of the PKC family including atypical isoforms (Akimoto et al. 1996; Nakanishi et al. 1993), p70 S6 kinase (Chung et al. 1994), JNK (Lopez-Ilasaca et al. 1997), and small GTPases of the Rho family (Nobes et al. 1995). Activation of the PI3K pathway by PDGFRs stimulates actin reorganization, directed cell movements, cell growth, and inhibition of apoptosis (Hu et al. 1995). PLC-γ binds PDGFRs, which results in its phosphorylation and thereby activation (for review, see (Tallquist and Kazlauskas 2004)). PLC-γ activation leads to mobilization of intracellular calcium ions and the activation of PKC (Berridge 1993a, b). The effects of PDGFR-β-mediated PLC-γ activation include promotion of cell growth and motility (Kundra et al. 1994). Several additional signaling molecules are engaged by PDGFRs, including enzymes, adaptors, and transcription factors. Activation of the Src TK promotes Myc transcription and mitogenic responses (for review, see (Erpel and Courtneidge 1995)). PKC-δ is phosphorylated by PDGFR-β, leading to its activation and translocation to the cell membrane. This in turn promotes cell differentiation (Li and Pierce 1996). STAT transcription factors may bind to

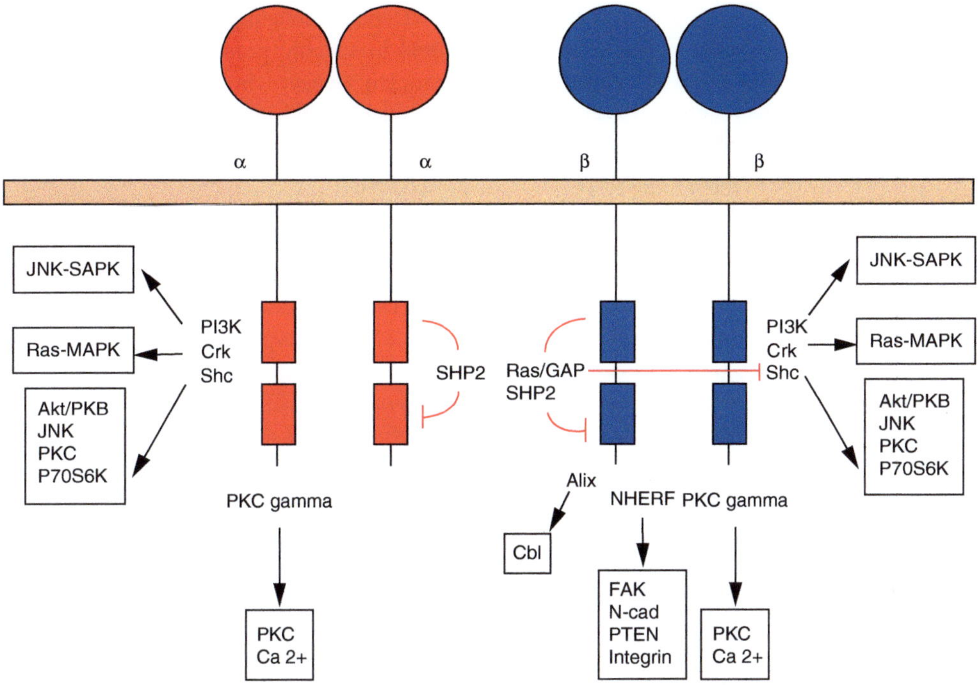

Fig. 5.5 PDGFR signal transduction: PDGFR α and β with intracellular domains. Negative feedback is illustrated in red. *Arrows* show linkage to important signaling pathways and effectors

PDGF receptors, causing their phosphorylation and activation (Darnell 1997). Interactions between PDGF receptors and integrins have been reported, and these interactions enhance cell proliferation, migration, and survival (Assoian 1997; Frisch and Ruoslahti 1997). PDGFR interaction with integrins helps localizing PDGFRs and interacting molecules at focal adhesions, which are sites where several signaling pathways initiate and cross-talk (Clark and Brugge 1995). Recently, Na^+/ H^+ exchanger regulatory factors (NHERFs) were observed to bind PDGFR-β and thereby cause a linkage with focal adherence kinase and the cortical actin cytoskeleton (James et al. 2004), as well as to N-cadherin (Theisen et al. 2007) and the phosphatase PTEN (Takahashi et al. 2006).

Feedback control mechanisms accurately regulate PDGF signaling. Stimulatory and inhibitory signals arise in a parallel way. The final response depends on the balance between these signals (Heldin et al. 1998). The SHP-2 tyrosine phosphatase binds PDGFR through its SH2 domain and dephosphorylates the receptor and its substrates (Lechleider et al. 1993). The negative regulator of Ras, Ras-GAP, also binds PDGFR-β through its SH2 domain (Fantl et al. 1992).

5.3.6 Cellular Responses to PDGFR Signaling

There are certain rapid cellular responses to PDGFs that proceed within seconds to minutes after PDGFR activation. These reactions are not dependent on gene expression and protein synthesis. There are similarities between responses caused by PDGFR-α and PDGFR-β, nevertheless the responses are not identical. Both receptors are able to promote the rearrangement of actin filaments, but only PDGFR-β causes the formation of circular ruffles. PDGFR-β also mobilizes calcium ions more efficiently than PDGFR-α does(Diliberto et al. 1992; Fatatis and Miller 1997). Inhibition of cell communication by phosphorylated gap junctions is observed to be caused by PDGFR-β (Hossain et al. 1998). It is unclear whether this ability is shared with PDGFR-α.

Like other RTKs, PDGFRs initiate fast transcriptional changes involving so-called immediate early genes (IEGs) (Cochran et al. 1983). IEGs are direct targets of the transcription factors, which get activated through various signaling pathways by posttranslational modification. The IEG responses seem to be necessary for many of the long-term effects of PDGFs in vitro and in vivo. The extent of specificity contributed to PDGFR signaling by IEG responses remains unclear. Different RTKs induce similar or even identical sets of IEGs (Fambrough et al. 1999). Furthermore, different signaling pathways activated by the same receptor (PDGFR-β) induce largely overlapping sets of IEGs in vitro (Fambrough et al. 1999). These studies implicate that quantitative rather than qualitative differences in the IEG responses are regulators for the specific responses to different RTKs and signaling pathways. In vivo analysis of an allelic series of pdgfrb tyrosine-to-phenylalanine mutations supports this view: it leads to disrupting connection to different substrates and signaling pathways. Mutations in single or multiple tyrosine residues caused quantitatively different but qualitatively similar developmental effects (Tallquist et al. 2003; Tallquist and Soriano 2003). In contrast, similar analyzes of PDGFR-α revealed a remarkable difference in the roles of the downstream signaling pathways. For PDGFR-β, there is no or only limited consequence from the disruption of signaling through PI3K alone (Heuchel et al. 1999; Tallquist et al. 2000). Quite contrary to this observation, PI3K is essential for PDGFR-α function during development (Klinghoffer et al. 2002). Deficient coupling to Src from PDGFR-α resulted in specific problems with the oligodendrocyte lineage. In contrast, other processes, such as skeletal development, remained normal.

There appears to be cooperation between different IEGs in their regulation of downstream cellular and developmental events. Analysis of gene trap mutants for >20 IEGs downstream from PDGFR signaling showed a striking degree of phenotypic overlap and genetic interaction. Different mutated IEGs produced qualitatively similar responses. Furthermore, the combination of mutations in several genes strengthened specific phenotypic outcomes known to depend on PDGFR signaling, such as craniofacial, cardiovascular, or kidney developmental processes (Schmahl et al. 2007).

The overlap and coincidence between signaling pathways, IEGs, and biological processes leads to a model in which specifity is determined by quantitative and spatial differences in dimension and duration of responses in the signaling cascade. Meanwhile, cell type- and context-specific PDGFR expression is the major reason for PDGFR specificity in developmental functions, and correlations between the expression patterns of the PDGFRs and their major sites of functions have been described (e.g., PDGFR-β is strongly expressed in pericyte progenitors). Lack of redundancy therefore depends in part on the different transcriptional regulation of the two pdgfr genes. If a PDGFR-β intracellular domain is knocked into the pdgfra gene, phenotypically normal animals are obtained, showing that PDGFR-β signaling might be a full substitute for PDGFR-α signaling if it is expressed in a spatially and temporally correct manner (Klinghoffer et al. 2001). In contrast, PDGFR-α signaling can only compensate for the loss of PDGFR-β signaling to some extent and targeted substitution in PDGFR-α with other RTK signaling domains also showed only partial rescue (Klinghoffer et al. 2001). Thus, specificity of PDGFR signaling might be obtained by a combination of cell type-specific expression and variable engagement of downstream signaling pathways.

Ligand occupancy of PDGFRs drives endocytotic receptor internalization, which is followed by lysosomal degradation, and according to this PDGFR signaling is temporally limited (Heldin et al. 1998; Sorkin et al. 1991). A lack of phosphatase TC-PTP, a negative regulator for PDGFR-β phosphorylation (Persson et al. 2004), signs for a recycling of PDGFR-β can be observed. PDGFR-α does not undergo such a recycling process (Karlsson et al. 2006). Trafficking toward lysosomal degradation of PDGFR-β depends on interactions with c-Cbl and receptor ubiquitination. Alix, an adapter protein which interacts with the C-terminal domain of PDGFR-β, facilitates ubiquitination and degradation of c-Cbl, and thus inhibits PDGFR-β-downregulation (Lennartsson et al. 2006).

5.3.7 PDGF and PDGFR in Malignancy

PDGF not only has an important role in many disease processes, but its role might even be causative, that is, in some malignancies, when genetic abnormalities cause uncontrolled PDGFR signaling in tumor cells. A functional role of PDGFR signaling has also been shown in various animal models by genetic or pharmacological loss-of-function-approaches, which implicates the reversibility of the disease process by PDGF pathway inhibitors. However, the limitation of this approach originates in the lack of specificity of all inhibitors currently available. Furthermore, it often remains unclear as to what degree the animal models are relevant for the corresponding human disease process. Considering these limitations, there is still a growing evidence for the involvement of PDGF signaling in several disease processes. Potent and nontoxic PDGFR inhibitors such as imatinib give augmenting possibilities to test theories about causative roles of PDGF signaling in malignancy in humans too.

In general, two types of cells have been described to respond in a pathological way to PDGFs – SMCs and fibroblasts – leading to vessel wall pathologies and tissue fibrosis. PDGFR-β appears to be the dominant PDGFR involved in vascular pathology, whereas growing evidence in contrast suggests a crucial role for PDGFR-α signaling in various types of mesenchymal cell/fibroblast-driven pathologies. Thus, there is a certain homology between the pathological roles of PDGFRs and their developmental roles in which PDGFR-β signaling has a key role in vascular mural cell formation, whereas PDGFR-α has both general and specific roles in the development of various mesenchymal and fibroblastic cell compartments.

Six acquired capabilities of cancer cells are described in the review on hallmarks of cancer by Hanahan and Weinberg – self-sufficiency in growth signals, insensitivity to antigrowth signals, escape from apoptosis, sustained angiogenesis, tissue invasion and metastasis, and limitless replicative potential (Hanahan and Weinberg 2000).

Several studies have recently shown that self-sufficiency in growth signals may be established for certain cell types via autocrine growth stimulatory loops involving PDGF-B/PDGFR-β signaling (Andrae et al. 2008; Heldin and Westermark 1999).

Autocrine PDGF signaling drives proliferative expansion of clones of genetically unstable or preneoplasitc cells, which then become malignant by further genetic alteration and thus contributes to tumorigenesis. Johnsson et al. demonstrated no difference between autocrine PDGF stimulation compared to exogenous PDGF stimulation (Johnsson et al. 1985). In addition, Uhrbom et al. showed that PDGF stimulation by injection of PDGF-B producing retroviruses into the mouse brain results in a malignant phenotype only by the additive induction of genetic changes by the retrovirus

(Uhrbom et al. 1998). PDGF expression and autocrine signaling has been described particularly in human gliomas (Hermansson et al. 1988; Lokker et al. 2002; Nister et al. 1988), and an overexpression is likely to cause the formation of glioma-like tumors (Newton 2003; Uhrbom et al. 1998). Subsequently, inhibition of PDGF signaling (e.g., by administration of imatinib which has also been tested in clinical trials (Newton 2003)) slows down the growth of glioma-like tumors (Lokker et al. 2002; Uhrbom et al. 2000). The mechanism by which PDGF signaling induces the formation of gliomas is not well understood yet, but there is evidence for a link between PDGF signaling and TGFβ signaling via Smad2/3/4. Futhermore, genetic alterations also lead to overexpression and/or altered gene products. Several different mechanisms cause genetic changes, for example, amplification, translocations, and activating mutation, which have all been described in human tumors with high PDGF expression. Upregulation of PDGFR-α is observed again in human gliomas of all malignant grades; the higher the expression, the more malignant is the tumor (Hermanson et al. 1996; Smith and Jenkins 2000; Smith et al. 2000). Gene amplifications have also been described in other tumor entities such as oesophageal squamous cell carcinoma (Arai et al. 2003), sarcomas (Zhao et al. 2002), and epithelial carcinomas (see later). Gastrointestinal stroma tumors (GISTs) carry activating mutations in the Kit receptor tyrosine kinase. In a subset of GISTs with wild-type Kit, gain-of-function mutations in PDGFR-A have been observed (Heinrich et al. 2003; Hirota et al. 2003). Kit and PDGFR-α mutations are mutually exclusive, but around 90% of all GISTs carry one of the two mutations. Constitutive activation of the receptor is a consequence of PDGFR-α mutation found either in the juxtamembrane region or in any of the two TK domains. Signaling via PI3K and STAT3 seems to be crucial for this activation (for review, see (Ali et al. 2007).

In leukemias and myeloid disorders, several different translocations of the PDGFR-B gene have been described by Sirvent et al. (2003), but since most of these translocations are very rare, their exact role in leukemogenesis remains to be elucidated. In epithelial carcinomas, PDGF signaling is mostly described as acting in a paracrine fashion (Heldin and Westermark 1999). There is evidence, however, that autocrine PDGF signaling is also important for tumorigenesis in carcinomas with ectopic onset of PDGFR expression (Heldin et al. 1988).

Beyond the consequences of autocrine PDGF signaling as a proliferative stimulus, it also seems to be of importance in invasion and metastasis of epithelial malignancies.

Paracrine PDGF signaling is necessary to recruit different stromal cells (e.g., vascular and fibroblastic stromal cells) and to regulate their functions (Abramsson et al. 2003; Forsberg et al. 1993; Furuhashi et al. 2004; Pietras et al. 2001; Skobe and Fusenig 1998). This seems to be an explanation for the frequently compromised drug delivery to tumors (e.g., due to high interstitial pressure caused by PDGF signaling). Tumor stroma is composed of nonneoplastic cells and extracellular matrix recruited from the circulation or from neighboring cells and makes up a variable proportion of the total tumor mass. The stroma composition itself is varied as well. In stromal cells of carcinomas, PDGFR expression is frequent and is found in lung, colorectal, breast, skin, and different other carcinomas (see (Andrae et al. 2008; Heldin and Westermark 1999; Ostman 2004) for further review).

In conclusion, PDGF signaling contributes to the causes for three of the six cancer cell traits summarized by Hanahan and Weinberg: self-sufficient growth, angiogenesis, and metastasis, and moreover is partly responsible for resistance to cytotoxic therapy.

Thus, VEGF and PDGF both play important roles in neovascularization, in particular in several human malignancies. Oxygen and nutrient support must be provided by vasculature to enable a tumor to grow beyond 1–2 mm diameter. VEGF and PDGF are causally involved in an angiogenic switch, which then provides vasculature for the tumor. Different factors precede and cause the upregulation of PDGF and VEGF in malignancy, for example, oncogene activation, inhibition of tumor supressors, release of growth factors and tumor hxpoxia, and necrosis, and furthermore, a certain protection against apoptotic signals is provided for tumor vasculature. The characteristics of both VEGF and PDGF make them a putative therapeutic target for anticancer strategies.

References

Abramsson A, Kurup S, Busse M, Yamada S, Lindblom P, Schallmeiner E, Stenzel D, Sauvaget D, Ledin J, Ringvall M, Landegren U, Kjellen L, Bondjers G, Li JP, Lindahl U, Spillmann D, Betsholtz C, Gerhardt H (2007) Defective N-sulfation of heparan sulfate proteoglycans limits PDGF-BB binding and pericyte recruitment in vascular development. Genes Dev 21:316–331

Abramsson A, Lindblom P, Betsholtz C (2003) Endothelial and nonendothelial sources of PDGF-B regulate pericyte recruitment and influence vascular pattern formation in tumors. J Clin Invest 112:1142–1151

Achen MG, Jeltsch M, Kukk E, Makinen T, Vitali A, Wilks AF, Alitalo K, Stacker SA (1998) Vascular endothelial growth factor D (VEGF-D) is a ligand for the tyrosine kinases VEGF receptor 2 (Flk1) and VEGF receptor 3 (Flt4). Proc Natl Acad Sci U S A 95:548–553

Afrakhte M, Nister M, Ostman A, Westermark B, Paulsson Y (1996) Production of cell-associated PDGF-AA by a human sarcoma cell line: evidence for a latent autocrine effect. Int J Cancer 68:802–809

Aguayo A, Kantarjian HM, Estey EH, Giles FJ, Verstovsek S, Manshouri T, Gidel C, O'Brien S, Keating MJ, Albitar M (2002) Plasma vascular endothelial growth factor levels have prognostic significance in patients with acute myeloid leukemia but not in patients with myelodysplastic syndromes. Cancer 95:1923–1930

Akimoto K, Takahashi R, Moriya S, Nishioka N, Takayanagi J, Kimura K, Fukui Y, Osada S, Mizuno K, Hirai S, Kazlauskas A, Ohno S (1996) EGF or PDGF receptors activate atypical PKClambda through phosphatidylinositol 3-kinase. EMBO J 15:788–798

Ali Y, Lin Y, Gharibo MM, Gounder MK, Stein MN, Lagattuta TF, Egorin MJ, Rubin EH, Poplin EA (2007) Phase I and pharmacokinetic study of imatinib mesylate (Gleevec) and gemcitabine in patients with refractory solid tumors. Clin Cancer Res 13:5876–5882

Alitalo K, Carmeliet P (2002) Molecular mechanisms of lymphangiogenesis in health and disease. Cancer Cell 1:219–227

Amaya H, Tanigawa N, Lu C, Matsumura M, Shimomatsuya T, Horiuchi T, Muraoka R (1997) Association of vascular endothelial growth factor expression with tumor angiogenesis, survival and thymidine phosphorylase/platelet-derived endothelial cell growth factor expression in human colorectal cancer. Cancer Lett 119:227–235

Andrae J, Gallini R, Betsholtz C (2008) Role of platelet-derived growth factors in physiology and medicine. Genes Dev 22:1276–1312

Arai H, Ueno T, Tangoku A, Yoshino S, Abe T, Kawauchi S, Oga A, Furuya T, Oka M, Sasaki K (2003) Detection of amplified oncogenes by genome DNA microarrays in human primary esophageal squamous cell carcinoma: comparison with conventional comparative genomic hybridization analysis. Cancer Genet Cytogenet 146:16–21

Arita Y, Kihara S, Ouchi N, Maeda K, Kuriyama H, Okamoto Y, Kumada M, Hotta K, Nishida M, Takahashi M, Nakamura T, Shimomura I, Muraguchi M, Ohmoto Y, Funahashi T, Matsuzawa Y (2002) Adipocyte-derived plasma protein adiponectin acts as a platelet-derived growth factor-BB-binding protein and regulates growth factor-induced common postreceptor signal in vascular smooth muscle cell. Circulation 105:2893–2898

Asano M, Yukita A, Matsumoto T, Kondo S, Suzuki H (1995) Inhibition of tumor growth and metastasis by an immunoneutralizing monoclonal antibody to human vascular endothelial growth factor/vascular permeability factor121. Cancer Res 55:5296–5301

Assoian RK (1997) Anchorage-dependent cell cycle progression. J Cell Biol 136:1–4

Ball SG, Shuttle CA, Kielty CM (2007) Mesenchymal stem cells and neovascularization: role of platelet-derived growth factor receptors. J Cell Mol Med 11:1012–1030

5

Bar-Sagi D, Feramisco JR (1986) Induction of membrane ruffling and fluid-phase pinocytosis in quiescent fibroblasts by ras proteins. Science 233:1061–1068

Bergsten E, Uutela M, Li X, Pietras K, Ostman A, Heldin CH, Alitalo K, Eriksson U (2001) PDGF-D is a specific, protease-activated ligand for the PDGF beta-receptor. Nat Cell Biol 3: 512–516

Berridge MJ (1993a) Cell signalling. A tale of two messengers. Nature 365:388–389

Berridge MJ (1993b) Inositol trisphosphate and calcium signalling. Nature 361:315–325

Betsholtz C (2004) Insight into the physiological functions of PDGF through genetic studies in mice. Cytokine Growth Factor Rev 15:215–228

Betsholtz C, Johnsson A, Heldin CH, Westermark B, Lind P, Urdea MS, Eddy R, Shows TB, Philpott K, Mellor AL et al (1986) cDNA sequence and chromosomal localization of human platelet-derived growth factor A-chain and its expression in tumour cell lines. Nature 320:695–699

Bonner JC, Badgett A, Hoffman M, Lindroos PM (1995) Inhibition of platelet-derived growth factor-BB-induced fibroblast proliferation by plasmin-activated alpha 2-macroglobulin is mediated via an alpha 2-macroglobulin receptor/low density lipoprotein receptor-related protein-dependent mechani. J Biol Chem 270:6389–6395

Bonner JC, Osornio-Vargas AR (1995) Differential binding and regulation of platelet-derived growth factor A and B chain isoforms by alpha 2-macroglobulin. J Biol Chem 270:16236–16242

Boocock CA, Charnock-Jones DS, Sharkey AM, McLaren J, Barker PJ, Wright KA, Twentyman PR, Smith SK (1995) Expression of vascular endothelial growth factor and its receptors flt and KDR in ovarian carcinoma. J Natl Cancer Inst 87:506–516

Borgstrom P, Bourdon MA, Hillan KJ, Sriramarao P, Ferrara N (1998) Neutralizing anti-vascular endothelial growth factor antibody completely inhibits angiogenesis and growth of human prostate carcinoma micro tumors in vivo. Prostate 35:1–10

Borgstrom P, Gold DP, Hillan KJ, Ferrara N (1999) Importance of VEGF for breast cancer angiogenesis in vivo: implications from intravital microscopy of combination treatments with an anti-VEGF neutralizing monoclonal antibody and doxorubicin. Anticancer Res 19:4203–4214

Borgstrom P, Hillan KJ, Sriramarao P, Ferrara N (1996) Complete inhibition of angiogenesis and growth of microtumors by anti-vascular endothelial growth factor neutralizing antibody: novel concepts of angiostatic therapy from intravital videomicroscopy. Cancer Res 56:4032–4039

Brown LF, Berse B, Jackman RW, Tognazzi K, Guidi AJ, Dvorak HF, Senger DR, Connolly JL, Schnitt SJ (1995) Expression of vascular permeability factor (vascular endothelial growth factor) and its receptors in breast cancer. Hum Pathol 26:86–91

Brown LF, Berse B, Jackman RW, Tognazzi K, Manseau EJ, Dvorak HF, Senger DR (1993a) Increased expression of vascular permeability factor (vascular endothelial growth factor) and its receptors in kidney and bladder carcinomas. Am J Pathol 143:1255–1262

Brown LF, Berse B, Jackman RW, Tognazzi K, Manseau EJ, Senger DR, Dvorak HF (1993b) Expression of vascular permeability factor (vascular endothelial growth factor) and its receptors in adenocarcinomas of the gastrointestinal tract. Cancer Res 53:4727–4735

Burgering BM, Coffer PJ (1995) Protein kinase B (c-Akt) in phosphatidylinositol-3-OH kinase signal transduction. Nature 376:599–602

Campbell JS, Seger R, Graves JD, Graves LM, Jensen AM, Krebs EG (1995) The MAP kinase cascade. Recent Prog Horm Res 50:131–159

Carmeliet P (1999) Developmental biology. Controlling the cellular brakes. Nature 401:657–658

Carmeliet P (2003) Blood vessels and nerves: common signals, pathways and diseases. Nat Rev Genet 4:710–720

Carmeliet P, Ferreira V, Breier G, Pollefeyt S, Kieckens L, Gertsenstein M, Fahrig M, Vandenhoeck A, Harpal K, Eberhardt C, Declercq C, Pawling J, Moons L, Collen D, Risau W, Nagy A (1996) Abnormal blood vessel development and lethality in embryos lacking a single VEGF allele. Nature 380:435–439

Carmeliet P, Ng YS, Nuyens D, Theilmeier G, Brusselmans K, Cornelissen I, Ehler E, Kakkar VV, Stalmans I, Mattot V, Perriard JC, Dewerchin M, Flameng W, Nagy A, Lupu F, Moons L, Collen D, D'Amore PA, Shima DT (1999) Impaired myocardial angiogenesis and ischemic cardiomyopathy in mice lacking the vascular endothelial growth factor isoforms VEGF164 and VEGF188. Nat Med 5:495–502

Cho NK, Keyes L, Johnson E, Heller J, Ryner L, Karim F, Krasnow MA (2002) Developmental control of blood cell migration by the Drosophila VEGF pathway. Cell 108:865–876

Chung J, Grammer TC, Lemon KP, Kazlauskas A, Blenis J (1994) PDGF- and insulin-dependent pp 70S6k activation mediated by phosphatidylinositol-3-OH kinase. Nature 370:71–75

Clark EA, Brugge JS (1995) Integrins and signal transduction pathways: the road taken. Science 268:233–239

Cochran BH, Reffel AC, Stiles CD (1983) Molecular cloning of gene sequences regulated by platelet-derived growth factor. Cell 33:939–947

Cohen T, Nahari D, Cerem LW, Neufeld G, Levi BZ (1996) Interleukin 6 induces the expression of vascular endothelial growth factor. J Biol Chem 271:736–741

Connolly DT, Heuvelman DM, Nelson R, Olander JV, Eppley BL, Delfino JJ, Siegel NR, Leimgruber RM, Feder J (1989a) Tumor vascular permeability factor stimulates endothelial cell growth and angiogenesis. J Clin Invest 84:1470–1478

Connolly DT, Olander JV, Heuvelman D, Nelson R, Monsell R, Siegel N, Haymore BL, Leimgruber R, Feder J (1989b) Human vascular permeability factor. Isolation from U937 cells. J Biol Chem 264:20017–20024

Cornali E, Zietz C, Benelli R, Weninger W, Masiello L, Breier G, Tschachler E, Albini A, Sturzl M (1996) Vascular endothelial growth factor regulates angiogenesis and vascular permeability in Kaposi's sarcoma. Am J Pathol 149: 1851–1869

Cunningham SA, Waxham MN, Arrate PM, Brock TA (1995) Interaction of the Flt-1 tyrosine kinase receptor with the p85 subunit of phosphatidylinositol 3-kinase. Mapping of a novel site involved in binding. J Biol Chem 270:20254–20257

Darnell JE Jr (1997) STATs and gene regulation. Science 277:1630–1635

de Vries C, Escobedo JA, Ueno H, Houck K, Ferrara N, Williams LT (1992) The fms-like tyrosine kinase, a receptor for vascular endothelial growth factor. Science 255:989–991

Dias S, Hattori K, Zhu Z, Heissig B, Choy M, Lane W, Wu Y, Chadburn A, Hyjek E, Gill M, Hicklin DJ, Witte L, Moore MA, Rafii S (2000) Autocrine stimulation of VEGFR-2 activates human leukemic cell growth and migration. J Clin Invest 106:511–521

Diliberto PA, Gordon GW, Yu CL, Earp HS, Herman B (1992) Platelet-derived growth factor (PDGF) alpha receptor activation modulates the calcium mobilizing activity of the PDGF beta receptor in Balb/c3T3 fibroblasts. J Biol Chem 267:11888–11897

Doolittle RF, Hunkapiller MW, Hood LE, Devare SG, Robbins KC, Aaronson SA, Antoniades HN (1983) Simian sarcoma virus onc gene, v-sis, is derived from the gene (or genes) encoding a platelet-derived growth factor. Science 221:275–277

Duchek P, Somogyi K, Jekely G, Beccari S, Rorth P (2001) Guidance of cell migration by the Drosophila PDGF/VEGF receptor. Cell 107:17–26

Eichmann A, Corbel C, Nataf V, Vaigot P, Breant C, Le Douarin NM (1997) Ligand-dependent development of the endothelial and hemopoietic lineages from embryonic mesodermal cells expressing vascular endothelial growth factor receptor 2. Proc Natl Acad Sci U S A 94:5141–5146

Ekman S, Thuresson ER, Heldin CH, Ronnstrand L (1999) Increased mitogenicity of an alphabeta heterodimeric PDGF receptor complex correlates with lack of RasGAP binding. Oncogene 18:2481–2488

Ellis LM, Takahashi Y, Fenoglio CJ, Cleary KR, Bucana CD, Evans DB (1998) Vessel counts and vascular endothelial growth factor expression in pancreatic adenocarcinoma. Eur J Cancer 34: 337–340

Erpel T, Courtneidge SA (1995) Src family protein tyrosine kinases and cellular signal transduction pathways. Curr Opin Cell Biol 7:176–182

Fambrough D, McClure K, Kazlauskas A, Lander ES (1999) Diverse signaling pathways activated by growth factor receptors induce broadly overlapping, rather than independent, sets of genes. Cell 97:727–741

Fantl WJ, Escobedo JA, Martin GA, Turck CW, del Rosario M, McCormick F, Williams LT (1992) Distinct phosphotyrosines on a growth factor receptor bind to specific molecules that mediate different signaling pathways. Cell 69:413–423

Fatatis A, Miller RJ (1997) Platelet-derived growth factor (PDGF)-induced Ca2+ signaling in the CG4 oligodendroglial cell line and in transformed oligodendrocytes expressing the beta-PDGF receptor. J Biol Chem 272:4351–4358

Ferrara N, Carver-Moore K, Chen H, Dowd M, Lu L, O'Shea KS, Powell-Braxton L, Hillan KJ, Moore MW (1996) Heterozygous embryonic lethality induced by targeted inactivation of the VEGF gene. Nature 380:439–442

Ferrara N, Chen H, Davis-Smyth T, Gerber HP, Nguyen TN, Peers D, Chisholm V, Hillan KJ, Schwall RH (1998) Vascular endothelial growth factor is essential for corpus luteum angiogenesis. Nat Med 4:336–340

Ferrara N, Davis-Smyth T (1997) The biology of vascular endothelial growth factor. Endocr Rev 18:4–25

Ferrara N, Gerber HP (2001) The role of vascular endothelial growth factor in angiogenesis. Acta Haematol 106:148–156

Ferrara N, Gerber HP, LeCouter J (2003) The biology of VEGF and its receptors. Nat Med 9:669–676

Feyzi E, Lustig F, Fager G, Spillmann D, Lindahl U, Salmivirta M (1997) Characterization of heparin and heparan sulfate domains binding to the long splice variant of platelet-derived growth factor A chain. J Biol Chem 272:5518–5524

Fiedler W, Mesters R, Tinnefeld H, Loges S, Staib P, Duhrsen U, Flasshove M, Ottmann OG, Jung W, Cavalli F, Kuse R, Thomalla J, Serve H, O'Farrell AM, Jacobs M, Brega NM, Scigalla P, Hossfeld DK, Berdel WE (2003) A phase 2 clinical study of SU5416 in patients with refractory acute myeloid leukemia. Blood 102:2763–2767

Folkman J (1971) Tumor angiogenesis: therapeutic implications. N Engl J Med 285:1182–1186

Folkman J, Merler E, Abernathy C, Williams G (1971) Isolation of a tumor factor responsible for angiogenesis. J Exp Med 133:275–288

Fong GH, Rossant J, Gertsenstein M, Breitman ML (1995) Role of the Flt-1 receptor tyrosine kinase in regulating the assembly of vascular endothelium. Nature 376:66–70

Forsberg K, Valyi-Nagy I, Heldin CH, Herlyn M, Westermark B (1993) Platelet-derived growth factor (PDGF) in oncogenesis: development of a vascular connective tissue stroma in xenotransplanted human melanoma producing PDGF-BB. Proc Natl Acad Sci U S A 90:393–397

Frank S, Hubner G, Breier G, Longaker MT, Greenhalgh DG, Werner S (1995) Regulation of vascular endothelial growth factor expression in cultured keratinocytes. Implications for normal and impaired wound healing. J Biol Chem 270:12607–12613

Franke TF, Yang SI, Chan TO, Datta K, Kazlauskas A, Morrison DK, Kaplan DR, Tsichlis PN (1995) The protein kinase encoded by the Akt proto-oncogene is a target of the PDGF-activated phosphatidylinositol 3-kinase. Cell 81:727–736

Fredriksson L, Li H, Eriksson U (2004) The PDGF family: four gene products form five dimeric isoforms. Cytokine Growth Factor Rev 15:197–204

Frisch SM, Ruoslahti E (1997) Integrins and anoikis. Curr Opin Cell Biol 9:701–706

Fruttiger M, Calver AR, Richardson WD (2000) Platelet-derived growth factor is constitutively secreted from neuronal cell bodies but not from axons. Curr Biol 10:1283–1286

Fuh G, Li B, Crowley C, Cunningham B, Wells JA (1998) Requirements for binding and signaling of the kinase domain receptor for vascular endothelial growth factor. J Biol Chem 273:11197–11204

Fukumura D, Xavier R, Sugiura T, Chen Y, Park EC, Lu N, Selig M, Nielsen G, Taksir T, Jain RK, Seed B (1998) Tumor induction of VEGF promoter activity in stromal cells. Cell 94:715–725

Furuhashi M, Sjoblom T, Abramsson A, Ellingsen J, Micke P, Li H, Bergsten-Folestad E, Eriksson U, Heuchel R, Betsholtz C, Heldin CH, Ostman A (2004) Platelet-derived growth factor production by B16 melanoma cells leads to increased pericyte abundance in tumors and an associated increase in tumor growth rate. Cancer Res 64:2725–2733

Gasparini G, Toi M, Gion M, Verderio P, Dittadi R, Hanatani M, Matsubara I, Vinante O, Bonoldi E, Boracchi P, Gatti C, Suzuki H, Tominaga T (1997) Prognostic significance of vascular endothelial growth factor protein in node-negative breast carcinoma. J Natl Cancer Inst 89:139–147

Gerber HP, Ferrara N (2003) The role of VEGF in normal and neoplastic hematopoiesis. J Mol Med 81:20–31

Gerber HP, Kowalski J, Sherman D, Eberhard DA, Ferrara N (2000) Complete inhibition of rhabdomyosarcoma xenograft growth and neovascularization requires blockade of both tumor and host vascular endothelial growth factor. Cancer Res 60:6253–6258

Gerber HP, McMurtrey A, Kowalski J, Yan M, Keyt BA, Dixit V, Ferrara N (1998) Vascular endothelial growth factor regulates endothelial cell survival through the phosphatidylinositol 3'-kinase/Akt signal transduction pathway. Requirement for Flk-1/KDR activation. J Biol Chem 273:30336–30343

Goldberg MA, Schneider TJ (1994) Similarities between the oxygen-sensing mechanisms regulating the expression of vascular endothelial growth factor and erythropoietin. J Biol Chem 269:4355–4359

Goldman CK, Kendall RL, Cabrera G, Soroceanu L, Heike Y, Gillespie GY, Siegal GP, Mao X, Bett AJ, Huckle WR, Thomas KA, Curiel DT (1998) Paracrine expression of a native soluble vascular endothelial growth factor receptor inhibits tumor growth, metastasis, and mortality rate. Proc Natl Acad Sci U S A 95:8795–8800

Goldmann E (1907) Growth of the malignant disease in man and the lower animals with special reference to vascular system. Lancet 170:1236–1240

Grugel S, Finkenzeller G, Weindel K, Barleon B, Marme D (1995) Both v-Ha-Ras and v-Raf stimulate expression of the vascular endothelial growth factor in NIH 3T3 cells. J Biol Chem 270:25915–25919

Grunstein J, Masbad JJ, Hickey R, Giordano F, Johnson RS (2000) Isoforms of vascular endothelial growth factor act in a coordinate fashion to recruit and expand tumor vasculature. Mol Cell Biol 20:7282–7291

Guidi AJ, Abu-Jawdeh G, Tognazzi K, Dvorak HF, Brown LF (1996) Expression of vascular permeability factor (vascular endothelial growth factor) and its receptors in endometrial carcinoma. Cancer 78:454–460

Hacker U, Nybakken K, Perrimon N (2005) Heparan sulphate proteoglycans: the sweet side of development. Nat Rev Mol Cell Biol 6:530–541

Hanahan D, Folkman J (1996) Patterns and emerging mechanisms of the angiogenic switch during tumorigenesis. Cell 86:353–364

Hanahan D, Weinberg RA (2000) The hallmarks of cancer. Cell 100:57–70

Hatva E, Kaipainen A, Mentula P, Jaaskelainen J, Paetau A, Haltia M, Alitalo K (1995) Expression of endothelial cell-specific receptor tyrosine kinases and growth factors in human brain tumors. Am J Pathol 146:368–378

Heinrich MC, Corless CL, Duensing A, McGreevey L, Chen CJ, Joseph N, Singer S, Griffith DJ, Haley A, Town A, Demetri GD, Fletcher CD, Fletcher JA (2003) PDGFRA activating mutations in gastrointestinal stromal tumors. Science 299:708–710

Heldin CH, Johnsson A, Wennergren S, Wernstedt C, Betsholtz C, Westermark B (1986) A human osteosarcoma cell line secretes a growth factor structurally related to a homodimer of PDGF A-chains. Nature 319:511–514

Heldin CH, Ostman A, Ronnstrand L (1998) Signal transduction via platelet-derived growth factor receptors. Biochim Biophys Acta 1378:F79–F113

Heldin CH, Westermark B (1999) Mechanism of action and in vivo role of platelet-derived growth factor. Physiol Rev 79:1283–1316

Heldin NE, Gustavsson B, Claesson-Welsh L, Hammacher A, Mark J, Heldin CH, Westermark B (1988) Aberrant expression of receptors for platelet-derived growth factor in an anaplastic thyroid carcinoma cell line. Proc Natl Acad Sci U S A 85:9302–9306

Hermanson M, Funa K, Koopmann J, Maintz D, Waha A, Westermark B, Heldin CH, Wiestler OD, Louis DN, von Deimling A, Nister M (1996) Association of loss of heterozygosity on chromosome 17p with high platelet-derived growth factor alpha receptor expression in human malignant gliomas. Cancer Res 56:164–171

Hermansson M, Nister M, Betsholtz C, Heldin CH, Westermark B, Funa K (1988) Endothelial cell hyperplasia in human glioblastoma: coexpression of mRNA for platelet-derived growth factor (PDGF) B chain and PDGF receptor suggests autocrine growth stimulation. Proc Natl Acad Sci U S A 85:7748–7752

Heuchel R, Berg A, Tallquist M, Ahlen K, Reed RK, Rubin K, Claesson-Welsh L, Heldin CH, Soriano P (1999) Platelet-derived growth factor beta receptor regulates interstitial fluid homeostasis through phosphatidylinositol-3' kinase signaling. Proc Natl Acad Sci U S A 96:11410–11415

Hirakawa S, Kodama S, Kunstfeld R, Kajiya K, Brown LF, Detmar M (2005) VEGF-A induces tumor and sentinel lymph node lymphangiogenesis and promotes lymphatic metastasis. J Exp Med 201:1089–1099

Hiratsuka S, Kataoka Y, Nakao K, Nakamura K, Morikawa S, Tanaka S, Katsuki M, Maru Y, Shibuya M (2005) Vascular endothelial growth factor A (VEGF-A) is involved in guidance of VEGF receptor-positive cells to the anterior portion of early embryos. Mol Cell Biol 25:355–363

Hiratsuka S, Maru Y, Okada A, Seiki M, Noda T, Shibuya M (2001) Involvement of Flt-1 tyrosine kinase (vascular endothelial growth factor receptor-1) in pathological angiogenesis. Cancer Res 61:1207–1213

Hiratsuka S, Minowa O, Kuno J, Noda T, Shibuya M (1998) Flt-1 lacking the tyrosine kinase domain is sufficient for normal development and angiogenesis in mice. Proc Natl Acad Sci U S A 95: 9349–9354

Hiratsuka S, Nakamura K, Iwai S, Murakami M, Itoh T, Kijima H, Shipley JM, Senior RM,

Shibuya M (2002) MMP9 induction by vascular endothelial growth factor receptor-1 is involved in lung-specific metastasis. Cancer Cell 2:289–300

Hirota S, Ohashi A, Nishida T, Isozaki K, Kinoshita K, Shinomura Y, Kitamura Y (2003) Gain-of-function mutations of platelet-derived growth factor receptor alpha gene in gastrointestinal stromal tumors. Gastroenterology 125:660–667

Hoch RV, Soriano P (2003) Roles of PDGF in animal development. Development 130:4769–4784

Holash J, Davis S, Papadopoulos N, Croll SD, Ho L, Russell M, Boland P, Leidich R, Hylton D, Burova E, Ioffe E, Huang T, Radziejewski C, Bailey K, Fandl JP, Daly T, Wiegand SJ, Yancopoulos GD, Rudge JS (2002) VEGF-Trap: a VEGF blocker with potent antitumor effects. Proc Natl Acad Sci U S A 99:11393–11398

Hossain MZ, Ao P, Boynton AL (1998) Platelet-derived growth factor-induced disruption of gap junctional communication and phosphorylation of connexin43 involves protein kinase C and mitogen-activated protein kinase. J Cell Physiol 176:332–341

Houck KA, Leung DW, Rowland AM, Winer J, Ferrara N (1992) Dual regulation of vascular endothelial growth factor bioavailability by genetic and proteolytic mechanisms. J Biol Chem 267:26031–26037

Hu Q, Klippel A, Muslin AJ, Fantl WJ, Williams LT (1995) Ras-dependent induction of cellular responses by constitutively active phosphatidylinositol-3 kinase. Science 268:100–102

Ide AG, Baker NH, Warren SL (1939) Vascularization of the Brown-Pearce rabbi epithelioma transplant as seen in the transparent ear chamber. Am J Radiol 42:891–899

Iliopoulos O, Levy AP, Jiang C, Kaelin WG Jr, Goldberg MA (1996) Negative regulation of hypoxia-inducible genes by the von Hippel-Lindau protein. Proc Natl Acad Sci U S A 93:10595–10599

Imoto H, Osaki T, Taga S, Ohgami A, Ichiyoshi Y, Yasumoto K (1998) Vascular endothelial growth factor expression in non-small-cell lung cancer: prognostic significance in squamous cell carcinoma. J Thorac Cardiovasc Surg 115:1007–1014

Ishigami SI, Arii S, Furutani M, Niwano M, Harada T, Mizumoto M, Mori A, Onodera H, Imamura M (1998) Predictive value of vascular endothelial growth factor (VEGF) in metastasis and prognosis of human colorectal cancer. Br J Cancer 78:1379–1384

Ishimaru S, Ueda R, Hinohara Y, Ohtani M, Hanafusa H (2004) PVR plays a critical role via JNK activation in thorax closure during Drosophila metamorphosis. EMBO J 23:3984–3994

Ito N, Huang K, Claesson-Welsh L (2001) Signal transduction by VEGF receptor-1 wild type and mutant proteins. Cell Signal 13:849–854

Jacobsen J, Grankvist K, Rasmuson T, Bergh A, Landberg G, Ljungberg B (2004) Expression of vascular endothelial growth factor protein in human renal cell carcinoma. BJU Int 93: 297–302

James MF, Beauchamp RL, Manchanda N, Kazlauskas A, Ramesh V (2004) A NHERF binding site links the betaPDGFR to the cytoskeleton and regulates cell spreading and migration. J Cell Sci 117:2951–2961

Johnsson A, Betsholtz C, von der Helm K, Heldin CH, Westermark B (1985) Platelet-derived growth factor agonist activity of a secreted form of the v-sis oncogene product. Proc Natl Acad Sci U S A 82:1721–1725

Johnsson A, Heldin CH, Westermark B, Wasteson A (1982) Platelet-derived growth factor: identification of constituent polypeptide chains. Biochem Biophys Res Commun 104:66–74

Joukov V, Pajusola K, Kaipainen A, Chilov D, Lahtinen I, Kukk E, Saksela O, Kalkkinen N, Alitalo K (1996) A novel vascular endothelial growth factor, VEGF-C, is a ligand for the Flt4 (VEGFR-3) and KDR (VEGFR-2) receptor tyrosine kinases. EMBO J 15:290–298

Kaetzel DM (2003) Transcription of the platelet-derived growth factor A-chain gene. Cytokine Growth Factor Rev 14:427–446

Kaipainen A, Korhonen J, Pajusola K, Aprelikova O, Persico MG, Terman BI, Alitalo K (1993) The related FLT4, FLT1, and KDR receptor tyrosine kinases show distinct expression patterns in human fetal endothelial cells. J Exp Med 178: 2077–2088

Kaplan RN, Riba RD, Zacharoulis S, Bramley AH, Vincent L, Costa C, MacDonald DD, Jin DK, Shido K, Kerns SA, Zhu Z, Hicklin D, Wu Y, Port JL, Altorki N, Port ER, Ruggero D, Shmelkov SV, Jensen KK, Rafii S, Lyden D (2005) VEGFR1-positive haematopoietic bone marrow progenitors initiate the pre-metastatic niche. Nature 438:820–827

Karlsson S, Kowanetz K, Sandin A, Persson C, Ostman A, Heldin CH, Hellberg C (2006) Loss of T-cell protein tyrosine phosphatase induces recycling of the platelet-derived growth factor (PDGF) beta-receptor but not the PDGF alpha-receptor. Mol Biol Cell 17:4846–4855

Kawasaki T, Kitsukawa T, Bekku Y, Matsuda Y, Sanbo M, Yagi T, Fujisawa H (1999) A requirement for neuropilin-1 in embryonic vessel formation. Development 126:4895–4902

Kazlauskas A, Cooper JA (1989) Autophosphorylation of the PDGF receptor in the kinase insert region regulates interactions with cell proteins. Cell 58:1121–1133

Keck PJ, Hauser SD, Krivi G, Sanzo K, Warren T, Feder J, Connolly DT (1989) Vascular permeability factor, an endothelial cell mitogen related to PDGF. Science 246:1309–1312

Kelly JD, Haldeman BA, Grant FJ, Murray MJ, Seifert RA, Bowen-Pope DF, Cooper JA, Kazlauskas A (1991) Platelet-derived growth factor (PDGF) stimulates PDGF receptor subunit dimerization and intersubunit trans-phosphorylation. J Biol Chem 266:8987–8992

Kelly JL, Sanchez A, Brown GS, Chesterman CN, Sleigh MJ (1993) Accumulation of PDGF B and cell-binding forms of PDGF A in the extracellular matrix. J Cell Biol 121:1153–1163

Kendall RL, Thomas KA (1993) Inhibition of vascular endothelial cell growth factor activity by an endogenously encoded soluble receptor. Proc Natl Acad Sci U S A 90:10705–10709

Keyt BA, Nguyen HV, Berleau LT, Duarte CM, Park J, Chen H, Ferrara N (1996) Identification of vascular endothelial growth factor determinants for binding KDR and FLT-1 receptors. Generation of receptor-selective VEGF variants by site-directed mutagenesis. J Biol Chem 271: 5638–5646

Kim KJ, Li B, Winer J, Armanini M, Gillett N, Phillips HS, Ferrara N (1993) Inhibition of vascular endothelial growth factor-induced angiogenesis suppresses tumour growth in vivo. Nature 362:841–844

Klein M, Vignaud JM, Hennequin V, Toussaint B, Bresler L, Plenat F, Leclere J, Duprez A, Weryha G (2001) Increased expression of the vascular endothelial growth factor is a pejorative prognosis marker in papillary thyroid carcinoma. J Clin Endocrinol Metab 86:656–658

Klinghoffer RA, Hamilton TG, Hoch R, Soriano P (2002) An allelic series at the PDGFalphaR locus indicates unequal contributions of distinct signaling pathways during development. Dev Cell 2:103–113

Klinghoffer RA, Mueting-Nelsen PF, Faerman A, Shani M, Soriano P (2001) The two PDGF receptors maintain conserved signaling in vivo despite divergent embryological functions. Mol Cell 7:343–354

Kohler N, Lipton A (1974) Platelets as a source of fibroblast growth-promoting activity. Exp Cell Res 87:297–301

Kong HL, Hecht D, Song W, Kovesdi I, Hackett NR, Yayon A, Crystal RG (1998) Regional suppression of tumor growth by in vivo transfer of a cDNA encoding a secreted form of the extracellular domain of the flt-1 vascular endothelial growth factor receptor. Hum Gene Ther 9:823–833

Kundra V, Soker S, Zetter BR (1994) Excess early signaling activity inhibits cellular chemotaxis toward PDGF-BB. Oncogene 9:1429–1435

Lechleider RJ, Sugimoto S, Bennett AM, Kashishian AS, Cooper JA, Shoelson SE, Walsh CT, Neel BG (1993) Activation of the SH2-containing phosphotyrosine phosphatase SH-PTP2 by its binding site, phosphotyrosine 1009, on the human platelet-derived growth factor receptor. J Biol Chem 268:21478–21481

Lee S, Chen TT, Barber CL, Jordan MC, Murdock J, Desai S, Ferrara N, Nagy A, Roos KP, Iruela-Arispe ML (2007) Autocrine VEGF signaling is required for vascular homeostasis. Cell 130: 691–703

Lennartsson J, Wardega P, Engstrom U, Hellman U, Heldin CH (2006) Alix facilitates the interaction between c-Cbl and platelet-derived growth factor beta-receptor and thereby modulates receptor down-regulation. J Biol Chem 281: 39152–39158

Leung DW, Cachianes G, Kuang WJ, Goeddel DV, Ferrara N (1989) Vascular endothelial growth factor is a secreted angiogenic mitogen. Science 246:1306–1309

Levy AP, Levy NS, Wegner S, Goldberg MA (1995) Transcriptional regulation of the rat vascular endothelial growth factor gene by hypoxia. J Biol Chem 270:13333–13340

Li J, Yen C, Liaw D, Podsypanina K, Bose S, Wang SI, Puc J, Miliaresis C, Rodgers L, McCombie R, Bigner SH, Giovanella BC, Ittmann M, Tycko B, Hibshoosh H, Wigler MH, Parsons R (1997) PTEN, a putative protein tyrosine phosphatase gene mutated in human brain, breast, and prostate cancer. Science 275:1943–1947

Li W, Pierce JH (1996) Protein kinase C-delta, an important signaling molecule in the platelet-derived

5

growth factor beta receptor pathway. Curr Top Microbiol Immunol 211:55–65

Li X, Ponten A, Aase K, Karlsson L, Abramsson A, Uutela M, Backstrom G, Hellstrom M, Bostrom H, Li H, Soriano P, Betsholtz C, Heldin CH, Alitalo K, Ostman A, Eriksson U (2000) PDGF-C is a new protease-activated ligand for the PDGF alpha-receptor. Nat Cell Biol 2:302–309

Lin ZH, Fukuda N, Suzuki R, Takagi H, Ikeda Y, Saito S, Matsumoto K, Kanmatsuse K, Mugishima H (2004) Adenovirus-encoded hammerhead ribozyme to PDGF A-chain mRNA inhibits neointima formation after arterial injury. J Vasc Res 41:305–313

Lindblom P, Gerhardt H, Liebner S, Abramsson A, Enge M, Hellstrom M, Backstrom G, Fredriksson S, Landegren U, Nystrom HC, Bergstrom G, Dejana E, Ostman A, Lindahl P, Betsholtz C (2003) Endothelial PDGF-B retention is required for proper investment of pericytes in the microvessel wall. Genes Dev 17:1835–1840

Liu Y, Cox SR, Morita T, Kourembanas S (1995) Hypoxia regulates vascular endothelial growth factor gene expression in endothelial cells. Identification of a 5' enhancer. Circ Res 77: 638–643

Lloyd RV, Scheithauer BW, Kuroki T, Vidal S, Kovacs K, Stefaneanu L (1999) Vascular endothelial growth factor (VEGF) expression in human pituitary adenomas and carcinomas. Endocr Pathol 10:229–235

Lokker NA, Sullivan CM, Hollenbach SJ, Israel MA, Giese NA (2002) Platelet-derived growth factor (PDGF) autocrine signaling regulates survival and mitogenic pathways in glioblastoma cells: evidence that the novel PDGF-C and PDGF-D ligands may play a role in the development of brain tumors. Cancer Res 62:3729–3735

Lopez-Ilasaca M, Li W, Uren A, Yu JC, Kazlauskas A, Gutkind JS, Heidaran MA (1997) Requirement of phosphatidylinositol-3 kinase for activation of JNK/SAPKs by PDGF. Biochem Biophys Res Commun 232:273–277

Lustig F, Hoebeke J, Simonson C, Ostergren-Lunden G, Bondjers G, Ruetchi U, Fager G (1999) Processing of PDGF gene products determines interactions with glycosaminoglycans. J Mol Recognit 12:112–120

Madan A, Curtin PT (1993) A 24-base-pair sequence 3' to the human erythropoietin gene contains a hypoxia-responsive transcriptional enhancer. Proc Natl Acad Sci U S A 90:3928–3932

Maeda K, Nishiguchi Y, Yashiro M, Yamada S, Onoda N, Sawada T, Kang SM, Hirakawa K (2000) Expression of vascular endothelial growth factor and thrombospondin-1 in colorectal carcinoma. Int J Mol Med 5:373–378

Maes C, Carmeliet P, Moermans K, Stockmans I, Smets N, Collen D, Bouillon R, Carmeliet G (2002) Impaired angiogenesis and endochondral bone formation in mice lacking the vascular endothelial growth factor isoforms VEGF164 and VEGF188. Mech Dev 111:61–73

Maglione D, Guerriero V, Viglietto G, Delli-Bovi P, Persico MG (1991) Isolation of a human placenta cDNA coding for a protein related to the vascular permeability factor. Proc Natl Acad Sci U S A 88:9267–9271

Maglione D, Guerriero V, Viglietto G, Ferraro MG, Aprelikova O, Alitalo K, Del Vecchio S, Lei KJ, Chou JY, Persico MG (1993) Two alternative mRNAs coding for the angiogenic factor, placenta growth factor (PlGF), are transcribed from a single gene of chromosome 14. Oncogene 8: 925–931

Matsumoto T, Claesson-Welsh L (2001) VEGF receptor signal transduction. Sci STKE 2001:RE21

Matthews W, Jordan CT, Gavin M, Jenkins NA, Copeland NG, Lemischka IR (1991) A receptor tyrosine kinase cDNA isolated from a population of enriched primitive hematopoietic cells and exhibiting close genetic linkage to c-kit. Proc Natl Acad Sci U S A 88:9026–9030

Melnyk O, Shuman MA, Kim KJ (1996) Vascular endothelial growth factor promotes tumor dissemination by a mechanism distinct from its effect on primary tumor growth. Cancer Res 56: 921–924

Mesiano S, Ferrara N, Jaffe RB (1998) Role of vascular endothelial growth factor in ovarian cancer: inhibition of ascites formation by immunoneutralization. Am J Pathol 153:1249–1256

Millauer B, Shawver LK, Plate KH, Risau W, Ullrich A (1994) Glioblastoma growth inhibited in vivo by a dominant-negative Flk-1 mutant. Nature 367:576–579

Millauer B, Wizigmann-Voos S, Schnurch H, Martinez R, Moller NP, Risau W, Ullrich A (1993) High affinity VEGF binding and developmental expression suggest Flk-1 as a major regulator of vasculogenesis and angiogenesis. Cell 72:835–846

Mueller MD, Vigne JL, Minchenko A, Lebovic DI, Leitman DC, Taylor RN (2000) Regulation of vascular endothelial growth factor (VEGF) gene transcription by estrogen receptors alpha and beta. Proc Natl Acad Sci U S A 97:10972–10977

Mueller MD, Vigne JL, Pritts EA, Chao V, Dreher E, Taylor RN (2003) Progestins activate vascular endothelial growth factor gene transcription in endometrial adenocarcinoma cells. Fertil Steril 79:386–392

Nakanishi S, Nakajima Y, Yokota Y (1993) Signal transduction and ligand-binding domains of the tachykinin receptors. Regul Pept 46:37–42

Newton HB (2003) Molecular neuro-oncology and development of targeted therapeutic strategies for brain tumors. Part 1: growth factor and Ras signaling pathways. Expert Rev Anticancer Ther 3:595–614

Nicol D, Hii SI, Walsh M, Teh B, Thompson L, Kennett C, Gotley D (1997) Vascular endothelial growth factor expression is increased in renal cell carcinoma. J Urol 157:1482–1486

Nister M, Hammacher A, Mellstrom K, Siegbahn A, Ronnstrand L, Westermark B, Heldin CH (1988) A glioma-derived PDGF A chain homodimer has different functional activities from a PDGF AB heterodimer purified from human platelets. Cell 52:791–799

Nobes CD, Hawkins P, Stephens L, Hall A (1995) Activation of the small GTP-binding proteins rho and rac by growth factor receptors. J Cell Sci 108(Pt 1):225–233

O'Byrne KJ, Koukourakis MI, Giatromanolaki A, Cox G, Turley H, Steward WP, Gatter K, Harris AL (2000) Vascular endothelial growth factor, platelet-derived endothelial cell growth factor and angiogenesis in non-small-cell lung cancer. Br J Cancer 82:1427–1432

Ogata Y, Fujita H, Yamana H, Sueyoshi S, Shirouzu K (2003) Expression of vascular endothelial growth factor as a prognostic factor in node-positive squamous cell carcinoma in the thoracic esophagus: long-term follow-up study. World J Surg 27: 584–589

Oku T, Tjuvajev JG, Miyagawa T, Sasajima T, Joshi A, Joshi R, Finn R, Claffey KP, Blasberg RG (1998) Tumor growth modulation by sense and antisense vascular endothelial growth factor gene expression: effects on angiogenesis, vascular permeability, blood volume, blood flow, fluorodeoxyglucose uptake, and proliferation of human melanoma intracerebral xenografts. Cancer Res 58:4185–4192

Olofsson B, Pajusola K, Kaipainen A, von Euler G, Joukov V, Saksela O, Orpana A, Pettersson RF, Alitalo K, Eriksson U (1996) Vascular endothelial growth factor B, a novel growth factor for endothelial cells. Proc Natl Acad Sci U S A 93:2576–2581

Olson TA, Mohanraj D, Carson LF, Ramakrishnan S (1994) Vascular permeability factor gene expression in normal and neoplastic human ovaries. Cancer Res 54:276–280

Ostman A (2004) PDGF receptors-mediators of autocrine tumor growth and regulators of tumor vasculature and stroma. Cytokine Growth Factor Rev 15:275–286

Paley PJ, Staskus KA, Gebhard K, Mohanraj D, Twiggs LB, Carson LF, Ramakrishnan S (1997) Vascular endothelial growth factor expression in early stage ovarian carcinoma. Cancer 80:98–106

Pan Q, Chanthery Y, Liang WC, Stawicki S, Mak J, Rathore N, Tong RK, Kowalski J, Yee SF, Pacheco G, Ross S, Cheng Z, Le Couter J, Plowman G, Peale F, Koch AW, Wu Y, Bagri A, Tessier-Lavigne M, Watts RJ (2007) Blocking neuropilin-1 function has an additive effect with anti-VEGF to inhibit tumor growth. Cancer Cell 11:53–67

Persson C, Savenhed C, Bourdeau A, Tremblay ML, Markova B, Bohmer FD, Haj FG, Neel BG, Elson A, Heldin CH, Ronnstrand L, Ostman A, Hellberg C (2004) Site-selective regulation of platelet-derived growth factor beta receptor tyrosine phosphorylation by T-cell protein tyrosine phosphatase. Mol Cell Biol 24:2190–2201

Pertovaara L, Kaipainen A, Mustonen T, Orpana A, Ferrara N, Saksela O, Alitalo K (1994) Vascular endothelial growth factor is induced in response to transforming growth factor-beta in fibroblastic and epithelial cells. J Biol Chem 269:6271–6274

Pietras K, Ostman A, Sjoquist M, Buchdunger E, Reed RK, Heldin CH, Rubin K (2001) Inhibition of platelet-derived growth factor receptors reduces interstitial hypertension and increases transcapillary transport in tumors. Cancer Res 61:2929–2934

Plate KH, Breier G, Weich HA, Risau W (1992) Vascular endothelial growth factor is a potential tumour angiogenesis factor in human gliomas in vivo. Nature 359:845–848

Prewett M, Huber J, Li Y, Santiago A, O'Connor W, King K, Overholser J, Hooper A, Pytowski B, Witte L, Bohlen P, Hicklin DJ (1999) Antivascular endothelial growth factor receptor (fetal liver kinase 1) monoclonal antibody inhibits tumor angiogenesis and growth of several mouse and human tumors. Cancer Res 59:5209–5218

5

Raines EW, Lane TF, Iruela-Arispe ML, Ross R, Sage EH (1992) The extracellular glycoprotein SPARC interacts with platelet-derived growth factor (PDGF)-AB and -BB and inhibits the binding of PDGF to its receptors. Proc Natl Acad Sci U S A 89:1281–1285

Raines EW, Ross R (1992) Compartmentalization of PDGF on extracellular binding sites dependent on exon-6-encoded sequences. J Cell Biol 116:533–543

Rak J, Mitsuhashi Y, Bayko L, Filmus J, Shirasawa S, Sasazuki T, Kerbel RS (1995) Mutant ras oncogenes upregulate VEGF/VPF expression: implications for induction and inhibition of tumor angiogenesis. Cancer Res 55:4575–4580

Reigstad LJ, Varhaug JE, Lillehaug JR (2005) Structural and functional specificities of PDGF-C and PDGF-D, the novel members of the platelet-derived growth factors family. FEBS J 272: 5723–5741

Risau W (1997) Mechanisms of angiogenesis. Nature 386:671–674

Ronnstrand L, Heldin CH (2001) Mechanisms of platelet-derived growth factor-induced chemotaxis. Int J Cancer 91:757–762

Ross R, Glomset J, Kariya B, Harker L (1974) A platelet-dependent serum factor that stimulates the proliferation of arterial smooth muscle cells in vitro. Proc Natl Acad Sci U S A 71:1207–1210

Ruhrberg C, Gerhardt H, Golding M, Watson R, Ioannidou S, Fujisawa H, Betsholtz C, Shima DT (2002) Spatially restricted patterning cues provided by heparin-binding VEGF-A control blood vessel branching morphogenesis. Genes Dev 16: 2684–2698

Sakurai Y, Ohgimoto K, Kataoka Y, Yoshida N, Shibuya M (2005) Essential role of Flk-1 (VEGF receptor 2) tyrosine residue 1173 in vasculogenesis in mice. Proc Natl Acad Sci U S A 102:1076–1081

Saleh M, Stacker SA, Wilks AF (1996) Inhibition of growth of C6 glioma cells in vivo by expression of antisense vascular endothelial growth factor sequence. Cancer Res 56:393–401

Sawano A, Takahashi T, Yamaguchi S, Shibuya M (1997) The phosphorylated 1169-tyrosine containing region of flt-1 kinase (VEGFR-1) is a major binding site for PLCgamma. Biochem Biophys Res Commun 238:487–491

Schmahl J, Raymond CS, Soriano P (2007) PDGF signaling specificity is mediated through multiple immediate early genes. Nat Genet 39:52–60

Senger DR, Asch BB, Smith BD, Perruzzi CA, Dvorak HF (1983) A secreted phosphoprotein marker for neoplastic transformation of both epithelial and fibroblastic cells. Nature 302:714–715

Shalaby F, Rossant J, Yamaguchi TP, Gertsenstein M, Wu XF, Breitman ML, Schuh AC (1995) Failure of blood-island formation and vasculogenesis in Flk-1-deficient mice. Nature 376:62–66

Shay-Salit A, Shushy M, Wolfovitz E, Yahav H, Breviario F, Dejana E, Resnick N (2002) VEGF receptor 2 and the adherens junction as a mechanical transducer in vascular endothelial cells. Proc Natl Acad Sci U S A 99:9462–9467

Shibuya M (1995) Role of VEGF-flt receptor system in normal and tumor angiogenesis. Adv Cancer Res 67:281–316

Shibuya M (2002) Vascular endothelial growth factor receptor family genes: when did the three genes phylogenetically segregate? Biol Chem 383:1573–1579

Shibuya M, Claesson-Welsh L (2006) Signal transduction by VEGF receptors in regulation of angiogenesis and lymphangiogenesis. Exp Cell Res 312:549–560

Shibuya M, Yamaguchi S, Yamane A, Ikeda T, Tojo A, Matsushime H, Sato M (1990) Nucleotide sequence and expression of a novel human receptor-type tyrosine kinase gene (flt) closely related to the fms family. Oncogene 5:519–524

Shih CH, Ozawa S, Ando N, Ueda M, Kitajima M (2000) Vascular endothelial growth factor expression predicts outcome and lymph node metastasis in squamous cell carcinoma of the esophagus. Clin Cancer Res 6:1161–1168

Shinkai A, Ito M, Anazawa H, Yamaguchi S, Shitara K, Shibuya M (1998) Mapping of the sites involved in ligand association and dissociation at the extracellular domain of the kinase insert domain-containing receptor for vascular endothelial growth factor. J Biol Chem 273:31283–31288

Shweiki D, Itin A, Soffer D, Keshet E (1992) Vascular endothelial growth factor induced by hypoxia may mediate hypoxia-initiated angiogenesis. Nature 359:843–845

Sirvent N, Maire G, Pedeutour F (2003) Genetics of dermatofibrosarcoma protuberans family of tumors: from ring chromosomes to tyrosine kinase inhibitor treatment. Genes Chromosomes Cancer 37:1–19

Skobe M, Fusenig NE (1998) Tumorigenic conversion of immortal human keratinocytes through

stromal cell activation. Proc Natl Acad Sci U S A 95:1050–1055
Smith JS, Jenkins RB (2000) Genetic alterations in adult diffuse glioma: occurrence, significance, and prognostic implications. Front Biosci 5:D213–D231
Smith JS, Wang XY, Qian J, Hosek SM, Scheithauer BW, Jenkins RB, James CD (2000) Amplification of the platelet-derived growth factor receptor-A (PDGFRA) gene occurs in oligodendrogliomas with grade IV anaplastic features. J Neuropathol Exp Neurol 59:495–503
Smolich BD, Yuen HA, West KA, Giles FJ, Albitar M, Cherrington JM (2001) The antiangiogenic protein kinase inhibitors SU5416 and SU6668 inhibit the SCF receptor (c-kit) in a human myeloid leukemia cell line and in acute myeloid leukemia blasts. Blood 97:1413–1421
Sorkin A, Westermark B, Heldin CH, Claesson-Welsh L (1991) Effect of receptor kinase inactivation on the rate of internalization and degradation of PDGF and the PDGF beta-receptor. J Cell Biol 112:469–478
Sowter HM, Corps AN, Evans AL, Clark DE, Charnock-Jones DS, Smith SK (1997) Expression and localization of the vascular endothelial growth factor family in ovarian epithelial tumors. Lab Invest 77:607–614
Soyombo AA, DiCorleto PE (1994) Stable expression of human platelet-derived growth factor B chain by bovine aortic endothelial cells. Matrix association and selective proteolytic cleavage by thrombin. J Biol Chem 269:17734–17740
Strawn LM, McMahon G, App H, Schreck R, Kuchler WR, Longhi MP, Hui TH, Tang C, Levitzki A, Gazit A, Chen I, Keri G, Orfi L, Risau W, Flamme I, Ullrich A, Hirth KP, Shawver LK (1996) Flk-1 as a target for tumor growth inhibition. Cancer Res 56:3540–3545
Stroobant P, Waterfield MD (1984) Purification and properties of porcine platelet-derived growth factor. EMBO J 3:2963–2967
Stupack DG, Cheresh DA (2004) Integrins and angiogenesis. Curr Top Dev Biol 64:207–238
Suzuki K, Hayashi N, Miyamoto Y, Yamamoto M, Ohkawa K, Ito Y, Sasaki Y, Yamaguchi Y, Nakase H, Noda K, Enomoto N, Arai K, Yamada Y, Yoshihara H, Tujimura T, Kawano K, Yoshikawa K, Kamada T (1996) Expression of vascular permeability factor/vascular endothelial growth factor in human hepatocellular carcinoma. Cancer Res 56:3004–3009
Takahashi T, Ueno H, Shibuya M (1999) VEGF activates protein kinase C-dependent, but Ras-independent Raf-MEK-MAP kinase pathway for DNA synthesis in primary endothelial cells. Oncogene 18:2221–2230
Takahashi T, Yamaguchi S, Chida K, Shibuya M (2001) A single autophosphorylation site on KDR/Flk-1 is essential for VEGF-A-dependent activation of PLC-gamma and DNA synthesis in vascular endothelial cells. EMBO J 20: 2768–2778
Takahashi Y, Morales FC, Kreimann EL, Georgescu MM (2006) PTEN tumor suppressor associates with NHERF proteins to attenuate PDGF receptor signaling. EMBO J 25:910–920
Tallquist M, Kazlauskas A (2004) PDGF signaling in cells and mice. Cytokine Growth Factor Rev 15:205–213
Tallquist MD, French WJ, Soriano P (2003) Additive effects of PDGF receptor beta signaling pathways in vascular smooth muscle cell development. PLoS Biol 1:E52
Tallquist MD, Klinghoffer RA, Heuchel R, Mueting-Nelsen PF, Corrin PD, Heldin CH, Johnson RJ, Soriano P (2000) Retention of PDGFR-beta function in mice in the absence of phosphatidylinositol 3'-kinase and phospholipase Cgamma signaling pathways. Genes Dev 14:3179–3190
Tallquist MD, Soriano P (2003) Cell autonomous requirement for PDGFRalpha in populations of cranial and cardiac neural crest cells. Development 130:507–518
Tanaka K, Yamaguchi S, Sawano A, Shibuya M (1997) Characterization of the extracellular domain in vascular endothelial growth factor receptor-1 (Flt-1 tyrosine kinase). Jpn J Cancer Res 88:867–876
Terman BI, Carrion ME, Kovacs E, Rasmussen BA, Eddy RL, Shows TB (1991) Identification of a new endothelial cell growth factor receptor tyrosine kinase. Oncogene 6:1677–1683
Theisen CS, Wahl JK 3rd, Johnson KR, Wheelock MJ (2007) NHERF links the N-cadherin/catenin complex to the platelet-derived growth factor receptor to modulate the actin cytoskeleton and regulate cell motility. Mol Biol Cell 18:1220–1232
Tischer E, Mitchell R, Hartman T, Silva M, Gospodarowicz D, Fiddes JC, Abraham JA (1991) The human gene for vascular endothelial growth factor. Multiple protein forms are encoded through alternative exon splicing. J Biol Chem 266:11947–11954

Toi M, Inada K, Suzuki H, Tominaga T (1995) Tumor angiogenesis in breast cancer: its importance as a prognostic indicator and the association with vascular endothelial growth factor expression. Breast Cancer Res Treat 36: 193–204

Tomisawa M, Tokunaga T, Oshika Y, Tsuchida T, Fukushima Y, Sato H, Kijima H, Yamazaki H, Ueyama Y, Tamaoki N, Nakamura M (1999) Expression pattern of vascular endothelial growth factor isoform is closely correlated with tumour stage and vascularisation in renal cell carcinoma. Eur J Cancer 35:133–137

Uchida S, Shimada Y, Watanabe G, Tanaka H, Shibagaki I, Miyahara T, Ishigami S, Imamura M (1998) In oesophageal squamous cell carcinoma vascular endothelial growth factor is associated with p53 mutation, advanced stage and poor prognosis. Br J Cancer 77:1704–1709

Uhrbom L, Hesselager G, Nister M, Westermark B (1998) Induction of brain tumors in mice using a recombinant platelet-derived growth factor B-chain retrovirus. Cancer Res 58:5275–5279

Uhrbom L, Hesselager G, Ostman A, Nister M, Westermark B (2000) Dependence of autocrine growth factor stimulation in platelet-derived growth factor-B-induced mouse brain tumor cells. Int J Cancer 85:398–406

Veikkola T, Jussila L, Makinen T, Karpanen T, Jeltsch M, Petrova TV, Kubo H, Thurston G, McDonald DM, Achen MG, Stacker SA, Alitalo K (2001) Signalling via vascular endothelial growth factor receptor-3 is sufficient for lymphangiogenesis in transgenic mice. EMBO J 20:1223–1231

Vincenti V, Cassano C, Rocchi M, Persico G (1996) Assignment of the vascular endothelial growth factor gene to human chromosome 6p21.3. Circulation 93:1493–1495

Volm M, Koomagi R, Mattern J (1997a) Prognostic value of vascular endothelial growth factor and its receptor Flt-1 in squamous cell lung cancer. Int J Cancer 74:64–68

Volm M, Koomagi R, Mattern J, Stammler G (1997b) Angiogenic growth factors and their receptors in non-small cell lung carcinomas and their relationships to drug response in vitro. Anticancer Res 17:99–103

Waltenberger J, Claesson-Welsh L, Siegbahn A, Shibuya M, Heldin CH (1994) Different signal transduction properties of KDR and Flt1, two receptors for vascular endothelial growth factor. J Biol Chem 269:26988–26995

Warren RS, Yuan H, Matli MR, Ferrara N, Donner DB (1996) Induction of vascular endothelial growth factor by insulin-like growth factor 1 in colorectal carcinoma. J Biol Chem 271:29483–29488

Warren RS, Yuan H, Matli MR, Gillett NA, Ferrara N (1995) Regulation by vascular endothelial growth factor of human colon cancer tumorigenesis in a mouse model of experimental liver metastasis. J Clin Invest 95:1789–1797

Wasteson A, Hook M, Westermark B (1976) Demonstration of a platelet enzyme, degrading heparan sulphate. FEBS Lett 64:218–221

Waterfield MD, Scrace GT, Whittle N, Stroobant P, Johnsson A, Wasteson A, Westermark B, Heldin CH, Huang JS, Deuel TF (1983) Platelet-derived growth factor is structurally related to the putative transforming protein p28sis of simian sarcoma virus. Nature 304:35–39

Wedge SR, Ogilvie DJ, Dukes M, Kendrew J, Curwen JO, Hennequin LF, Thomas AP, Stokes ES, Curry B, Richmond GH, Wadsworth PF (2000) ZD4190: an orally active inhibitor of vascular endothelial growth factor signaling with broad-spectrum antitumor efficacy. Cancer Res 60:970–975

Wizigmann-Voos S, Breier G, Risau W, Plate KH (1995) Up-regulation of vascular endothelial growth factor and its receptors in von Hippel-Lindau disease-associated and sporadic hemangioblastomas. Cancer Res 55:1358–1364

Wood JM, Bold G, Buchdunger E, Cozens R, Ferrari S, Frei J, Hofmann F, Mestan J, Mett H, O'Reilly T, Persohn E, Rosel J, Schnell C, Stover D, Theuer A, Towbin H, Wenger F, Woods-Cook K, Menrad A, Siemeister G, Schirner M, Thierauch KH, Schneider MR, Drevs J, Martiny-Baron G, Totzke F (2000) PTK787/ZK 222584, a novel and potent inhibitor of vascular endothelial growth factor receptor tyrosine kinases, impairs vascular endothelial growth factor-induced responses and tumor growth after oral administration. Cancer Res 60:2178–2189

Yamamoto S, Konishi I, Mandai M, Kuroda H, Komatsu T, Nanbu K, Sakahara H, Mori T (1997) Expression of vascular endothelial growth factor (VEGF) in epithelial ovarian neoplasms: correlation with clinicopathology and patient survival, and analysis of serum VEGF levels. Br J Cancer 76:1221–1227

Yoshiji H, Gomez DE, Shibuya M, Thorgeirsson UP (1996) Expression of vascular endothelial growth factor, its receptor, and other angiogenic factors in human breast cancer. Cancer Res 56:2013–2016

Zhao J, Roth J, Bode-Lesniewska B, Pfaltz M, Heitz PU, Komminoth P (2002) Combined comparative genomic hybridization and genomic microarray for detection of gene amplifications in pulmonary artery intimal sarcomas and adrenocortical tumors. Genes Chromosomes Cancer 34:48–57

Zundel W, Schindler C, Haas-Kogan D, Koong A, Kaper F, Chen E, Gottschalk AR, Ryan HE, Johnson RS, Jefferson AB, Stokoe D, Giaccia AJ (2000) Loss of PTEN facilitates HIF-1-mediated gene expression. Genes Dev 14:391–396

Vascular Integrins: Therapeutic and Imaging Targets of Tumor Angiogenesis

6

Curzio Rüegg and Gian Carlo Alghisi

Abstract Cells, including endothelial cells, continuously sense their surrounding environment and rapidly adapt to changes in order to assure tissues and organs homeostasis. The extracellular matrix (ECM) provides a physical scaffold for cell positioning and represents an instructive interface allowing cells to communicate over short distances. Cell surface receptors of the integrin family emerged through evolution as essential mediators and integrators of ECM-dependent communication. In preclinical studies, pharmacological inhibition of vascular integrins suppressed angiogenesis and inhibited tumor progression. $\alpha_V\beta_3$ and $\alpha_V\beta_5$ were the first integrins targeted to suppress tumor angiogenesis. Subsequently, additional integrins, in particular $\alpha_1\beta_1$, $\alpha_2\beta_1$, $\alpha_5\beta_1$, and $\alpha_6\beta_4$, emerged as potential therapeutic targets. Integrin inhibitors are currently tested in clinical trials for their safety and antiangiogenic/antitumor activity. In this chapter, we review the role of integrins in angiogenesis and present recent advances in the use of integrin antagonists as potential therapeutics in cancer and discuss future perspectives.

C. Rüegg (✉)
Division of Experimental Oncology,
Centre Pluridisciplinaire d'Oncologie,
155, Chemin des Boveresses,
CH1066 Epalinges, Switzerland
e-mail: curzio.ruegg@unil.ch

6.1 Integrin Structure

Integrins comprise a family of cell surface heterodimeric complexes formed by the noncovalent association of two subunits, α and β (Takada et al. 2007). There are 18 α and 8 β subunits capable of forming 24 different functional heterodimers. The αβ composition of the heterodimer largely determines the ligand specificity, although some ligands can bind directly to individual subunits, such as collagens, to the I-domain on the α subunit. Each individual subunit consists of a large extracellular domain (about 750 amino acids for the β subunits and around to 1000 amino acids for the α subunits), a single transmembrane domain (22–24 amino acids), and a short cytoplasmic tail (15–58 amino acids, except for the β_4 subunit, which contains over 1000 intracellular residues). The cytoplasmic domain is essential for the regulation of integrin activity and function: on the one side it controls extracellular ligand-binding activity of the complex ("inside-out" signaling), while on the other, it initiates cellular responses upon ligand binding ("outside-in" signaling) (Ginsberg et al. 2005). In resting, nonligated integrins, the β subunit cytoplasmic domain interacts with the α subunit cytoplasmic domain, thereby maintaining the receptor in its inactive state

R. Liersch et al. (eds.), *Angiogenesis Inhibition,* Recent Results in Cancer Research,
DOI: 10.1007/978-3-540-78281-0_6, © Springer Verlag Berlin Heidelberg 2010

(Luo et al. 2007). Binding of the cytoplasmic protein talin to the β subunit cytoplasmic domain disrupts this interaction, resulting in a conformational change of the extracellular domain leading to a high affinity ligand-binding state (affinity maturation). The "released" β cytoplasmic tail interacts with additional intracellular structural (e.g., paxillin, vinculin), adaptor (e.g., Shc, Cas), and signaling (e.g., FAK, ILK) proteins, thereby initiating cytoskeletal rearrangement and cell signaling events. Ligated integrins can cluster to form small focal contacts at the cell periphery, large focal adhesions retracted from the cell border, or fibrillar adhesions located underneath the cell body along actin stress fibers (Romer et al. 2006).

6.2 Integrin Functions

6.2.1 Cell Adhesion

Integrins are the main cell adhesion receptors for ECM proteins for virtually every cell, including endothelial cells (Hynes 2007). A particular feature of integrins is their ability to recognize short amino acid sequences on exposed loops of their cognate ligands, the tripeptide RGD being the best known and studied. In addition, integrins also bind matricellular proteins, such as thrombospondins, and cell surface molecules, such as ICAMs (for a comprehensive detailed list of ligands, see (Takada et al. 2007)). Ligand binding specificity is promiscuous and redundant: that is, one integrin can bind several different ligands, and many different integrins can bind to the same ligand. Redundancy may be an advantage when the cellular response needed in a particular context (e.g., survival or migration during matrix remodeling) is more important than the nature of the ECM protein eliciting. For example integrin $\alpha_V\beta_3$ binds to many ECM proteins present at sites of inflammation, coagulation, and tissue remodeling. Promiscuity may reflect the need to initiate different signaling events and cellular responses from the same ECM. For example, integrin $\alpha_5\beta_1$ and $\alpha_V\beta_6$ bind to fibronectin, but $\alpha_5\beta_1$ suppresses cell migration, while $\alpha_V\beta_6$ stimulates it (Coutifaris et al. 2005; Scott et al. 2004). More recently, integrins have been reported to bind to a multitude of noncanonical ligands, which themselves are known modulators of vascular functions, including VEGF (Vlahakis et al. 2007), FGF (Murakami et al. 2008), angiopoietins (Camenisch et al. 2002), or matrix-bound VEGFR-1 (Orecchia et al. 2003). These observations open the intriguing possibility that angiogenic growth factors, when associated to the ECM, may modulate endothelial cell functions by signaling through integrins in complement to their activities mediated by their canonical receptors.

6.2.2 Cell Signaling

Integrin ligation also initiates signaling cascades, modulating complex cell functions like spreading, migration, survival, proliferation, or differentiation (Alghisi and Ruegg 2006; Stupack 2007) (Fig. 6.1). As integrins do not have intrinsic enzymatic activity, they need to recruit cytoplasmic structural (e.g., α-actinin, talin, vinculin) and signaling (e.g., FAK, paxillin, and Src family kinases) proteins at adhesion complexes to initiate signal transduction (Luo et al. 2007; Romer et al. 2006). Many signaling pathways activated by integrins are also activated by growth factor receptors, and maximal signal transduction is achieved when integrins and growth factor receptors are concomitantly engaged. Signaling pathways activated by integrins, including in angiogenesis, comprise: MAPK, Akt/PKB, Rho family GTPases, and NF-κB (Mahabeleshwar et al. 2006).

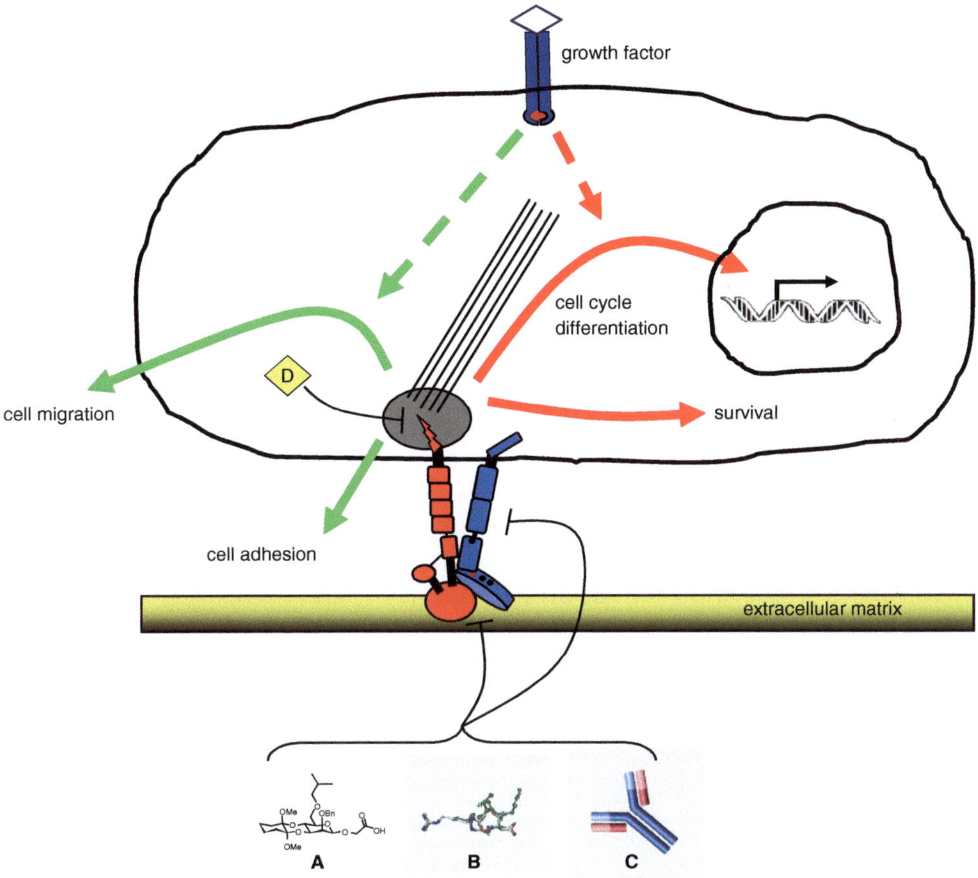

Fig. 6.1 Integrin functions and how to inhibit them. Integrins act as cell adhesion and motility mediators (*green arrows*) or as signal transducers (*red arrows*). These functions can be modulated by growth factors and their receptors (*green and red dashed arrows*). On one hand, the inhibition or integrin function can be achieved extracellularly by the action of peptidomimetics (**a**), peptides, most frequently RGD-based, but also as noncanonical peptides (**b**) or antibodies (**c**). These three classes of inhibitors could also be used as imaging tools if they are labeled with a detectable tracers. On the other hand, peptides disrupting or blocking the interaction between the β integrin cytoplasmic tail with cytoplasmic adaptor or signaling proteins inhibit integrin function and may be developed in the future as therapeutic tools (**d**)

A pathway activated by integrin, particularly relevant to vascular biology and angiogenesis, is the COX-2/prostaglandin pathway. Integrin-mediated adhesion and binding of soluble ligands induce COX-2 mRNA expression and stabilize COX-2 protein in endothelial cells resulting in enhanced prostaglandin production (Zaric and Ruegg 2005). In turn, prostaglandins activate the adenylcyclase via prostane receptor signaling, resulting in PKA activation, accelerated $\alpha_V\beta_3$-dependent cell adhesion, spreading, and migration in a Rac1-dependent manner (Dormond and Ruegg 2003). Consistent with these findings, COX-2 inhibitors inhibit $\alpha_V\beta_3$-dependent endothelial cell spreading and migration in vitro and angiogenesis in vivo.

6

6.3 Integrins in Tumor Angiogenesis

- Integrin $\alpha_V\beta_3$ was the first integrin associated with angiogenesis (Brooks et al. 1994). $\alpha_V\beta_3$ is highly expressed in angiogenic endothelial cells in granulation tissue and in malignant tumors, but is virtually absent from quiescent endothelial cells (Hynes 2007). Inhibition of $\alpha_V\beta_3$ with a function-blocking monoclonal antibody, or RGD-based peptides, or peptidomimetics suppressed corneal neovascularization (Klotz et al. 2000), hypoxia-induced retinal neovascularization (Hammes et al. 1996), tumor angiogenesis, and tumor progression in various in vivo models (MacDonald et al. 2001; Reinmuth et al. 2003), and endothelial cell sprouting and angiogenesis in an in vitro 3D model of angiogenesis (Nisato et al. 2004). Importantly, quiescent and pre-existing vessels were not perturbed by these treatments. The results obtained with pharmacological antagonists of integrins $\alpha_V\beta_3/\alpha_V\beta_5$ contrast with results obtained through genetic approaches. Mice deficient in α_V integrins and lacking $\alpha_V\beta_1$, $\alpha_V\beta_3$, $\alpha_V\beta_5$, $\alpha_V\beta_6$, and $\alpha_V\beta_8$ expression, were still able to undergo extensive developmental vasculogenesis and angiogenesis, although they died in utero or shortly after birth (Bader et al. 1998). Analysis of the phenotype of individual β integrin knock-out mice showed that the β_8 knock-out was the only one to reproduce the α_V knock-out phenotype (Zhu et al. 2002), thereby revealing a role for $\alpha_V\beta_8$ in the association between cerebral microvessels and brain parenchymal cells. Deletion of the β_3 subunit did not significantly disrupt vascular development, although some embryos died in utero due to placenta defects, while others died postnatally due to bleeding and anemia (Hodivala-Dilke et al. 1999). β_3-deficiency reproduce the inherited human bleeding disorder known as Glanzmann thrombasthenia due to the concomitant lack of $\alpha_{IIb}\beta_3$ (Tomiyama 2000). Paradoxically, mice lacking $\alpha_V\beta_3$ integrins had enhanced pathological angiogenesis, including tumor angiogenesis (Reynolds et al. 2002), associated with enhanced VEGFR-2 signaling (Reynolds et al. 2004). The reason for the divergence of the results obtained with pharmacological inhibition vs. genetic deletion of $\alpha_V\beta_3$ are not yet fully clear (Hynes 2002).
- More recently, β_1 integrins (i.e., $\alpha_1\beta_1$, $\alpha_2\beta_1$, $\alpha_3\beta_1$, $\alpha_4\beta_1$, $\alpha_5\beta_1$, $\alpha_V\beta_1$), $\alpha_V\beta_8$, and $\alpha_6\beta_4$ have also been shown to promote angiogenesis (Alghisi and Ruegg 2006; Serini et al. 2006). β_1 integrin expression on vascular endothelial cells is dispensable for vasculogenesis, but crucial for embryonic angiogenesis (Tanjore et al. 2007). Deletion of the α_5 gene is embryonically lethal and is associated with vascular and cardiac defects (Francis et al. 2002). $\alpha_5\beta_1$ is up regulated in angiogenesis and blocking anti-α_5 antibodies suppressed VEGF-induced tumor angiogenesis in both chick embryo and murine models (Collo and Pepper 1999; Kim et al. 2000). An $\alpha_5\beta_1$ antagonist in combination with chemotherapy reduced metastasis and suppressed angiogenesis at metastatic lesions (Stoeltzing et al. 2003).
- Integrins $\alpha_1\beta_1$ and $\alpha_2\beta_1$ are highly upregulated by VEGF in cultured endothelial cells, resulting in enhanced cell spreading on collagen I, while anti-$\alpha_1\beta_1$ and anti-$\alpha_2\beta_1$ antibodies inhibited VEGF-driven angiogenesis in vivo. Combined administration of anti-$\alpha_1\beta_1$ and anti-$\alpha_2\beta_1$ antibodies to mice bearing squamous cell carcinoma xenografts, resulted in reduced tumor angiogenesis and tumor growth (Hong et al. 2004; Perruzzi et al. 2003; Senger et al. 2002). The role of $\alpha_2\beta_1$ for the regulation of murine wound angiogenesis was confirmed in a genetic approach (Zweers et al. 2007).
- $\alpha_6\beta_4$ promotes an invasive endothelial cell phenotype at the early phase of angiogenesis in response to growth factors (FGF-2, VEGF)

(Nikolopoulos et al. 2004). Genetic studies have revealed that $\alpha_6\beta_4$ signaling promotes both angiogenesis and tumorigenesis. Importantly, $\alpha_6\beta_4$ combines with multiple receptor tyrosine kinases, including ErbB2, EGF-R and c-Met, and enhances their signaling function (Giancotti 2007).

6.4 Integrin Antagonists with Antiangiogenic Activities

Four different types of integrin antagonists have been developed: antibodies, endogenous inhibitors, peptides, and nonpeptidic antagonists. We describe here the main representative drugs within each class that have shown antiangiogenic activity in preclinical models, with particular emphasis on drugs that entered clinical testing. These and additional inhibitors are summarized in Table 6.1.

6.4.1 Antibodies

- *LM609/MEDI-522/Vitaxin.* The anti-$\alpha_V\beta_3$ monoclonal antibody LM609 blocked endothelial cell adhesion, migration, and sprouting in vitro and angiogenesis in vivo in the CAM assay (Brooks et al. 1994). Subsequently, LM609 was humanized and affinity maturated allowing the isolation of an antibody with a 90-fold improved affinity (MEDI-522 or Vitaxin) (Wu et al. 1998). Phase I studies demonstrated that treatment was well tolerated with little or no toxicity. The most common side effect was infusion-related fevers. Doses of 1 mg/kg/week or more produced plasma concentrations sufficient to saturate $\alpha_V\beta_3$ in vitro. Vitaxin demonstrated a half-life longer than five days with no tendency to accumulation. One partial response and several stable diseases were observed (Posey et al. 2001). Combination of Vitaxin with chemotherapy was well tolerated. There was possible effect on tumor perfusion detected by dynamic computed tomography imaging, but no objective antitumor responses (McNeel et al. 2005). In treated patients, there was evidence of reduced FAK phosphorylation in skin wound vessels, consistent with inhibition of $\alpha_V\beta_3$ signaling (Zhang et al. 2007). Vitaxin has entered Phase II trials mostly on hormone-refractory prostate cancers or metastatic melanoma (www.clinicaltrials.gov).
- *CNTO 95.* CNTO 95 is a pan anti-α_V fully humanized antibody. In a human melanoma xenograft model, wherein CNTO 95 recognized $\alpha_V\beta_3$ and $\alpha_V\beta_5$ on human tumor cells but not mouse cells, CNTO 95 treatment inhibited tumor growth by 80%. In a nude rat, human skin xenograft tumor model where CNTO 95 blocks $\alpha_V\beta_3$ and $\alpha_V\beta_5$ on both human tumor cells and human skin endothelial cells, treatment reduced final tumor weight by >99% (Trikha et al. 2004). The antibody did not show any adverse effects in monkeys (Martin et al. 2005) and entered Phase I clinical trials in various solid tumors, including ovarian, colorectal, melanoma, and renal cell carcinoma. Results on these patients showed that CNTO 95 was well tolerated up to weekly doses of 10 mg/kg (www.asco.org). CNTO 95 is now in Phase I/II in combination with other chemotherapeutic drugs in Stage IV melanoma or metastatic HRPC.
- *M200/Volociximab.* M200 is an affinity maturated humanized chimeric monoclonal antibody blocking $\alpha_5\beta_1$ integrin. It inhibited tumor angiogenesis and tumor growth in a rabbit syngenic tumor model (M200 does not bind to rodent $\alpha_5\beta_1$) despite a 20-fold lower affinity for rabbit integrin, relative to human (Bhaskar et al. 2007a). A function blocking rat-anti-mouse $\alpha_5\beta_1$ antibody with features similar to M200 was shown to inhibit angiogenesis and suppress tumor growth and metastasis in mice (Bhaskar et al. 2007b;

6

Table 6.1 Integrin antagonists in clinical trials

	Inhibitor	Targeted integrins	Clinical development	References
Antibodies	LM609, MEDI-522, vitaxin®	$\alpha_V\beta_3$	Passed phase I In phase II	(Gutheil et al. 2000; McNeel et al. 2005; Posey et al. 2001)
	Volociximab, M200	$\alpha_5\beta_1$	Passed phase I, currently in phase II	(Kuwada 2007; Ramakrishnan et al. 2006) www.pdl.com
	CNTO 95	α_V family, strong affinity for $\alpha_V\beta_3$ and $\alpha_V\beta_5$	Phase I or phaseI/II	(Mullamitha et al. 2007; Trikha et al. 2004) www.clinicaltrials.gov
	17E6	α_V family, strong affinity for $\alpha_V\beta_3$, $\alpha_V\beta_5$ and $\alpha_V\beta_1$		(Mitjans et al. 1995, 2000)
	7E3, abciximab, ReoPro	$\alpha_{IIb}\beta_3$ primarily but also $\alpha_V\beta_3$ and $\alpha_M\beta_2$ (Mac-1)	Passed phase I and II. Currently in phase III for the prevention of restenosis	(Nakada et al. 2006; Varner et al. 1999)
	Ha 31/8	$\alpha_1\beta_1$		(Senger et al. 1997, 2002)
	Ha 1/29	$\alpha_2\beta_1$		(Senger et al. 1997, 2002)
	NKI-SAM-1, JBS5 or IIA1	$\alpha_5\beta_1$		(Francis et al. 2002; Kim et al. 2000)
Endogenous inhibitors	Endostatin (C-terminal fragment of collagen XVIII)	$\alpha_5\beta_1$	Phase I	(Herbst et al. 2002), www.clinicaltrials.gov
	Tumstatin (C-terminal fragment of collagen IV)	$\alpha_V\beta_3$		(Hamano and Kalluri 2005; Maeshima et al. 2002)
	Endorepellin (C-terminal module of perlecan)	$\alpha_2\beta_1$		(Woodall et al., 2008)
	Angiocidin	$\alpha_2\beta_1$		(Sabherwal et al. 2006)
	PEX (MMP-2 proteolytic fragment)	$\alpha_V\beta_3$		(Bello et al. 2001; Pfeifer et al. 2000)
	Fastatin (FAS1 domain of βig-h3	$\alpha_V\beta_3$		(Nam et al. 2005)

Table 6.1 (continued)

	Inhibitor	Targeted integrins	Clinical development	References
Synthetic peptides	EMD121974, cilengitide	$\alpha_V\beta_3$	Passed phase I Phase II	(Eskens et al. 2003; Nabors et al. 2007) www.clinicaltrials.gov
	TP508 (thrombospondin derived peptide)	$\alpha_V\beta_3$		(Tsopanoglou et al. 2004)
	S247	$\alpha_V\beta_3$		(Abdollahi et al. 2005)
	ATN-161	$\alpha_5\beta_1$	Phase I Phase II	(Cianfrocca et al. 2006) www.clinicaltrials.gov
	CRRETAWAC (fibronectin peptide)	$\alpha_5\beta_1$		(Koivunen et al. 1994; Mould et al. 1998)
Peptidomimetics	SCH221153	$\alpha_V\beta_3$ and $\alpha_V\beta_5$		(Kumar et al. 2001)
	BCH-14661 BCH-15056	$\alpha_V\beta_3$ and $\alpha_V\beta_5$		(Meerovitch et al. 2003)
	ST1646	$\alpha_V\beta_3$ and $\alpha_V\beta_5$		(Belvisi et al. 2005)
	Thiolutin	$\alpha_V\beta_3$ (indirect), decreases paxillin levels		(Minamiguchi et al. 2001)
	SJ749	$\alpha_5\beta_1$		(Kim et al. 2000; Marinelli et al. 2005)
	JSM6427	$\alpha_5\beta_1$		(Umeda et al. 2006)

A nonexhaustive list of available antibody, peptide and peptidomimetic antagonists of integrins with anti-angiogenic activities developed so far is presented (some compounds are further described in the text)

Ramakrishnan et al. 2006). Based on this activity profile, Volociximab was tested in Phase I trials in various refractory solid tumors including renal cell carcinoma and metastatic melanoma. The study data showed that adverse events were generally mild to moderate in intensity and there were no dose limiting toxicities. Volociximab is currently evaluated in Phase II trials as a single agent (Kuwada 2007). Combination trials with chemotherapy are planned.

- *c7E3/Abciximab/ReoPro*. c7E3 is a humanized monoclonal antibody Fab fragment approved for use as adjunct therapy to prevent cardiac ischemic complications in patients undergoing coronary angioplasty (Cohen et al. 2000). c7E3 also interacts with integrins $\alpha_V\beta_3$ and Mac-1 ($\alpha_M\beta_2$). In animal models, c7E3 inhibited tumor growth and angiogenesis (Nakada et al. 2006).

6.4.2 Endogenous Antagonists

- *Endostatin* is a carboxyl-terminal fragment of Collagen XVIII inhibiting endothelial cell proliferation in vitro and angiogenesis and tumor growth in vivo (O'Reilly et al. 1997). The generation of endostatin from Collagen XII is mediated by various proteases (e.g., cathepsin L and MMPs). The antiangiogenic activity of endostatin is due, at least in part, to binding to integrin $\alpha_5\beta_1$ and caveolin-1 on endothelial cells, causing downregulation of RhoA activity and Src family kinase-dependent disassembly of focal adhesions and actin stress fibers, resulting in decreased matrix deposition and migration (Wickstrom et al. 2005). Recombinant human endostatin entered clinical testing and was found to be safe and well tolerated (Hansma et al. 2005; Herbst et al. 2002).

- *Tumstatin* consists of the carboxyl-terminal noncollagenous 1 (NC1) domain of the α3 chain of Collagen IV. It inhibited in vivo neovascularization in Matrigel plug assays, suppressed tumor growth in xenograft models, and induced endothelial cell apoptosis (Hamano and Kalluri 2005). Tumstatin binds to $\alpha_V\beta_3$ integrin in endothelial cells, and selectively inhibits protein synthesis by suppressing mTOR (Maeshima et al. 2002).

6.4.3 Peptides

- *EMD121974/Cilengitide.* The discovery that many integrins recognize their ligands through short amino acid sequences, most notably RGD, led to the development of small peptides that competitively blocked ligand–receptor interaction. Cyclized peptides were up to 100-fold more selective than linear counterparts, and cyclic pentapeptides that possessed two hydrophobic amino acids next to the recognition sequence proved to be highly active and selective for $\alpha_V\beta_3/\alpha_V\beta_5$. The cyclic pentapeptide cyclo(-Arg-Gly-Asp-D-Phe-Val-) (EMD66203 Merck KGaA) showed nanomolar inhibition of vitronectin binding to the $\alpha_V\beta_3$ integrin without interfering with $\alpha_{IIb}\beta_3$ integrin (Haubner et al. 1996). Modification of the amino acids flanking the RGD sequence led to the synthesis of EMD121974 (Cilengitide) inhibiting $\alpha_V\beta_3$ integrin binding to vitronectin with an IC_{50} of 0.6 nM versus 900 nM for the $\alpha_{IIb}\beta_3$ integrin (Smith 2003). Cilengitide showed antitumor effects in brain, melanoma, head and neck, and brain tumors (MacDonald et al. 2001; Mitjans et al. 2000; Raguse et al. 2004; Taga et al. 2002). In Phase I, studies of cilengitide were well tolerated with no dose-limiting toxicities, and showed evidence of activity in recurrent malignant gliomas (Nabors et al. 2007). Cilengitide is now in Phase II clinical trials, alone and in combination with radio and chemotherapies, in solid tumors, leukemia, and lymphoma (Stupp and Ruegg 2007).
- *ATN-161* is a peptide derived from the $\alpha_5\beta_1$-binding sequence PHSRN present in fibronectin (Livant et al. 2000). Chemical modifications of this sequence led to the synthesis of ATN-161 (Ac-PHSCN-NH_2) that, in contrast to other integrin antagonist peptides, is not a RGD-based peptide. ATN-161 possesses antitumorigenic antiangiogenic activities in mice in the absence of toxicities (Livant et al. 2000). ATN-161 was tested in a Phase I study in patients with advanced solid tumors for up to 14 cycles of 4 weeks and was well tolerated at all dose levels. Approximately, one-third of the treated patients manifested prolonged stable disease (Cianfrocca et al. 2006).

6.4.4 Non-peptidic Inhibitors

Peptidomimetics are compounds containing non-peptidic structural elements mimicking the action(s) of a natural parent peptide. Peptidomimetics can be administered orally, are insensitive to protease-mediated degradation, and have longer stability (Cacciari and Spalluto 2005).

- *SCH221153* was obtained by screening and further modifying an RGD-based peptidomimetic library. It targets $\alpha_V\beta_3$ and $\alpha_V\beta_5$ integrins with IC_{50} of 3.2 and 1.7 nM, respectively. SCH221153 inhibited endothelial cell adhesion to vitronectin and suppressed angiogenesis in a CAM assay (Kumar et al. 2001).
- *BCH-14661* and *BCH-15046* are integrin antagonists that induce cell detachment and apoptosis of angiogenic endothelial grown on RGD-based matrices (i.e., vitronectin and fibronectin). BCH-14661 is specific for $\alpha_V\beta_3$, while BCH-15046 antagonizes $\alpha_V\beta_3$, $\alpha_V\beta_5$ and $\alpha_5\beta_1$ (Meerovitch et al. 2003). BCH-15046 was also capable to induce endothelial cell apoptosis independently of cell detachment.
- *Thiolutin* is a non-peptidic antagonist of cell adhesion interfering with integrin-post-receptor events (Minamiguchi et al. 2001). The antiadhesive effect of thiolutin is due to decreased paxillin protein expression, disruption of focal adhesions, and cell detachment.
- *SJ749*, which structure mimics RGD-based sequences, is a potent inhibitor of $\alpha_5\beta_1$ integrin (IC_{50} around 0.8 nM), and it inhibited angiogenesis in the CAM assay (Kim et al. 2000). The structure of this non-peptidic compound bound to the head of the $\alpha_5\beta_1$ integrin has been resolved, thereby opening new perspectives in rational design to improve its specificity and binding constant (Marinelli et al. 2005).
- *JSM6427* is another $\alpha_5\beta_1$-specific peptidomimetic inhibitor with antiangiogenic activities (Umeda et al. 2006). Interestingly, JSM6427 inhibited inflammatory lymphangiogenesis (Dietrich et al. 2007) suggesting the possibility of combined targeting angiogenesis and lymphangiogenesis by targeting one integrin.

6.5 Open Questions and Current Developments

Preclinical studies suggest that vascular integrins are valuable targets for antiangiogenic treatments. Results obtained in Phase I clinical trials have shown that the integrin antagonists tested so far are well tolerated and hint some antitumor activity. Phase II trials aimed at demonstrating antiangiogenic/antitumor activities are ongoing (Stupp and Ruegg 2007). Important basic questions on the role of integrins in angiogenesis and their therapeutic targeting, however, have remained unanswered and new ones have emerged. In this section we review some of the open outstanding questions.

6.5.1 Most Relevant Targets

Endothelial cells can express up to 12 integrins ($\alpha_V\beta_3$, $\alpha_V\beta_5$, $\alpha_5\beta_1$, $\alpha_1\beta_1$, $\alpha_2\beta_1$, $\alpha_6\beta_4$, $\alpha_3\beta_1$, $\alpha_4\beta_1$, $\alpha_6\beta_1$, $\alpha_8\beta_1$, $\alpha_V\beta_1$, and $\alpha_V\beta_8$) (Alghisi and Ruegg 2006). At this point, we do not know which one of these integrins is the best therapeutic target for antiangiogenic treatments, and if angiogenic vessels in different tumors or at different stages of development may use different integrins. More preclinical work is needed to test and compare the suitability of individual integrins as therapeutic target and to evaluate the possibility of combined targeting.

6.5.2 Combination Therapies

Combined treatment with integrin antagonists and chemotherapy or radiotherapy has shown enhanced therapeutic efficacy in preclinical models (Ruegg and Mutter 2007). Since combination therapy appears to be a general rule for antiangiogenic treatments in humans, the critical issue is to define the best combination in term of drug association, timing, and schedule.

- *Radiotherapy.* Integrin antagonists enhance efficacy of radiotherapy. Radiation was found to upregulate $\alpha_V\beta_3$ expression in endothelial cells and to induce activation of Akt/PKB, possibly as a mechanism for the tumor vasculature to escape or recover from radiation-induced injury. Inhibitors of $\alpha_V\beta_3$ integrin suppressed radiation-induced Akt/PKB phosphorylation, increased cell death and enhanced antiangiogenic and antitumor effects in xenograft models (Abdollahi et al. 2005; Ning et al. 2007). Using a different model, cilengitide sensitized tumors to radioimmunotherapy (Burke et al. 2002). These results reinforce the rationale of combining vascular integrin antagonists with radiotherapy.
- *Chemotherapy.* Combination of ATN-161 ($\alpha_5\beta_1$ antagonist) with 5-fluoroacil synergized the reduction of the number of liver metastases and tumor burden of CT26 colon cancer cells in mice (Stoeltzing et al. 2003). Liver tumors in the ATN-161 and ATN-161/5-FU groups had significantly fewer microvessels than tumors in the control or 5-FU-treated groups.
- *Tumor Necrosis Factor (TNF).* TNF is used in combination with high dose chemotherapy in an isolation limb perfusion setting to treat advanced cancers of the limbs (Lejeune et al. 2006). The mechanism by which TNF exerts its antitumor activity involves detachment and death of angiogenic endothelial cells expressing $\alpha_V\beta_3$ (Ruegg et al. 1998). Integrin-mediated adhesion is required for TNF-induced Akt/PKB activation, an event essential for the survival of TNF-stimulated endothelial cells (Bieler et al. 2007). Consistent with these results, cilengitide sensitizes endothelial cells to TNF-induced death in vitro. Thus, combined administration of cilengitide may open new perspectives to the therapeutic use of TNF as anticancer agent.
- Tyrosine Kinase Inhibitors (TKI). Since integrins facilitate signaling from several receptor tyrosine kinases, including ErbB2, VEGFR-2, EGF-R, and Met, it is reasonable to hypothesize that integrin inhibition may sensitize endothelial cells to currently available TKI antiangiogenic drugs (e.g., bevacizumab, sorafenib, sunitinib, temsirolimus) or to other TKI with antiangiogenic activities, such as EGFR antagonists (e.g., cetuximab or gefitinib), or PDGFRs inhibitors (e.g., Imatinib). Indeed, combined administration of cilengitide and SU5416, a VEGR-2 TKI reduced tumoral vessel density and intratumoral blood flow compared to single drug treatments (Strieth et al. 2006). $\alpha_6\beta_4$ might be an interesting integrin to target in combination with ErbB2, EGFR, and Met inhibitors, since, in addition to antiangiogenic effects, it may also have direct antitumor activity, as $\alpha_6\beta_4$ and ErbB2, EGF-R and Met are expressed on many carcinoma cells (Giancotti 2007). The endogenous antiangiogenic peptide tumstatin was shown to exert direct antitumoral effects in $\alpha_V\beta_{3,}$ expressing glioma cells in vitro and in vivo by suppressing $\alpha_V\beta_3$-dependent Akt and mTOR signaling (Kawaguchi et al. 2006), suggesting the possibility that a combination strategy may be chosen in a way to target angiogenic endothelial cells and tumor cells.

6.5.3 Drug Targeting

Vascular integrins expressed on tumoral vessels, such as $\alpha_V\beta_3$ have been used to target drugs to tumors. Cationic nanoparticles coupled with an integrin $\alpha_V\beta_3$-targeting ligand were used to deliver a dominant-negative mutant Raf gene to angiogenic blood vessels in tumor-bearing mice, resulting in apoptosis of the tumor vessels and regression of established primary and metastatic tumors (Hood et al. 2002). Paclitaxel

(Taxol), an antitumor drug commonly used for the treatment of advanced metastatic breast cancer, conjugated with an RGD-based peptide had a better uptake kinetic in vivo compared to free paclitaxel (i.e., 4 h for free PTX vs. 2 h for the PTX-RGD conjugate), although it did not show enhanced potency at the cellular level(Chen et al. 2005). These experiments demonstrate the feasibility of integrin-based targeted drug delivery to tumors. More recently, several studies reported that conjugation of $\alpha_V\beta_3$-targeting RGD peptides or peptidomimetics to carrier proteins (e.g., antibody), synthetic scaffold structures, or micelles (e.g., PEG-polyLys-associated with plasmid DNA) resulted in improved pharmacokinetics, retention in the tumor tissue, and cellular uptake (Mitra et al. 2006; Oba et al. 2007; Shin et al. 2007). $\alpha_V\beta_3$-integrin-targeted nanoparticles rapidly taken up by $\alpha_V\beta_3$-positive angiogenic vessels and tumors were developed for delivery and imaging purposes (Xie et al. 2007).

6.5.4 Tumor Imaging

Vascular integrins upregulated in angiogenic vessels have also been explored for noninvasive tumor imaging purposes. Most approaches have targeted $\alpha_V\beta_3$ in combination with positron emission tomography (PET) and Magnetic Resonance Imaging (MRI) imaging techniques (Choe and Lee 2007). The proof of concept experiment was reported already in 1998, where gadolinium-labeled LM609 was used to detect angiogenesis in a rabbit tumor model.

Before this approach be successfully translated into the clinic, however, substantial gains in sensitivity brought about by improved coils, pulse sequences, and contrast agents were needed (Barrett et al. 2007). Thanks to its high sensitivity, PET technology has been preferred and used in animal models and in humans to detect $\alpha_V\beta_3$ using ^{18}F-labeled monomeric or multimeric RGD peptides. The level of expression $\alpha_V\beta_3$ detected by PET, correlated with the level of $\alpha_V\beta_3$ determined by immunohistochemistry, suggesting that this approach may be used for the noninvasive measurement of $\alpha_V\beta_{3,}$ and monitoring antiangiogenic therapy in patients (Beer et al. 2006). ^{64}Cu-DOTA-labeled Vitaxin (Abegrin) were used in animal models and showed high levels of late tumor activity accumulation (i.e., 71 h) post injection (Cai et al. 2006). Similarly, ^{99m}Tc-labeled RGD peptides were used to image tumors and angiogenic vascular beds by gamma camera (Decristoforo et al. 2006) or single photon emission computed tomography (SPECT) in experimental models (Liu et al. 2007). Recently, near-infrared fluorescence imaging coupled with 3D optical imaging systems have been used to image $\alpha_V\beta_3$-positive tumor vessels and tumor cells in mice using Cy5.5-RGD peptides (Hsu et al. 2006). Taken together, these results illustrate the potential of employing integrin-targeted molecular probes to image tumor vasculature and monitoring response to therapy.

6.6 Future Directions

6.6.1 New Generation of Extracellular Antagonists

While most efforts have been focused on the generation of small molecular inhibitors based on the RGD sequence or the ligand-binding pocket, recent studies have reported inhibitors acting in a RGD-independent manner, such as tumstatin (Maeshima et al. 2000) or ATN-161 (Livant et al. 2000). The resolution of the 3D structure of cilengitide-$\alpha_V\beta_3$ complex (Xiong et al. 2002) and of SJ749-$\alpha_5\beta_1$ complex (Marinelli et al. 2005), allows for the exploration of additional regions of the receptor for binding of novel inhibitory molecules, "*in silico*" design and virtual screenings of improved or fully novel antagonists (Zhou et al. 2006). Furthermore, "broad spectrum" inhibitors blocking several angiogenic integrins (e.g., β_1 and β_3) may be developed, as suggested by the recent report of BCH-15046, a $\alpha_V\beta_3$, $\alpha_V\beta_5$ and $\alpha_5\beta_1$ antagonist (Meerovitch et al. 2003).

6.6.2 Targeting the Integrin Intracellular Domains

Interaction of the cytoplasmic tail of the β subunit is essential for integrin function (Travis et al. 2003). Expression of isolated β integrin subunit cytoplasmic and transmembrane domains in adherent endothelial cells caused cell detachment and death in vitro and in vivo (Hasmim et al. 2005; Oguey et al. 2000), consistent with the notion that overexpression of isolated β-cytoplasmic domain competes for binding of essential cytoplasmic adaptor proteins (e.g., talin), resulting in "mechanical uncoupling"of the integrins from focal adhesions and cytoskeletal structures. These results also suggest the possibility of targeting the cytoplasmic domain for therapeutic purposes. Two main problems need to be addressed: the first one concerns integrin specificity (current constructs that do not differentiate between β_1 and β_3 integrins). The second problem concerns intracellular delivery: to allow penetration into the cell, an inhibitory peptide has to be fused to cytoplasmic transduction peptides (Kim et al. 2006). Alternatively, non-peptidic drugs may be developed to disrupt β_3-tail interaction with structural or signaling cytoplasmic proteins.

6.6.3 Targeting Angiogenic Precursor Cells and Inflammatory Cells

Bone marrow cells are mobilized during tumor growth and recruited at tumor sites to promote tumor angiogenesis. While some of the cells include true endothelial precursors giving rise to mature endothelial cells, most of them are of monocyte/macrophage lineage (De Palma and Naldini 2006). Monocyte/macrophage is very sensitive to hypoxia and produces angiogenic factors and chemokines that stimulate tumor angiogenesis, progression, and metastasis (Condeelis and Pollard 2006). Since leukocytes and inflammatory cells use integrins to extravasate and migrate through the stroma, such as $\alpha_L\beta_2$, $\alpha_4\beta_1$, $\alpha_M\beta_2$, $\alpha_V\beta_3$, or $\alpha_5\beta_1$, it may be reasonable to inhibit their recruitment to tumor sites by targeting their integrins (Ulbrich et al. 2003). For example, antagonists of integrin $\alpha_4\beta_1$ blocked extravasation of monocytes into tumor tissue and prevented monocyte macrophage colonization of tumors and tumor angiogenesis (Jin et al. 2006). Since it is also possible that some of the antiangiogenic effects observed with $\alpha_V\beta_3$ or $\alpha_5\beta_1$ antagonists may be due to the inhibition of leukocyte recruitment, in future experimental and clinical studies it will be important to monitor the effect of integrin inhibitors on the recruitment of inflammatory cells to tumor sites. Of note is the observation that Cilengitide inhibited proliferation and differentiation of human endothelial progenitor cells in vitro (Loges et al. 2007).

6.7 Conclusions

Preclinical evidence indicates that integrins expressed in angiogenic endothelial cells are potentially relevant targets for antiangiogenic therapies in cancer. Early clinical trials have provided initial evidence of activity in human cancers, and ongoing clinical trials tell us whether they may bring benefits to human cancer treatment. If this is the case, besides further clinical trials, there will be a race to generate novel, more potent, and orally bioavailable "second generation" antagonists as well as to define the best combination strategy. The possibility of coupling the use of integrin antagonists for therapeutic purposes with non-invasive imaging of vascular integrins would open the possibility to select patients expressing high levels of the target, and therefore those who are most likely to benefit from the treatment.

Acknowledgments Work in our laboratory was supported by funds from the Molecular Oncology Program of the National Center for Competence in Research (NCCR), a research instrument of the Swiss National Science Foundation, the Swiss Cancer League/Oncosuisse, the Swiss National Science Foundation, and the Medic Foundation. We apologize to those colleagues whose work could not be cited due to space limitations.

References

Abdollahi A, Griggs DW, Zieher H, Roth A, Lipson KE, Saffrich R, Grone H-J, Hallahan DE, Reisfeld RA, Debus J, Niethammer AG, Huber PE (2005) Inhibition of alpha(v)beta3 integrin survival signaling enhances antiangiogenic and antitumor effects of radiotherapy. Clin Cancer Res 11: 6270–6279

Alghisi GC, Ruegg C (2006) Vascular integrins in tumor angiogenesis: mediators and therapeutic targets. Endothelium 13:113–135

Bader B, Rayburn H, Crowley D, Hynes R (1998) Extensive vasculogenesis, angiogenesis, and organogenesis precede lethality in mice lacking all alpha v integrins. Cell 95:507–519

Barrett T, Brechbiel M, Bernardo M, Choyke PL (2007) MRI of tumor angiogenesis. J Magn Reson Imaging 26:235–249

Beer AJ, Haubner R, Sarbia M, Goebel M, Luderschmidt S, Grosu AL, Schnell O, Niemeyer M, Kessler H, Wester HJ, Weber WA, Schwaiger M (2006) Positron emission tomography using [18F]Galacto-RGD identifies the level of integrin alpha(v)beta3 expression in man. Clin Cancer Res 12:3942–3949

Bello L, Lucini V, Carrabba G, Giussani C, Machluf M, Pluderi M, Nikas D, Zhang J, Tomei G, Villani RM, Carroll RS, Bikfalvi A, Black PM (2001) Simultaneous inhibition of glioma angiogenesis, cell proliferation, and invasion by a naturally occurring fragment of human metalloproteinase-2. Cancer Res 61: 8730–8736

Belvisi L, Riccioni T, Marcellini M, Vesci L, Chiarucci I, Efrati D, Potenza D, Scolastico C, Manzoni L, Lombardo K, Stasi MA, Orlandi A, Ciucci A, Nico B, Ribatti D, Giannini G, Presta M, Carminati P, Pisano C (2005) Biological and molecular properties of a new alpha(v)beta3/alpha(v)beta5 integrin antagonist. Mol Cancer Ther 4:1670–1680

Bhaskar V, Fox M, Breinberg D, Wong MH, Wales PE, Rhodes S, Dubridge RB, Ramakrishnan V (2007a) Volociximab, a chimeric integrin alpha5beta1 antibody, inhibits the growth of VX2 tumors in rabbits. Invest New Drugs 26(1):7–12

Bhaskar V, Zhang D, Fox M, Seto P, Wong MH, Wales PE, Powers D, Chao DT, Dubridge RB, Ramakrishnan V (2007b) A function blocking anti-mouse integrin alpha5beta1 antibody inhibits angiogenesis and impedes tumor growth in vivo. J Transl Med 5:61

Bieler G, Hasmim M, Monnier Y, Imaizumi N, Ameyar M, Bamat J, Ponsonnet L, Chouaib S, Grell M, Goodman SL, Lejeune F, Ruegg C (2007) Distinctive role of integrin-mediated adhesion in TNF-induced PKB/Akt and NF-kappaB activation and endothelial cell survival. Oncogene 26: 5722–5732

Brooks PC, Clark RA, Cheresh DA (1994) Requirement of vascular integrin alpha v beta 3 for angiogenesis. Science 264:569–571

Burke PA, DeNardo SJ, Miers LA, Lamborn KR, Matzku S, DeNardo GL (2002) Cilengitide targeting of alpha(v)beta3 integrin receptor synergizes with radioimmunotherapy to increase efficacy and apoptosis in breast cancer xenografts. Cancer Res 62:4263–4272

Cacciari B, Spalluto G (2005) Non peptidic alphavbeta3 antagonists: recent developments. Curr Med Chem 12:51–70

Cai W, Wu Y, Chen K, Cao Q, Tice DA, Chen X (2006) In vitro and in vivo characterization of 64Cu-labeled Abegrin, a humanized monoclonal antibody against integrin alpha v beta 3. Cancer Res 66:9673–9681

Camenisch G, Pisabarro MT, Sherman D, Kowalski J, Nagel M, Hass P, Xie MH, Gurney A, Bodary S, Liang XH, Clark K, Beresini M, Ferrara N, Gerber HP (2002) ANGPTL3 stimulates endothelial cell adhesion and migration via integrin alpha vbeta 3 and induces blood vessel formation in vivo. J Biol Chem 277: 17281–17290

Chen X, Plasencia C, Hou Y, Neamati N (2005) Synthesis and biological evaluation of dimeric RGD peptide-paclitaxel conjugate as a model for integrin-targeted drug delivery. J Med Chem 48:1098–1106

Choe YS, Lee KH (2007) Targeted in vivo imaging of angiogenesis: present status and perspectives. Curr Pharm Des 13:17–31

Cianfrocca ME, Kimmel KA, Gallo J, Cardoso T, Brown MM, Hudes G, Lewis N, Weiner L, Lam GN, Brown SC, Shaw DE, Mazar AP, Cohen RB (2006) Phase 1 trial of the antiangiogenic peptide ATN-161 (Ac-PHSCN-NH(2)), a beta integrin antagonist, in patients with solid tumours. Br J Cancer 94:1621–1626

Cohen S, Trikha M, Mascelli M (2000) Potential future clinical applications for the GPIIb/IIIa antagonist, abciximab in thrombosis, vascular and oncological indications. Pathol Oncol Res 6: 163–174

Collo G, Pepper MS (1999) Endothelial cell integrin alpha5beta1 expression is modulated by cytokines and during migration in vitro. J Cell Sci 112: 569–578

Condeelis J, Pollard JW (2006) Macrophages: obligate partners for tumor cell migration, invasion, and metastasis. Cell 124:263–266

Coutifaris C, Omigbodun A, Coukos G (2005) The fibronectin receptor alpha5 integrin subunit is upregulated by cell-cell adhesion via a cyclic AMP-dependent mechanism: implications for human trophoblast migration. Am J Obstet Gynecol 192:1240–1253; discussion 1253–1255

De Palma M, Naldini L (2006) Role of haematopoietic cells and endothelial progenitors in tumour angiogenesis. Biochim Biophys Acta 1766: 159–166

Decristoforo C, Faintuch-Linkowski B, Rey A, von Guggenberg E, Rupprich M, Hernandez-Gonzales I, Rodrigo T, Haubner R (2006) [99mTc]HYNIC-RGD for imaging integrin alphavbeta3 expression. Nucl Med Biol 33:945–952

Dietrich T, Onderka J, Bock F, Kruse FE, Vossmeyer D, Stragies R, Zahn G, Cursiefen C (2007) Inhibition of inflammatory lymphangiogenesis by integrin alpha5 blockade. Am J Pathol 171: 361–372

Dormond O, Ruegg C (2003) Regulation of endothelial cell integrin function and angiogenesis by COX-2, cAMP and protein kinase A. Thromb Haemost 90:577–585

Eskens FALM, Dumez H, Hoekstra R, Perschl A, Brindley C, Bottcher S, Wynendaele W, Drevs J, Verweij J, van Oosterom AT (2003) Phase I and pharmacokinetic study of continuous twice weekly intravenous administration of Cilengitide (EMD 121974), a novel inhibitor of the integrins [alpha]v[beta]3 and [alpha]v[beta]5 in patients with advanced solid tumours. Eur J Cancer 39: 917–926

Francis SE, Goh KL, Hodivala-Dilke K, Bader BL, Stark M, Davidson D, Hynes RO (2002) Central roles of alpha5beta1 integrin and fibronectin in vascular development in mouse embryos and embryoid bodies. Arterioscler Thromb Vasc Biol 22:927–933

Giancotti FG (2007) Targeting integrin beta4 for cancer and anti-angiogenic therapy. Trends Pharmacol Sci 28:506–511

Ginsberg MH, Partridge A, Shattil SJ (2005) Integrin regulation. Curr Opin Cell Biol 17:509–516

Gutheil JC, Campbell TN, Pierce PR, Watkins JD, Huse WD, Bodkin DJ, Cheresh DA (2000) Targeted antiangiogenic therapy for cancer using vitaxin: a humanized monoclonal antibody to the integrin aVb3. Clin Cancer Res 6:3056–3061

Hamano Y, Kalluri R (2005) Tumstatin, the NC1 domain of alpha3 chain of type IV collagen, is an endogenous inhibitor of pathological angiogenesis and suppresses tumor growth. Biochem Biophys Res Commun 333:292–298

Hammes H, Brownlee M, Jonczyk A, Sutter A, Preissner K (1996) Subcutaneous injection of a cyclic peptide antagonist of vitronectin receptor-type integrins inhibits retinal neovascularization. Nat Med 2:529–533

Hansma AHG, Broxterman HJ, van der Horst I, Yuana Y, Boven E, Giaccone G, Pinedo HM, Hoekman K (2005) Recombinant human endostatin administered as a 28-day continuous intravenous infusion, followed by daily subcutaneous injections: a phase I and pharmacokinetic study in patients with advanced cancer. Ann Oncol 16: 1695–1701

Hasmim M, Vassalli G, Alghisi G, Bamat J, Ponsonnet L, Bieler G, Bonnard C, Paroz C, Oguey D, Rüegg C (2005) Expressed isolated integrin b1 subunit cytodomain induces endothelial cell death secondary to detachment. Thromb Haemost 94: 1060–1070

Haubner R, Gratias R, Diefenbach B, Goodman SL, Jonczyk A, Kessler H (1996) Structural and functional aspects of rgd-containing cyclic pentapeptides as highly potent and selective integrin αvβ3 antagonists. J. Am. Chem. Soc. 118:7461–7472

Herbst RS, Hess KR, Tran HT, Tseng JE, Mullani NA, Charnsangavej C, Madden T, Davis DW, McConkey DJ, O'Reilly MS, Ellis LM, Pluda J, Hong WK, Abbruzzese JL (2002) Phase I study of recombinant human endostatin in patients with advanced solid tumors. J Clin Oncol 20: 3792–3803

Hodivala-Dilke KM, McHugh KP, Tsakiris DA, Rayburn H, Crowley D, Ullman-Cullere M, Ross FP, Coller BS, Teitelbaum S, Hynes RO (1999) β3-integrin–deficient mice are a model for Glanzmann thrombasthenia showing placental defects and reduced survival. J Clin Invest 103:229–238

Hong YK, Lange-Asschenfeldt B, Velasco P, Hirakawa S, Kunstfeld R, Brown LF, Bohlen P, Senger DR, Detmar M (2004) VEGF-A promotes tissue repair-associated lymphatic vessel formation via VEGFR-2 and the alpha1beta1 and alpha2beta1 integrins. Faseb J 18: 1111–1113

Hood JD, Bednarski M, Frausto R, Guccione S, Reisfeld RA, Xiang R, Cheresh DA (2002) Tumor regression by targeted gene delivery to the neovasculature. Science 296:2404–2407

Hsu AR, Hou LC, Veeravagu A, Greve JM, Vogel H, Tse V, Chen X (2006) In vivo near-infrared fluorescence imaging of integrin alphavbeta3 in an orthotopic glioblastoma model. Mol Imaging Biol 8:315–323

Hynes RO (2002) A reevaluation of integrins as regulators of angiogenesis. Nat Med 8:918–921

Hynes RO (2007) Cell-matrix adhesion in vascular development. J Thromb Haemost 5(Suppl 1): 32–40

Jin H, Su J, Garmy-Susini B, Kleeman J, Varner J (2006) Integrin alpha4beta1 promotes monocyte trafficking and angiogenesis in tumors. Cancer Res 66:2146–2152

Kawaguchi T, Yamashita Y, Kanamori M, Endersby R, Bankiewicz KS, Baker SJ, Bergers G, Pieper RO (2006) The PTEN/Akt pathway dictates the direct alphaVbeta3-dependent growth-inhibitory action of an active fragment of tumstatin in glioma cells in vitro and in vivo. Cancer Res 66:11331–11340

Kim D, Jeon C, Kim JH, Kim MS, Yoon CH, Choi IS, Kim SH, Bae YS (2006) Cytoplasmic transduction peptide (CTP): new approach for the delivery of biomolecules into cytoplasm in vitro and in vivo. Exp Cell Res 312:1277–1288

Kim S, Bell K, Mousa SA, Varner JA (2000) Regulation of angiogenesis in vivo by ligation of integrin a5b1 with the central cell-binding domain of fibronectin. Am J Pathol 156: 1345–1362

Klotz O, Park JK, Pleyer U, Hartmann C, Baatz H (2000) Inhibition of corneal neovascularization by alpha(v)-integrin antagonists in the rat. Graefes Arch Clin Exp Ophthalmol 238:88–93

Koivunen E, Wang B, Ruoslahti E (1994) Isolation of a highly specific ligand for the alpha 5 beta 1 integrin from a phage display library. J Cell Biol 124:373–380

Kumar CC, Malkowski M, Yin Z, Tanghetti E, Yaremko B, Nechuta T, Varner J, Liu M, Smith EM, Neustadt B, Presta M, Armstrong L (2001) Inhibition of angiogenesis and tumor growth by SCH221153, a dual avb3 and avb5 integrin receptor antagonist. Cancer Res 61:2232–2238

Kuwada SK (2007) Drug evaluation: volociximab, an angiogenesis-inhibiting chimeric monoclonal antibody. Curr Opin Mol Ther 9:92–98

Lejeune FJ, Lienard D, Matter M, Ruegg C (2006) Efficiency of recombinant human TNF in human cancer therapy. Cancer Immun 6:6

Liu S, Hsieh WY, Jiang Y, Kim YS, Sreerama SG, Chen X, Jia B, Wang F (2007) Evaluation of a (99m)Tc-labeled cyclic RGD tetramer for noninvasive imaging integrin alpha(v)beta3-positive breast cancer. Bioconjug Chem 18:438–446

Livant DL, Brabec RK, Pienta KJ, Allen DL, Kurachi K, Markwart S, Upadhyaya A (2000) Anti-invasive, antitumorigenic, and antimetastatic activities of the PHSCN sequence in prostate carcinoma. Cancer Res 60:309–320

Loges S, Butzal M, Otten J, Schweizer M, Fischer U, Bokemeyer C, Hossfeld DK, Schuch G, Fiedler W (2007) Cilengitide inhibits proliferation and differentiation of human endothelial progenitor cells in vitro. Biochem Biophys Res Commun 357:1016–1020

Luo BH, Carman CV, Springer TA (2007) Structural basis of integrin regulation and signaling. Annu Rev Immunol 25:619–647

MacDonald T, Taga T, Shimada H, Tabrizi P, Zlokovic B, Cheresh D, Laug W (2001) Preferential susceptibility of brain tumors to the antiangiogenic effects of an alpha(v) integrin antagonist. Neurosurgery 48:151–157

Maeshima Y, Colorado PC, Torre A, Holthaus KA, Grunkemeyer JA, Ericksen MB, Hopfer H, Xiao Y, Stillman IE, Kalluri R (2000) Distinct antitumor properties of a Type IV collagen domain derived from basement membrane. J Biol Chem 275:21340–21348

Maeshima Y, Sudhakar A, Lively JC, Ueki K, Kharbanda S, Kahn CR, Sonenberg N, Hynes RO, Kalluri R (2002) Tumstatin, an endothelial cell-specific inhibitor of protein synthesis. Science 295:140–143

Mahabeleshwar GH, Feng W, Phillips DR, Byzova TV (2006) Integrin signaling is critical for pathological angiogenesis. J Exp Med 203: 2495–2507

Marinelli L, Meyer A, Heckmann D, Lavecchia A, Novellino E, Kessler H (2005) Ligand binding analysis for human alpha5beta1 integrin: strategies for designing new alpha5beta1 integrin antagonists. J Med Chem 48:4204–4207

Martin PL, Jiao Q, Cornacoff J, Hall W, Saville B, Nemeth JA, Schantz A, Mata M, Jang H, Fasanmade AA, Anderson L, Graham MA, Davis HM, Treacy G (2005) Absence of adverse effects in cynomolgus macaques treated with CNTO 95, a fully human anti-av integrin monoclonal antibody, despite widespread tissue binding. Clin Cancer Res 11:6959–6965

McNeel DG, Eickhoff J, Lee FT, King DM, Alberti D, Thomas JP, Friedl A, Kolesar J, Marnocha R, Volkman J, Zhang J, Hammershaimb L, Zwiebel JA, Wilding G (2005) Phase I trial of a monoclonal antibody specific for avb3 integrin (MEDI-522) in patients with advanced malignancies, including an assessment of effect on tumor perfusion. Clin Cancer Res 11:7851–7860

Meerovitch K, Bergeron F, Leblond L, Grouix B, Poirier C, Bubenik M, Chan L, Gourdeau H, Bowlin T, Attardo G (2003) A novel RGD antagonist that targets both alphavbeta3 and alpha5beta1 induces apoptosis of angiogenic endothelial cells on type I collagen. Vascul Pharmacol 40:77–89

Minamiguchi K, Kumagai H, Masuda T, Kawada M, Ishizuka M, Takeuchi T (2001) Thiolutin, an inhibitor of HUVEC adhesion to vitronectin, reduces paxillin in HUVECs and suppresses tumor cell-induced angiogenesis. Int J Cancer 93:307–316

Mitjans F, Sander D, Adan J, Sutter A, Martinez JM, Jaggle CS, Moyano JM, Kreysch HG, Piulats J, Goodman SL (1995) An anti-alpha v-integrin antibody that blocks integrin function inhibits the development of a human melanoma in nude mice. J Cell Sci 108:2825–2838

Mitjans F, Meyer T, Fittschen C, Goodman S, Jonczyk A, Marshall J, Reyes G, Piulats J (2000) In vivo therapy of malignant melanoma by means of antagonists of alphav integrins. Int J Cancer 87: 716–723

Mitra A, Coleman T, Borgman M, Nan A, Ghandehari H, Line BR (2006) Polymeric conjugates of mono- and bi-cyclic alphaVbeta3 binding peptides for tumor targeting. J Control Release 114:175–183

Mould AP, Burrows L, Humphries MJ (1998) Identification of amino acid residues that form part of the ligand-binding pocket of integrin alpha 5beta 1. J. Biol. Chem. 273:25664–25672

Mullamitha SA, Ton NC, Parker GJ, Jackson A, Julyan PJ, Roberts C, Buonaccorsi GA, Watson Y, Davies K, Cheung S, Hope L, Valle JW, Radford JA, Lawrance J, Saunders MP, Munteanu MC, Nakada MT, Nemeth JA, Davis HM, Jiao Q, Prabhakar U, Lang Z, Corringham RE, Beckman RA, Jayson GC (2007) Phase I evaluation of a fully human anti-alphav integrin monoclonal antibody (CNTO 95) in patients with advanced solid tumors. Clin Cancer Res 13:2128–2135

Murakami M, Elfenbein A, Simons M (2008) Non-canonical fibroblast growth factor signaling in angiogenesis. Cardiovasc Res 78(2):223–231

Nabors LB, Mikkelsen T, Rosenfeld SS, Hochberg F, Akella NS, Fisher JD, Cloud GA, Zhang Y, Carson K, Wittemer SM, Colevas AD, Grossman SA (2007) Phase I and correlative biology study of cilengitide in patients with recurrent malignant glioma. J Clin Oncol 25:1651–1657

Nakada MT, Cao G, Sassoli PM, DeLisser HM (2006) c7E3 Fab inhibits human tumor angiogenesis in a SCID mouse human skin xenograft model. Angiogenesis 9:171–176

Nam JO, Jeong HW, Lee BH, Park RW, Kim IS (2005) Regulation of tumor angiogenesis by fastatin, the fourth FAS1 domain of betaig-h3, via alphavbeta3 integrin. Cancer Res 65:4153–4161

Nikolopoulos SN, Blaikie P, Yoshioka T, Guo W, Giancotti FG (2004) Integrin [beta]4 signaling promotes tumor angiogenesis. Cancer Cell 6:471–483

Ning S, Chen Z, Dirks A, Husbeck B, Hsu M, Bedogni B, O'Neill M, Powell MB, Knox SJ (2007) Targeting integrins and PI3K/Akt-mediated signal transduction pathways enhances radiation-induced anti-angiogenesis. Radiat Res 168: 125–133

Nisato RE, Tille J-C, Jonczyk A, Goodman SL, Pepper MS (2004) alphav beta3 and alphav beta5 integrin antagonists inhibit angiogenesis in vitro. Angiogenesis 6:105–119

O'Reilly MS, Boehm T, Shing Y, Fukai N, Vasios G, Lane WS, Flynn E, Birkhead JR, Olsen BR, Folkman J (1997) Endostatin: an endogenous inhibitor of angiogenesis and tumor growth. Cell 88:277–285

Oba M, Fukushima S, Kanayama N, Aoyagi K, Nishiyama N, Koyama H, Kataoka K (2007) Cyclic RGD peptide-conjugated polyplex micelles as a targetable gene delivery system directed to cells possessing alphavbeta3 and alphavbeta5 integrins. Bioconjug Chem 18:1415–1423

Oguey D, George P, Ruegg C (2000) Disruption of integrin-dependent adhesion and survival of endothelial cells by recombinant adenovirus expressing isolated beta integrin cytoplasmic domains. Gene Ther 7:1292–1303

Orecchia A, Lacal PM, Schietroma C, Morea V, Zambruno G, Failla CM (2003) Vascular endothelial growth factor receptor-1 is deposited in the extracellular matrix by endothelial cells and is a ligand for the alpha 5 beta 1 integrin. J Cell Sci 116:3479–3489

Perruzzi CA, de Fougerolles AR, Koteliansky VE, Whelan MC, Westlin WF, Senger DR (2003) Functional overlap and cooperativity among alphav and beta1 integrin subfamilies during skin angiogenesis. J Invest Dermatol 120: 1100–1109

Pfeifer A, Kessler T, Silletti S, Cheresh DA, Verma IM (2000) Suppression of angiogenesis by lentiviral delivery of PEX, a noncatalytic fragment of matrix metalloproteinase 2. PNAS 97:12227–12232

Posey J, Khazaeli M, DelGrosso A, Saleh M, Lin C, Huse W, LoBuglio A (2001) A pilot trial of Vitaxin, a humanized anti-vitronectin receptor (anti alpha v beta 3) antibody in patients with metastatic cancer. Cancer Biother Radiopharm 16:125–132

Raguse J-D, Gath HJ, Bier J, Riess H, Oettle H (2004) Cilengitide (EMD 121974) arrests the growth of a heavily pretreated highly vascularised head and neck tumour. Oral Oncol 40:228–230

Ramakrishnan V, Bhaskar V, Law DA, Wong MH, DuBridge RB, Breinberg D, O'Hara C, Powers DB, Liu G, Grove J, Hevezi P, Cass KM, Watson S, Evangelista F, Powers RA, Finck B, Wills M, Caras I, Fang Y, McDonald D, Johnson D, Murray R, Jeffry U (2006) Preclinical evaluation of an anti-alpha5beta1 integrin antibody as a novel anti-angiogenic agent. J Exp Ther Oncol 5: 273–286

Reinmuth N, Liu W, Ahmad SA, Fan F, Stoeltzing O, Parikh AA, Bucana CD, Gallick GE, Nickols MA, Westlin WF, Ellis LM (2003) Alphavbeta3 integrin antagonist S247 decreases colon cancer metastasis and angiogenesis and improves survival in mice. Cancer Res 63:2079–2087

Reynolds AR, Reynolds LE, Nagel TE, Lively JC, Robinson SD, Hicklin DJ, Bodary SC, Hodivala-Dilke KM (2004) Elevated Flk1 (vascular endothelial growth factor receptor 2) signaling mediates enhanced angiogenesis in b3-integrin-deficient mice. Cancer Res 64:8643–8650

Reynolds L, Wyder L, Lively J, Taverna D, Robinson S, Huang X, Sheppard D, Hynes R, Hodivala-Dilke K (2002) Enhanced pathological angiogenesis in mice lacking beta3 integrin or beta3 and beta5 integrins. Nat Med 8:27–34

Romer LH, Birukov KG, Garcia JG (2006) Focal adhesions: paradigm for a signaling nexus. Circ Res 98:606–616

Ruegg C, Yilmaz A, Bieler G, Bamat J, Chaubert P, Lejeune FJ (1998) Evidence for the involvement of endothelial cell integrin alphaVbeta3 in the disruption of the tumor vasculature induced by TNF and IFN-gamma. Nat Med 4:408–414

Ruegg C, Mutter N (2007) Anti-angiogenic therapies in cancer: achievements and open questions. Bull Cancer 94:753–762

Sabherwal Y, Rothman VL, Dimitrov S, L'Heureux DZ, Marcinkiewicz C, Sharma M, Tuszynski GP (2006) Integrin alpha2beta1 mediates the anti-angiogenic and anti-tumor activities of angiocidin, a novel tumor-associated protein. Exp Cell Res 312: 2443–2453

Scott KA, Arnott CH, Robinson SC, Moore RJ, Thompson RG, Marshall JF, Balkwill FR (2004) TNF-alpha regulates epithelial expression of MMP-9 and integrin alphavbeta6 during tumour promotion. A role for TNF-alpha in keratinocyte migration? Oncogene 23:6954–6966

Senger DR, Claffey KP, Benes JE, Perruzzi CA, Sergiou AP, Detmar M (1997) Angiogenesis promoted by vascular endothelial growth factor: regulation through alpha 1beta 1 and alpha 2beta 1 integrins. Proc Natl Acad Sci 94: 13612–13617

Senger DR, Perruzzi CA, Streit M, Koteliansky VE, de Fougerolles AR, Detmar M (2002) The a1b1 and a2b1 integrins provide critical support for vascular endothelial growth factor signaling, endothelial cell migration, and tumor angiogenesis. Am J Pathol 160:195–204

Serini G, Valdembri D, Bussolino F (2006) Integrins and angiogenesis: a sticky business. Exp Cell Res 312(5):651–658
Shin IS, Jang BS, Danthi SN, Xie J, Yu S, Le N, Maeng JS, Hwang IS, Li KC, Carrasquillo JA, Paik CH (2007) Use of antibody as carrier of oligomers of peptidomimetic alphavbeta3 antagonist to target tumor-induced neovasculature. Bioconjug Chem 18:821–828
Smith JW (2003) Cilengitide Merck. Curr Opin Investig Drugs 4:741–745
Stoeltzing O, Liu W, Reinmuth N, Fan F, Parry G, Parikh A, McCarty M, Bucana C, Mazar A, Ellis L (2003) Inhibition of integrin alpha5beta1 function with a small peptide (ATN-161) plus continuous 5-FU infusion reduces colorectal liver metastases and improves survival in mice. Int J Cancer 104:496–503
Strieth S, Eichhorn ME, Sutter A, Jonczyk A, Berghaus A, Dellian M (2006) Antiangiogenic combination tumor therapy blocking alpha(v)-integrins and VEGF-receptor-2 increases therapeutic effects in vivo. Int J Cancer 119:423–431
Stupack DG (2007) The biology of integrins. Oncology (Williston Park) 21:6–12
Stupp R, Ruegg C (2007) Integrin inhibitors reaching the clinic. J Clin Oncol 25:1637–1638
Taga T, Suzuki A, Gonzalez-Gomez I, Gilles FH, Stins M, Shimada H, Barsky L, Weinberg KI, Laug WE (2002) Alphav-Integrin antagonist EMD 121974 induces apoptosis in brain tumor cells growing on vitronectin and tenascin. Int J Cancer 98:690–697
Takada Y, Xiaojing X, Scott S (2007) The integrins. Genome Biol 8:215
Tanjore H, Zeisberg EM, Gerami-Naini B, Kalluri R (2007) Beta1 integrin expression on endothelial cells is required for angiogenesis but not for vasculogenesis. Dev Dyn 237:75–82
Tomiyama Y (2000) Glanzmann thrombasthenia: integrin alpha IIb beta 3 deficiency. Int J Hematol 72:448–454
Travis MA, Humphries JD, Humphries MJ (2003) An unraveling tale of how integrins are activated from within. Trends Pharmacol Sci 24:192–197
Trikha M, Zhou Z, Nemeth J, Chen Q, Sharp C, Emmell E, Giles-Komar J, Nakada M (2004) CNTO 95, a fully human monoclonal antibody that inhibits av integrins, has antitumor and antiangiogenic activity in vivo. Int J Cancer 110:326–335
Tsopanoglou NE, Papaconstantinou ME, Flordellis CS, Maragoudakis ME (2004) On the mode of action of thrombin-induced angiogenesis: thrombin peptide, TP508, mediates effects in endothelial cells via alphavbeta3 integrin. Thromb Haemost 92: 846–857
Ulbrich H, Eriksson EE, Lindbom L (2003) Leukocyte and endothelial cell adhesion molecules as targets for therapeutic interventions in inflammatory disease. Trends Pharmacol Sci 24:640–647
Umeda N, Kachi S, Akiyama H, Zahn G, Vossmeyer D, Stragies R, Campochiaro PA (2006) Suppression and regression of choroidal neovascularization by systemic administration of an alpha5beta1 integrin antagonist. Mol Pharmacol 69:1820–1828
Varner JA, Nakada MT, Jordan RE, Coller BS (1999) Inhibition of angiogenesis and tumor growth by murine 7E3, the parent antibodyof c7E3 Fab (abciximab; ReoProTM). Angiogenesis 3:53–60
Vlahakis NE, Young BA, Atakilit A, Hawkridge AE, Issaka RB, Boudreau N, Sheppard D (2007) Integrin alpha9beta1 directly binds to vascular endothelial growth factor (VEGF)-A and contributes to VEGF-A-induced angiogenesis. J Biol Chem 282:15187–15196
Wickstrom SA, Alitalo K, KeskiOja J (2005) Endostatin signaling and regulation of endothelial cell-matrix interactions. Adv Cancer Res 94:197–229
Woodall BP, Nystrom A, Iozzo RA, Eble JA, Niland S, Krieg T, Eckes B, Pozzi A, Iozzo RV (2008) Integrin alpha 2beta 1 is the required receptor for endorepellin angiostatic activity. J Biol Chem 283(4):2335–2343
Wu H, Beuerlein G, Nie Y, Smith H, Lee BA, Hensler M, Huse WD, Watkins JD (1998) Stepwise in vitro affinity maturation of Vitaxin, an alpha vbeta 3-specific humanized mAb. Proc Natl Acad Sci 95:6037–6042
Xie J, Shen Z, Li KC, Danthi N (2007) Tumor angiogenic endothelial cell targeting by a novel integrin-targeted nanoparticle. Int J Nanomed 2:479–485
Xiong JP, Stehle T, Zhang R, Joachimiak A, Frech M, Goodman SL, Arnaout MA (2002) Crystal structure of the extracellular segment of integrin alpha

Vbeta3 in complex with an Arg-Gly-Asp ligand. Science 296:151–155
Zaric J, Ruegg C (2005) Integrin-mediated adhesion and soluble ligand binding stabilize COX-2 protein levels in endothelial cells by inducing expression and preventing degradation. J Biol Chem 280:1077–1085
Zhang D, Pier T, McNeel DG, Wilding G, Friedl A (2007) Effects of a monoclonal anti-alphavbeta3 integrin antibody on blood vessels – a pharmacodynamic study. Invest New Drugs 25:49–55
Zhou Y, Peng H, Ji Q, Qi J, Zhu Z, Yang C (2006) Discovery of small molecule inhibitors of integrin alphavbeta3 through structure-based virtual screening. Bioorg Med Chem Lett 16: 5878–5882
Zhu J, Motejlek K, Wang D, Zang K, Schmidt A, Reichardt LF (2002) β8 integrins are required for vascular morphogenesis in mouse embryos. Development 129:2891–2903
Zweers MC, Davidson JM, Pozzi A, Hallinger R, Janz K, Quondamatteo F, Leutgeb B, Krieg T, Eckes B (2007) Integrin alpha2beta1 is required for regulation of murine wound angiogenesis but is dispensable for reepithelialization. J Invest Dermatol 127:467–478

PDGF and Vessel Maturation

7

Carina Hellberg, Arne Östman, and C.-H. Heldin

Abstract Pericytes are smooth muscle-like cells found in close contact with the endothelium in capillaries, where they regulate the morphology and function of the vessels. During vessel formation, platelet-derived growth factor-BB (PDGF-BB) is required for the recruitment and differentiation of pericytes. Tumor vessels display abnormal morphology and increased endothelial proliferation, resulting in leaky, tortuous vessels that are often poorly perfused. These vessels typically display decreased pericyte density, and the tumor-associated pericytes often express abnormal markers and show abnormal morphology. Anti-angiogenic therapy targeting pro-angiogenic growth factor pathways has been applied to a broad range of solid tumors with varying results. Studies utilizing mouse models indicate that the presence of pericytes protect endothelial cells against inhibition of vascular endothelial growth factor (VEGF) signaling. Simultaneous inhibition of PDGF receptors on pericytes therefore improves the effect of VEGF inhibitors on endothelial cells and enhances anti-angiogenic therapy.

C.-H. Heldin (✉)
Ludwig Institute for Cancer Research,
Uppsala University, S-751 24, Uppsala, Sweden
e-mail: C-H.Heldin@LICR.uu.e

7.1 Introduction

Newly formed capillaries are stabilized through the recruitment of a specialized form of mural cells termed pericytes. In addition to providing physical stabilization, the presence of pericytes reduces endothelial cell proliferation and promotes differentiation, a process termed vascular maturation. During this process, activation of the platelet-derived growth factor (PDGF) β-receptor plays a crucial role in the recruitment of pericytes to the newly formed vessels. In the present communication, we review the role of PDGF in vessel maturation.

7.2 The PDGF Family

The PDGF family of growth factors is composed of disulfide-bonded homodimers of four polypeptide chains, the classical PDGF-A and -B chains and the more recently described PDGF-C and -D chains (Fredriksson et al. 2004). In addition, the A and B chains heterodimerize to form PDGF-AB. PDGF isoforms exert their biological effects through the

R. Liersch et al. (eds.), *Angiogenesis Inhibition,* Recent Results in Cancer Research,
DOI: 10.1007/978-3-540-78281-0_7, © Springer Verlag Berlin Heidelberg 2010

activation of two tyrosine kinase receptors, PDGF α- and β-receptors (Heldin et al. 1998).

PDGF family are major mitogens for a number of cell types, including mesenchymal cells such as fibroblasts and smooth muscle cells. During the embryonal development, PDGF isoforms are important for the development of mesenchymal cells of different organs, such as mesangial cells of the kidney, alveolar smooth muscle cells of the lung, smooth muscle cells and pericytes of blood vessels, and glial cells of the central nervous system. Overactivity of PDGF has been linked to atherosclerosis, fibrotic diseases, and malignancies. In certain types of rather rare solid tumors, PDGF is involved in autocrine stimulation of tumor cell growth. In addition, PDGF is commonly involved in paracrine recruitment of tumor stroma fibroblasts and stimulation of angiogenesis (Ostman and Heldin 2007).

7.3 Pericytes

7.3.1 Role of Pericytes

Mature blood vessels are composed of endothelial cells and mural cells, including pericytes and smooth muscle cells. Arteries and veins are surrounded by vascular smooth muscle cells, whereas pericytes are present on capillaries, postcapillary venules, and collecting venules throughout the body. Pericytes are smooth muscle-like single cells found in close contact with endothelial cells within the basement membrane, where they are wrapped around the vessel sending out long protrusions that make contact with a number of endothelial cells and other pericytes (Fig. 7.1) (Bergers and Song 2005). The presence of pericytes on these vessel types is plastic, and varies between tissues.

PDGF made by endothelial cells has a crucial role in the recruitment of pericytes to vessels (Betsholtz 2004). Moreover, a basic retention motif in the common C-terminus of PDGF-BB is crucial for this process, since it makes contact with sulfated heparan proteoglycans and ensures that PDGF-BB remains in the close environment of the producing endothelial cells (Lindblom et al. 2003; Abramsson et al. 2007). Since pericytes are contractile cells they presumably exert parts of their morphogenic control of capillary diameter through PDGF-BB-induced pericyte contractility. In addition, pericytes also regulate capillary diameter by regulating endothelial proliferation and differentiation. Absence of pericytes in PDGF-B/PDGF β-receptor null mice coincides with endothelial hyperplasia, suggesting that pericytes negatively control endothelial proliferation (Hellstrom et al. 2001). Absence of pericytes also leads to defects in endothelial junction formation, suggesting that pericytes control endothelial differentiation in vivo.

7.3.2 Identification of Pericytes

Despite their physiological importance, pericytes still remain an understudied cell type. Part of the problem when studying pericytes is the difficulty in identifying them, since there is no convenient pan-pericyte marker. Pericytes reside within the basement membrane; thus morphological identification by electron microscopy remains the most reliable means of identifying a pericyte in mature tissues (Baluk et al. 2005). However, during angiogenic sprouting and vascular remodeling, the basement membrane is not fully developed, making this method of identification more difficult to apply (Baluk et al. 2003). Therefore, several marker proteins are used for studying pericytes during angiogenesis (Bergers and Song 2005).

As expected from its importance for the recruitment of pericytes, the PDGF β-receptor is one of the most widely used markers for pericytes. However, this receptor is also expressed

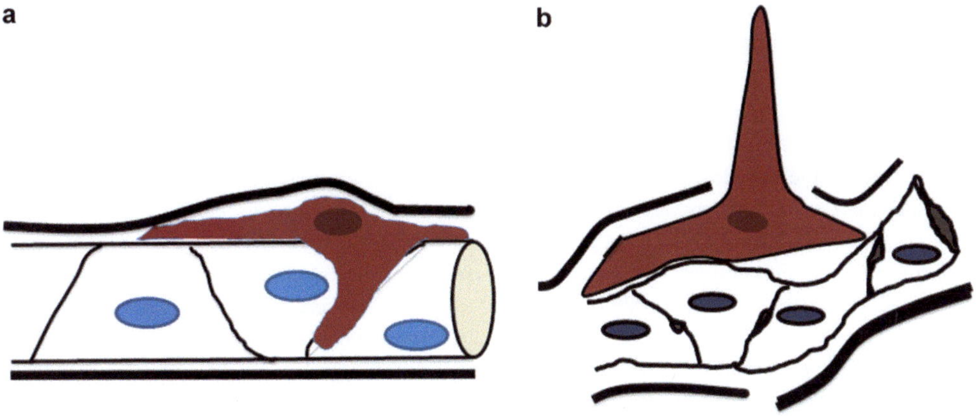

Fig. 7.1 (**a**) Morphology of capillaries of normal tissues. The pericytes reside between the basement membrane and the endothelial cells. Each pericyte makes contact with several endothelial cells and wraps itself around the vessel. (**b**) Morphology of capillaries of tumors. The tumor vessels are contorted and often flattened. Pericytes make contact with the endothelium, but are often partly dethatched and often extend protrusions away from the vessel. The basement membrane varies in thickness and has gaps in it.

on other stromal cells such as smooth muscle cells, fibroblasts and myofibroblasts. Another commonly used marker is α-smooth muscle actin (ASMA) that is expressed by pericytes, smooth muscle cells, and myofibroblasts. The expression of ASMA by pericytes is primarily restricted to sites of vascular remodeling. Desmin is a component of intermediate filaments, and is found in mature skeletal, cardiac, and smooth muscle cells. On pericytes, its expression appears to be restricted to differentiated cells in close physical contact with the endothelium. The expression of ASMA and desmin is likely to reflect the role of pericytes as contractile cells that participate in the regulation of capillary blood flow. The NG2 chondroitin sulfate proteoglycan (also known as high-molecular-weight melanoma-associated antigen, or sometimes AN2 in mice) is expressed on the surface of activated pericytes during vasculogenesis and angiogenesis. The regulator of G-protein signaling-5 (RGS-5), a regulator of signaling pathways downstream of heterotrimeric G-protein coupled receptors, was recently described as a marker for developing pericytes. Its expression overlaps with the expression of NG2 and the PDGF β-receptor.

Not much is known about the regulation of the expression of these markers, and they may represent either distinct or overlapping populations of pericytes. The expressions of pericyte markers are dynamic, and their expression varies, depending on the species and tissue studied. When addressing the involvement of pericytes in vessel maturation, the difficulty to identify pericytes still present a problem, and most studies therefore contain the analysis of several marker proteins.

7.3.3 The Origin of Pericytes

During embryonic development, pericytes and smooth muscle cells, as well as endothelial cells, are believed to be derived from mesenchymal precursors (Bergers and Song 2005). During this process, PDGF-BB/PDGF β-receptor signaling is essential for the recruitment and differentiation of pericytes. Postnatally, pericytes are presumed to either migrate with the endothelial sprouts during the initiation of angiogenesis, or to differentiate from a local source of mesenchymal cells in response to PDGF and/or transforming growth factor β (TGF-β). However, recent studies have also described the existence of bone marrow-derived pericyte progenitor cells (Lamagna and Bergers 2006) and tissue-specific pericyte progenitors (Howson et al. 2005; Dore-Duffy et al. 2006; Tamaki et al. 2007).

The adult bone marrow contains both hematopoietic and mesenchymal stem and progenitor cells. Therefore, the recruitment of bone marrow-derived progenitors into tumors supports the initiation of tumor angiogenesis by incorporating endothelial and pericyte progenitor cells into the newly formed vessels. It has been proposed that the release of cytokines from tumors induces the mobilization of hematopoietic bone marrow stem cells (Petit et al. 2007). The recruitment of endothelial progenitor cells and their incorporation into tumor vessels have been demonstrated in a number of studies (Lyden et al. 2001; Shirakawa et al. 2002), and was recently shown to have an important role in the vascularization of at least two types of lung metastases. Circulating progenitor cells positive for PDGF β-receptor, the stem cell antigen-1 (Sca-1) and CD11b have been demonstrated to incorporate into blood vessels and to mature into NG2-, ASMA- and desmin-positive pericytes (Song et al. 2005). Circulating cells positive for CD11b and CD45 have also been shown to incorporate into vessels as pericyte-like cells, although these cells only expressed NG2 (Rajantie et al. 2004).

Several studies have also demonstrated the presence of pericyte progenitor cells in various other tissues, which appear to contribute to postnatal vasculogenesis and angiogenesis. Since these progenitor cells give rise to cell populations expressing different pericyte markers (see later in the text), it is unclear as to what extent the presence of these cells on vessels stabilizes the vascular function. Thus, the neonatal rat aorta contains cells positive for the PDGF β-receptor, Tie2 and CD34, but negative for endothelial markers (Howson et al. 2005). These cells differentiates into pericytes when cocultured with endothelial cells or aorta ring explants in vitro. In the microvasculature of the adult rat CNS, cells positive for nestin and NG2 that has the capacity to differentiate into pericyte-like cells in vitro were identified (Dore-Duffy et al. 2006). In mice, skeletal muscle-derived stem cells negative for CD31 and CD45 were reported to differentiate into pericytes, endothelial cells, and smooth muscle in vivo (Tamaki et al. 2007). Although these studies indicate the presence of cells with the capability to differentiate into pericytes in adult tissues, most of the studies were performed in vitro. Information is still scarce about differentiation of tissue pericytes in vivo during vascular remodeling, or during tumor angiogenesis. Further studies addressing the physiological function of vessels that contain pericytes recruited from different sources are required.

7.4 Vessel Maturation

7.4.1 Normal Vessels

During embryonic development, the nascent vascular network is formed through de novo vessel formation from angioblasts or stem cells, a process termed vasculogenesis. From these vessels, new vessels sprout and form bridges by angiogenesis. The vessels are then stabilized through the recruitment of mural cells, and through generation of the basal membrane. The final patterning of the vascular network is determined by signals provided by soluble angiogenesis factors as well as components of the basement membrane and ECM, which stimulates proliferation, survival, migration, and differentiation of endothelial and mural cells. As already described, PDGF-BB is secreted by the endothelial cells during angiogenesis, presumably in response to vascular endothelial growth factor (VEGF), which facilitates the recruitment of mural cells. The endothelial differentiation sphingolipid G-protein coupled receptor 1 (EDG1 or $S1P_1$) (Allende and Proia 2002), which is activated by sphingosine 1-phosphate, appears to be important for mural-cell migration, and its genetic ablation in mouse led to a similar phenotype as that of PDGF ko mice. It remains to be investigated whether these signals are unrelated or if the EDG1 receptor signals downstream of the PDGF β-receptor.

Angiopoietin (Ang) 1 and 2 both act through the Tie2 receptor, but with different outcomes (Morisada et al. 2006). Ang1 stabilizes the physical contacts between endothelial cells and pericytes, thereby making the vessels less leaky. The role of Ang2 appears to be contextual. When VEGF is absent, Ang2 destabilizes vessels by inhibiting Ang1 signaling, but in the presence of VEGF Ang2 facilitates vascular sprouting. TGF-β is expressed by both endothelial and mural cells. It promotes vessel maturation not only by inducing differentiation of mesenchymal cells to mural cells, but also by stimulating ECM production. As with Ang2, TGF-β can be either pro- or antiangiogenic, depending on the context (Bertolino et al. 2005).

The presence of pericytes on the capillary bed is necessary for normal vessel function. Genetic studies in mice showed that loss of PDGF-BB or the PDGF β-receptor leads to a severe deficiency in pericyte recruitment, causing microvascular leakage and hemorrhage (Lindahl et al. 1997; Hellstrom et al. 1999). When investigating animals chimaeric for the PDGF β-receptor, it was evident that only PDGF β-receptor positive cells populated the vascular smooth muscle and pericyte compartment, directly demonstrating a need for PDGF signaling for the development of these cells (Crosby et al. 1998).

During angiogenic sprouting, PDGF-B is expressed by the endothelial tip cell (Gerhardt et al. 2003). Tissue-specific knockout of PDGF-BB in endothelial cells resulted in a similar phenotype as that of PDGF β-receptor ko, indicating that paracrine signaling between the endothelium and pericytes is required in the process of pericyte recruitment (Bjarnegard et al. 2004). When examining animals chimaeric for endothelial PDGF-BB, they displayed a variation in pericyte coverage and morphology of individual brain capillaries indicative of segments of PDGF-BB, expressing endothelium with normal recruitment of pericytes (Bjarnegard et al. 2004). The PDGF-BB molecule contains a short, basic sequence that functions as a retention motif allowing the secreted growth factor to remain on the tip cell. Mutational loss of the retention sequence resulted in partial detachment of the pericytes from the angiogenic sprout, presumably due to diffusion of PDGF-BB into the surrounding tissue (Lindblom et al. 2003). These findings highlight the need for a paracrine PDGF signal and a physical contact with endothelial cells for pericyte recruitment and differentiation.

Although PDGF β-receptor ko mice die from bleedings due to microaneurysms and a lack of mural cells, loss of pericytes in all tissues is not complete (Hellstrom et al. 1999). It thus appears as if PDGF is critical for the proliferation and migration of both pericytes and vascular smooth muscle cells, but that the initial formation of these cell types can also be induced by other factors. It is presently unclear where these cells originate from and what are the factors that induce their differentiation. It has been proposed that endothelial cells only express PDGF-BB at the sites of the vessels where pericyte recruitment occurs (Lindahl et al. 1997; Hellstrom et al. 1999). This is supported by the finding that in the developing CNS, PDGF-BB is mainly expressed by the endothelial cells situated at the tip of the sprouting vessels (Gerhardt et al. 2003).

7

7.4.2 Tumor Vessels

The growth of large, solid tumors is directly dependent on the presence of a tumor vasculature (Folkman 1971). As the tumor grows, hypoxia induces the expression of VEGF by tumor cells. This induces angiogenesis by activating the endothelial cells on surrounding vessels, thereby stimulating the branching and growth of new blood vessels into the tumor (Bergers and Benjamin 2003) (Fig. 7.2). During this process, the connections between the endothelial cells are loosened. Matrix metalloproteases are activated, leading to the degradation of the basement membrane. This serves two purposes. First, it allows the detachment of both endothelial cells and pericytes from the basement membrane, facilitating their migration into the tumor. Second, it may also activate proangiogenic factors within the basement membrane. Endothelial cells and pericytes migrate into the tumor tissue, where they proliferate and reconnect to form new vessels. Although most studies suggest that the endothelial cells lead the formation of new vessels, there are also studies suggesting that the pericytes migrate into the tissue first.

Tumor blood vessels have a number of structural and functional abnormalities (Jain 2003). They are dynamic, and vessels are continuously being initiated, remodeled, and regressed. The vessels are irregular in size and shape, tortuous and lack the normal hierarchical arrangement of arterioles, capillaries, and venules. The structure of the vessel wall is also abnormal. The tumor vessel diameter varies greatly, and the endothelial cells form an imperfect lining and contain a large number of fenestrations (Baluk et al. 2005). Although the presence of a basement membrane surrounding tumor vessels have been reported, it appears to be morphologically and functionally altered due to the vessel remodeling (Baluk et al. 2003). As a result of the

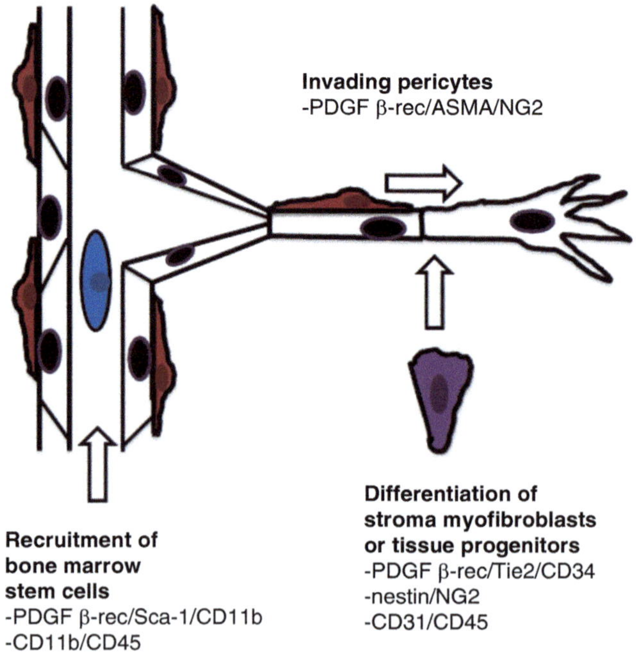

Fig. 7.2 Angiogenic sprouting. A new capillary is formed as a tip cell leads the sprouting capillary into the tissue. Pericytes may be recruited through the invasion and proliferation of pericytes from the mother vessel, by differentiation of stromal precursors, or through the recruitment of bone marrow precursor cells. Different molecular markers described for pericytes derived from mother vessels (Gerhardt et al., 2003), bone marrow-derived progenitors (Song et al., 2005; Rajantie et al., 2004, respectively) and tissue progenitors (Dore-Duffy et al., 2006; Howson et al., 2005; Tamaki et al., 2007, respectively) are given.

abnormal organization and ultrastructure of the vessels, the blood flow in the tumor vessels is chaotic and the vessels are leaky (Hashizume et al. 2000), resulting in an increase the interstitial fluid pressure (IFP) in the tumor. Furthermore, because of continuous remodeling of the vasculature, the blood flow and permeability varies not only between tumors, but also between regions of the same tumor, between the same region over time, and between the tumor and metastases. This is at least partly due to an imbalance between various pro- and antiangiogenic factors such as VEGF and Ang1/2. Taken together, the vessel abnormalities render the tumor vasculature inefficient at delivering not only oxygen and nutrients, but also drugs.

The density of pericytes covering normal capillaries varies between tissues, which is the case also for the pericyte coverage of tumor vessels (Baluk et al. 2005). In some studies no pericytes were found around the tumor capillaries, whereas other studies found the vessels covered to varying extents. It is unclear as to what extent these variations are due to differences between the tissues or the tumor types studied. Since PDGF-BB expression by endothelial cells is heterogeneous (Hellstrom et al. 1999), this may explain the uneven pericyte coverage of tumor vessels. Also, as discussed earlier, there may also be differences in the expression of the various molecular markers between tumor types, making an accurate pericyte count difficult. It is not just the pericyte density that is abnormal. Tumor-associated pericytes often display both an abnormal expression of markers, as well as abnormal morphology (Baluk et al. 2005). In tumors, pericytes are often found to express both ASMA and NG2, which are known to be expressed during vascular remodeling. Where normal pericytes are in close contact with the endothelium and reside within the basement membrane, tumor pericytes are often loosely associated with the endothelium, and may extend long protrusions into the surrounding tissue. At present, it is not clear whether the cells displaying the abnormal morphology are truly pericytes, if they are in the process of differentiation from myofibroblasts, or if they represent pericytes that are partially detaching from the endothelium to divide. Furthermore, it is unclear as to what extent these pericytes are able to participate in vessel function.

There are several sources described for pericyte progenitors during normal vascular remodeling, but it is currently unclear where tumor pericytes originate from. In angiogenesis in the retina, pericytes have been shown to migrate along the angiogenic sprout in response to the PDGF-BB expressed by the endothelial cells (Gerhardt et al. 2003). In tumors, it is also possible that components of the tumor microenvironment induce the differentiation of fibroblasts into myofibroblasts. Such cues may be TGF-β or PDGF expressed by tumor cells or the surrounding stroma. The incorporation of bone marrow-derived circulating pericyte progenitors into tumors have also been described (Song et al. 2005). The relative importance of these sources of pericytes is yet to be determined.

7.5 Tumor Therapy Targeting PDGF Receptors on the Vasculature

The genetic instability of tumor cells poses a serious problem when developing specific drugs targeting mutated proteins in tumors. Tumors that initially respond well to targeted therapies often develop resistance to the therapy, partly because of the enrichment of cells with new mutations. It has been proposed that targeting of tumor stroma, tumor vessels, and fibroblasts could be a means to avoid drug resistance since these tissues are more genetically stable (Hofmeister et al. 2008). Given the importance of PDGF in tumor stroma formation, the PDGF receptors are interesting targets in antistromal therapy.

7.5.1 Antiangiogenic Therapy Targeting Pericytes

Targeting of tumor angiogenesis has long been an attractive idea for the treatment of solid tumors (Folkman 1971; Cao 2004). Although therapies targeting the VEGF pathway are efficient in mouse tumor models, the results of several clinical trials suggests that therapies targeting VEGF alone may not be enough for efficient antiangiogenic therapy (Cobleigh et al. 2003; Yang et al. 2003).

When revisiting the mouse models, studies indicated that the response to VEGF-targeting therapy may be dependent on the maturity of the tumor vessels. Established, mature tumor vessels with richer pericyte coverage appear to be less sensitive to the antiangiogenic therapy than vessels with fewer pericytes. The notion that PDGF-BB may protect endothelial cells from antiangiogenic therapy was further supported by a study by Huang et al. (Huang et al. 2004), where an increased expression of PDGF-BB was detected around vessels that became resistant to anti-VEGF therapy. These observations initiated the idea that antiangiogenic therapy may be more efficient if both endothelial cells and pericytes are targeted using both VEGF receptor and PDGF receptor kinase inhibitors. This notion has recently been corroborated in a study of vessels in a nonmalignant tissue, chicken chorioallantoic membranes, displaying different stages of vascular maturity during development (Hlushchuk et al. 2007). In tumors, this type of combination therapy have been shown to give synergistic antiangiogenic and antitumor effects (Bergers et al. 2003; Erber et al. 2004; Hasumi et al. 2007), although the magnitude of the effect of PDGF inhibitors on the vasculature may be contextual (Sennino et al. 2007). It is currently not known why tumor pericytes are targeted during this treatment, while the vast majority of mural cells in the body are unaffected. It is possible that only a subset of abnormal, activated pericytes that are in the process of being remodeled, are targeted while more mature subsets are unaffected (Hasumi et al. 2007).

7.5.2 Improving the Efficacy of Conventional Therapies

As a consequence of the poor perfusion and abnormal functions of tumor vessels, the delivery of nutrients and oxygen into the tumor is poor (Jain 2005). This also affects the therapeutic outcome of both chemotherapy and radiotherapy. In the clinic, hypoxia strongly correlates with tumor radioresistance (Moeller et al. 2007), and preclinical data showed that increased tumor oxygenation improved the response to radiation therapy. Different approaches to modify the tumor vasculature have been taken to correct for this problem.

The abnormal tumor vasculature and stroma results in an elevated IFP in tumors compared to normal tissues. In addition to forming a barrier to transcapillary transport of nutrients and oxygen, the elevated IFP also results in inefficient uptake of therapeutic agents, especially macromolecules such as liposomes and antibodies (Heldin et al. 2004). Thus, lowering of IFP could be used to improve the therapeutic efficiency of both chemotherapy and radiation therapy. There are several factors affecting the IFP in tumors. The excess VEGF produced by hypoxic tumor cells induce capillary leakiness, resulting in an increased outflow of plasma proteins into the interstitium. Tumors are typically void of functional lymph vessels, which impair the fluid drainage from the tumor. Also, fibrosis and contraction of interstitial matrix mediated by stroma fibroblasts participates in the elevation of tumor IFP. PDGF contributes to the regulation of IFP through the phosphatidylinositol-3' kinase (PI3K) signaling pathway (Heuchel et al. 1999). Activation of PDGF β-receptors on stromal fibroblasts induce $\alpha v\beta 3$ intergrin-mediated contraction of the extracellular matrix thereby controlling the dermal IFP (Liden et al. 2006). The PDGF β-receptor may also participate in the regulation of vessel leakiness by recruiting pericytes that stabilizes the capillaries (Lindahl et al. 1997). Lowering of IFP by VEGF inhibitors (Lee et al. 2000; Tong et al. 2004) as well as PDGF inhibitors (Pietras et al. 2001) have been demonstrated. At present, it is not clear if the PDGF inhibitors reduce IFP by acting on pericytes or fibroblasts, or on both cell types. The reduction in IFP has been correlated to increased drug uptake (Pietras et al. 2001; Willett et al. 2004) and increased effect of chemotherapy (Pietras et al. 2002).

It has been proposed that restoring the balance between pro-and antiangiogenic factors could temporary normalize the vasculature, allowing for drug delivery (Jain 2005). According to this notion, removal of VEGF signaling would target the immature vasculature, pruning the less functional vessels and promoting the blood flow through the remaining vessels. Part of the normalization of vessel function seen after anti-VEGF therapy can be explained by decreased vessel leakiness, which reduces the osmotic pressure of the interstitium and consequently reduces the tumor IFP. The reported effects of anti-VEGF therapy have been transient, which would be expected if prolonged treatment disrupt also mature vessel function. Studies have demonstrated that targeting VEGF receptors alters vessel morphology (Miller et al. 2005; Taguchi et al. 2008), with temporary improvements in tumor oxygenation and response to radiotherapy (Dings et al. 2007). Another study demonstrated decreased effects of chemotherapy on glioblastomas, presumably due to restoration of the blood–brain barrier (Claes et al. 2008).

7.6 Future Perspectives

It is increasingly clear that the properties of the tumor vasculature are important for the outcome of both antiangiogenic targeted therapies and conventional cancer therapies. The presence of pericytes on the vessels gives structural stability to capillaries, resulting in improved perfusion, and provides endothelial cells with protection to anti-angiogenic therapy targeting the VEGF pathway. Understanding the precise mechanisms underlying vascular maturation should provide cues for refining therapies targeting the vasculature, whether to inhibit tumor angiogenesis or to normalize the vascular function for more efficient drug delivery. To achieve this, further studies evaluating the effects of antiangiogenic inhibitors on vessel function, both in animal models and in patients, are needed. The approval of several PDGF receptor inhibitors for use in the clinic (Ostman and Heldin 2007) will be important for further validation of the concept of vascular normalization after antiangiogenic therapy and the concomitant increase in drug uptake in patients. Such studies should reveal the extent to which different tumor types vary regarding their response to the combined targeting of VEGF- and PDGF receptor signaling, and may provide markers for the prediction of the therapeutic outcome in subsets of tumors.

The pericytes on tumor vessels are abnormal, both in the expression of molecular markers and in morphology. Nevertheless, B16 mouse melanoma tumors expressing PDGF-BB display increased pericyte coverage of the vessels, and an increased growth rate (Furuhashi et al. 2004), which correlates to an increased perfusion of small vessels and increased blood-flow rate (Robinson et al. 2008), indicating that the presence of abnormal pericytes exert effects on tumor vessel function. So how do these pericytes differ from the function of a fully differentiated pericyte? Further studies are required to understand the molecular mechanisms underlying pericyte differentiation and their interactions with endothelial cells. It will also be important to determine the source of tumor pericytes and the signaling pathways involved in their recruitment into the tumor vasculature. These studies require further development of more refined methods for studying vessel function in vivo.

7

References

Abramsson A, Kurup S, Busse M, Yamada S, Lindblom P, Schallmeiner E, Stenzel D, Sauvaget D, Ledin J, Ringvall M, Landegren U, Kjellen L, Bondjers G, Li JP, Lindahl U, Spillmann D, Betsholtz C, Gerhardt H (2007) Defective N-sulfation of heparan sulfate proteoglycans limits PDGF-BB binding and pericyte recruitment in vascular development. Genes Dev 21:316–331

Allende ML, Proia RL (2002) Sphingosine-1-phosphate receptors and the development of the vascular system. Biochim Biophys Acta 1582: 222–227

Baluk P, Hashizume H, McDonald DM (2005) Cellular abnormalities of blood vessels as targets in cancer. Curr Opin Genet Dev 15:102–111

Baluk P, Morikawa S, Haskell A, Mancuso M, McDonald DM (2003) Abnormalities of basement membrane on blood vessels and endothelial sprouts in tumors. Am J Pathol 163: 1801–1815

Bergers G, Benjamin LE (2003) Tumorigenesis and the angiogenic switch. Nat Rev Cancer 3: 401–410

Bergers G, Song S (2005) The role of pericytes in blood-vessel formation and maintenance. Neuro-Oncol 7:452–464

Bergers G, Song S, Meyer-Morse N, Bergsland E, Hanahan D (2003) Benefits of targeting both pericytes and endothelial cells in the tumor vasculature with kinase inhibitors. J Clin Invest 111:1287–1295

Bertolino P, Deckers M, Lebrin F, ten Dijke P (2005) Transforming growth factor-beta signal transduction in angiogenesis and vascular disorders. Chest 128:585S–590S

Betsholtz C (2004) Insight into the physiological functions of PDGF through genetic studies in mice. Cytokine Growth Factor Rev 15:215–228

Bjarnegard M, Enge M, Norlin J, Gustafsdottir S, Fredriksson S, Abramsson A, Takemoto M, Gustafsson E, Fässler R, Betsholtz C (2004) Endothelium-specific ablation of PDGFB leads to pericyte loss and glomerular, cardiac and placental abnormalities. Development 131:1847–1857

Cao Y (2004) Antiangiogenic cancer therapy. Semin Cancer Biol 14:139–145

Claes A, Wesseling P, Jeuken J, Maass C, Heerschap A, Leenders WP (2008) Antiangiogenic compounds interfere with chemotherapy of brain tumors due to vessel normalization. Mol Cancer Ther 7:71–78

Cobleigh MA, Langmuir VK, Sledge GW, Miller KD, Haney L, Novotny WF, Reimann JD, Vassel A (2003) A phase I/II dose-escalation trial of bevacizumab in previously treated metastatic breast cancer. Semin Oncol 30:117–124

Crosby JR, Seifert RA, Soriano P, Bowen-Pope DF (1998) Chimaeric analysis reveals role of Pdgf receptors in all muscle lineages. Nat Genet 18:385–388

Dings RP, Loren M, Heun H, McNiel E, Griffioen AW, Mayo KH, Griffin RJ (2007) Scheduling of radiation with angiogenesis inhibitors anginex and Avastin improves therapeutic outcome via vessel normalization. Clin Cancer Res 13:3395–3402

Dore-Duffy P, Katychev A, Wang X, Van Buren E (2006) CNS microvascular pericytes exhibit multipotential stem cell activity. J Cereb Blood Flow Metab 26:613–624

Erber R, Thurnher A, Katsen AD, Groth G, Kerger H, Hammes HP, Menger MD, Ullrich A, Vajkoczy P (2004) Combined inhibition of VEGF and PDGF signaling enforces tumor vessel regression by interfering with pericyte-mediated endothelial cell survival mechanisms. FASEB J 18:338–340

Folkman J (1971) Tumor angiogenesis: therapeutic implications. N Engl J Med 285:1182–1186

Fredriksson L, Li H, Eriksson U (2004) The PDGF family: four gene products form five dimeric isoforms. Cytokine Growth Factor Rev 15:197–204

Furuhashi M, Sjöblom T, Abramsson A, Ellingsen J, Micke P, Li H, Bergsten-Folestad E, Eriksson U, Heuchel R, Betsholtz C, Heldin CH, Östman A (2004) Platelet-derived growth factor production by B16 melanoma cells leads to increased pericyte abundance in tumors and an associated increase in tumor growth rate. Cancer Res 64: 2725–2733

Gerhardt H, Golding M, Fruttiger M, Ruhrberg C, Lundkvist A, Abramsson A, Jeltsch M, Mitchell C, Alitalo K, Shima D, Betsholtz C (2003) VEGF guides angiogenic sprouting utilizing endothelial tip cell filopodia. J Cell Biol 161:1163–1177

Hashizume H, Baluk P, Morikawa S, McLean JW, Thurston G, Roberge S, Jain RK, McDonald DM (2000) Openings between defective endothelial cells explain tumor vessel leakiness. Am J Pathol 156:1363–1380

Hasumi Y, Klosowska-Wardega A, Furuhashi M, Östman A, Heldin CH, Hellberg C (2007) Identification of a subset of pericytes that respond to combination therapy targeting PDGF and VEGF signaling. Int J Cancer 121:2606–2614

Heldin CH, Rubin K, Pietras K, Östman A (2004) High interstitial fluid pressure – an obstacle in cancer therapy. Nat Rev Cancer 4:806–813

Heldin CH, Östman A, Rönnstrand L (1998) Signal transduction via platelet-derived growth factor receptors. Biochim Biophys Acta 1378:F79–F113

Hellström M, Gerhardt H, Kalen M, Li X, Eriksson U, Wolburg H, Betsholtz C (2001) Lack of pericytes leads to endothelial hyperplasia and abnormal vascular morphogenesis. J Cell Biol 153:543–553

Hellström M, Kalén M, Lindahl P, Abramsson A, Betsholtz C (1999) Role of PDGF-B and PDGFR-beta in recruitment of vascular smooth muscle cells and pericytes during embryonic blood vessel formation in the mouse. Development 126: 3047–3055

Heuchel R, Berg A, Tallquist M, Åhlen K, Reed RK, Rubin K, Claesson-Welsh L, Heldin CH, Soriano P (1999) Platelet-derived growth factor beta receptor regulates interstitial fluid homeostasis through phosphatidylinositol-3' kinase signaling. Proc Natl Acad Sci U S A 96:11410–11415

Hlushchuk R, Baum O, Gruber G, Wood J, Djonov V (2007) The synergistic action of a VEGF-receptor tyrosine-kinase inhibitor and a sensitizing PDGF-receptor blocker depends upon the stage of vascular maturation. Microcirculation 14:813–825

Hofmeister V, Schrama D, Becker JC (2008) Anti-cancer therapies targeting the tumor stroma. Cancer Immunol Immunother 57:1–17

Howson KM, Aplin AC, Gelati M, Alessandri G, Parati EA, Nicosia RF (2005) The postnatal rat aorta contains pericyte progenitor cells that form spheroidal colonies in suspension culture. Am J Physiol Cell Physiol 289:C1396–C1407

Huang J, Soffer SZ, Kim ES, McCrudden KW, New T, Manley CA, Middlesworth W, O'Toole K, Yamashiro DJ, Kandel JJ (2004) Vascular remodeling marks tumors that recur during chronic suppression of angiogenesis. Mol Cancer Res 2:36–42

Jain RK (2003) Molecular regulation of vessel maturation. Nat Med 9:685–693

Jain RK (2005) Normalization of tumor vasculature: an emerging concept in antiangiogenic therapy. Science 307:58–62

Lamagna C, Bergers G (2006) The bone marrow constitutes a reservoir of pericyte progenitors. J Leukoc Biol 80:677–681

Lee CG, Heijn M, di Tomaso E, Griffon-Etienne G, Ancukiewicz M, Koike C, Park KR, Ferrara N, Jain RK, Suit HD, Boucher Y (2000) Anti-vascular endothelial growth factor treatment augments tumor radiation response under normoxic or hypoxic conditions. Cancer Res 60:5565–5570

Liden A, Berg A, Nedrebo T, Reed RK, Rubin K (2006) Platelet-derived growth factor BB-mediated normalization of dermal interstitial fluid pressure after mast cell degranulation depends on beta3 but not beta1 integrins. Circ Res 98:635–641

Lindahl P, Johansson BR, Leveen P, Betsholtz C (1997) Pericyte loss and microaneurysm formation in PDGF-B-deficient mice. Science 277: 242–245

Lindblom P, Gerhardt H, Liebner S, Abramsson A, Enge M, Hellström M, Bäckstrom G, Fredriksson S, Landegren U, Nystrom HC, Bergström G, Dejana E, Ostman A, Lindahl P, Betsholtz C (2003) Endothelial PDGF-B retention is required for proper investment of pericytes in the microvessel wall. Genes Dev 17:1835–1840

Lyden D, Hattori K, Dias S, Costa C, Blaikie P, Butros L, Chadburn A, Heissig B, Marks W, Witte L, Wu Y, Hicklin D, Zhu Z, Hackett NR, Crystal RG, Moore MA, Hajjar KA, Manova K, Benezra R, Rafii S (2001) Impaired recruitment of bone-marrow-derived endothelial and hematopoietic precursor cells blocks tumor angiogenesis and growth. Nat Med 7: 1194–1201

Miller DW, Vosseler S, Mirancea N, Hicklin DJ, Bohlen P, Volcker HE, Holz FG, Fusenig NE (2005) Rapid vessel regression, protease inhibition, and stromal normalization upon short-term vascular endothelial growth factor receptor 2 inhibition in skin carcinoma heterotransplants. Am J Pathol 167:1389–1403

Moeller BJ, Richardson RA, Dewhirst MW (2007) Hypoxia and radiotherapy: opportunities for improved outcomes in cancer treatment. Cancer Metastasis Rev 26:241–248

Morisada T, Kubota Y, Urano T, Suda T, Oike Y (2006) Angiopoietins and angiopoietin-like proteins in angiogenesis. Endothelium 13:71–79

Östman A, Heldin CH (2007) PDGF receptors as targets in tumor treatment. Adv Cancer Res 97: 247–274

Petit I, Jin D, Rafii S (2007) The SDF-1-CXCR4 signaling pathway: a molecular hub modulating neo-angiogenesis. Trends Immunol 28:299–307

Pietras K, Östman A, Sjöquist M, Buchdunger E, Reed RK, Heldin CH, Rubin K (2001) Inhibition of platelet-derived growth factor receptors reduces interstitial hypertension and increases transcapillary transport in tumors. Cancer Res 61:2929–2934

Pietras K, Rubin K, Sjöblom T, Buchdunger E, Sjöquist M, Heldin CH, Östman A (2002)

Inhibition of PDGF receptor signaling in tumor stroma enhances antitumor effect of chemotherapy. Cancer Res 62:5476–5484

Rajantie I, Ilmonen M, Alminaite A, Ozerdem U, Alitalo K, Salven P (2004) Adult bone marrow-derived cells recruited during angiogenesis comprise precursors for periendothelial vascular mural cells. Blood 104:2084–2086

Robinson SP, Ludwig C, Paulsson J, Östman A (2008) The effects of tumor-derived platelet-derived growth factor on vascular morphology and function in vivo revealed by susceptibility MRI. Int J Cancer 122:1548–1556

Sennino B, Falcon BL, McCauley D, Le T, McCauley T, Kurz JC, Haskell A, Epstein DM, McDonald DM (2007) Sequential loss of tumor vessel pericytes and endothelial cells after inhibition of platelet-derived growth factor B by selective aptamer AX102. Cancer Res 67: 7358–7367

Shirakawa K, Shibuya M, Heike Y, Takashima S, Watanabe I, Konishi F, Kasumi F, Goldman CK, Thomas KA, Bett A, Terada M, Wakasugi H (2002) Tumor-infiltrating endothelial cells and endothelial precursor cells in inflammatory breast cancer. Int J Cancer 99:344–351

Song S, Ewald AJ, Stallcup W, Werb Z, Bergers G (2005) PDGFRbeta+ perivascular progenitor cells in tumours regulate pericyte differentiation and vascular survival. Nat Cell Biol 7:870–879

Taguchi E, Nakamura K, Miura T, Shibuya M, Isoe T (2008) Anti-tumor activity and tumor vessel normalization by the vascular endothelial growth factor receptor tyrosine kinase inhibitor KRN951 in a rat peritoneal disseminated tumor model. Cancer Sci 99(3):623–630

Tamaki T, Okada Y, Uchiyama Y, Tono K, Masuda M, Wada M, Hoshi A, Akatsuka A (2007) Synchronized reconstitution of muscle fibers, peripheral nerves and blood vessels by murine skeletal muscle-derived CD34(-)/45 (-) cells. Histochem Cell Biol 128:349–360

Tong RT, Boucher Y, Kozin SV, Winkler F, Hicklin DJ, Jain RK (2004) Vascular normalization by vascular endothelial growth factor receptor 2 blockade induces a pressure gradient across the vasculature and improves drug penetration in tumors. Cancer Res 64:3731–3736

Willett CG, Boucher Y, di Tomaso E, Duda DG, Munn LL, Tong RT, Chung DC, Sahani DV, Kalva SP, Kozin SV, Mino M, Cohen KS, Scadden DT, Hartford AC, Fischman AJ, Clark JW, Ryan DP, Zhu AX, Blaszkowsky LS, Chen HX, Shellito PC, Lauwers GY, Jain RK (2004) Direct evidence that the VEGF-specific antibody bevacizumab has antivascular effects in human rectal cancer. Nat Med 10:145–147

Yang JC, Haworth L, Sherry RM, Hwu P, Schwartzentruber DJ, Topalian SL, Steinberg SM, Chen HX, Rosenberg SA (2003) A randomized trial of bevacizumab, an anti-vascular endothelial growth factor antibody, for metastatic renal cancer. N Engl J Med 349:427–434

Lymphangiogenesis in Cancer: Current Perspectives

8

Rüediger Liersch, Christoph Biermann, Rolf M. Mesters, and Wolfgang E. Berdel

Abstract Although the lymphatic system has been initially described in the sixteenth century, basic research has been limited. Despite its importance for the maintenance of tissue fluid homeostasis and for the afferent immune response, research of the molecular mechanisms of lymphatic vessel formation and function has for a long time been hampered. One reason could be because of the difficulties of visibility due to the lack of lymphatic markers. But since the discovery of several molecules specifically expressed in lymphatic endothelial cells, a rediscovery of the lymphatic vasculature has taken place. New scientific insights has facilitated detailed analysis of the nature and organization of the lymphatic system in physiological and pathophysiological conditions, such as in chronic inflammation and metastatic cancer spread. Knowledge about the molecules that control lymphangiogenesis and tumor-associated lymphangiogenesis is now expanding, allowing better opportunities for the development of drugs interfering with the relevant signaling pathways. Advances in our understanding of the mechanisms have translated into a number of novel therapeutic studies.

R. Liersch (✉)
Department of Medicine, Hematology/Oncology,
University Hospital Münster,
Albert-Schweitzer-Str. 33, 48129,
Münster, Germany
e-mail: rliersch@uni-muenster.de

8.1 Introduction

The lymphatic vasculature develops separately, but is functionally related to the blood vascular system. While the blood vascular system is a closed circulatory system, the lymphatic system is open-ended. It collects the interstitial fluid in the periphery and drains the absorbed lymph in the nuchal region into the subclavian veins. This loop controls the balance of various factors and 10% of the body fluid volume. Next to the transport of interstitial fluid, the lymphatic system plays an essential role in the circulation of macromolecules, dietary fats, lymphocytes, and antigen-presenting cells. In the immune-regulatory network, the lymphatic system directs the trafficking of cytokines and immune cells. However, the lymphatic system is also a common pathway for lymphatic metastasis, and therefore plays an essential role for overall survival of cancer patients.

R. Liersch et al. (eds.), *Angiogenesis Inhibition,* Recent Results in Cancer Research,
DOI: 10.1007/978-3-540-78281-0_8,

8.2 Embryonic Lymphatic Development

The lymphatic system develops in parallel with the blood vascular system, but although major progress has been made, it remains controversial as to whether the lymphatic vasculature is developing from embryonic veins, from lymphangioblasts, or from both (Wilting et al. 1999). In 1902, Florence Sabin proposed the most widely accepted theory that the lymphatic vasculature develops from embryonic veins (Sabin 1902; Sabin 1904) and that the peripheral lymphatic system expands from the primary lymph sacs, originates from vascular endothelial cells, and then spreads by endothelial sprouting, forming capillaries. Upon the formation of the vascular system, Lyve-1 (lymphatic vessel endothelial hyaluron receptor) starts to be expressed in venous endothelial cells of the cardinal vein, and endothelial cells become competent to respond to lymphatic signals (lymphatic competence). Induced by a so far unknown signal almost at the same time, Prox-1 expression occurs in restricted areas of the cardinal vein, determining the lymphatic fate (lymphatic bias) of budding endothelial cells. Homebox gene Prox-1 is a transcription factor related to the Drosophila gene prospero, and expressing endothelial cells are detected in a polarized manner in a subset of cells of the cardinal vein, leading to budding of endothelial cells, initially in the jugular and mesonephric regions (Wigle and Oliver 1999). The analysis of Prox-1 null mice revealed that Prox-1 is required to promote lymphangiogenesis in a specific subpopulation in the embryonic vein. The importance becomes evident by the fact that in Prox-1 null mice the lymphatics do not develop, whereas the blood vessels seem to be unaffected (Wigle and Oliver 1999). Prox-1 promotes the lymphatic differentiation and leads to the downregulation of blood vessel markers (Wigle et al. 2002).

The vascular endothelial growth factor (VEGF)-C plays another essential role during lymphatic development. Binding of its receptor, the VEGF-Receptor-3 (VEGFR-3), expressed on early blood vessels and on lymphatic endothelium is required for migration and budding. In VEGF-C knockout mice, endothelial cells commit to the lymphatic lineage but do not sprout to form lymph vessels (Karkkainen et al. 2004). Xenopus tadpoles with VEGF-C knockdown had lymphatic commitment but impaired the directional migration and budding (Ny et al. 2005). Taken together, these results suggest that Prox-1 activity is required for the commitment of the venous endothelial cells to lymphatic differentiation, whereas VEGF-C/VEGFR-3 signaling provides essential signals for sprouting (Karkkainen et al. 2004; Wigle and Oliver 1999). The development of the lymphatic vasculature during embryogenesis lags behind that of the blood vessels, and these vessels at a later point in time develop Prox-1, Lyve-1, and CD31 positive vessel structures. Vascular endothelial growth factor–A and –C, but not basic FGF-2 (basic FGF), hepatocyte growth factor (HGF), and hypoxia, stimulate the development of early lymphatics (Kreuger et al. 2006; Liersch et al. 2006). Additional molecules, including the mucin-type glycoprotein podoplanin, Neuropilin-2 (Nrp-2), and angiopoietin-2 (Ang2) play major roles in the further maturation of the developing lymphatic system. Integrin $\alpha 9\beta 1$ is required for the development of the fully functional lymphatic system and is involved in mediating the effects of VEGF-C and VEGF-D via VEGFR-3. Mice deficient in the integrin $\alpha 9$-subunit show edema and chylothorax, and die shortly after birth.

An alternative model suggested that the primary lymphatics develop in the mesenchyme from precursor cells, so-called lymphangioblasts, independent from veins, and only later establish connections with the venous system (Huntington and McClure 1910). This was supported by the findings obtained in birds, where the lymph sacs develop by sprouting and form the embryonic mesenchyme (Schneider et al. 1999). Recently it has been shown in the tadpole model that both mechanisms can also contribute to lymph vessel development (Ny et al. 2005). Evidence for both models has been recently found in murine embroid bodies. In these

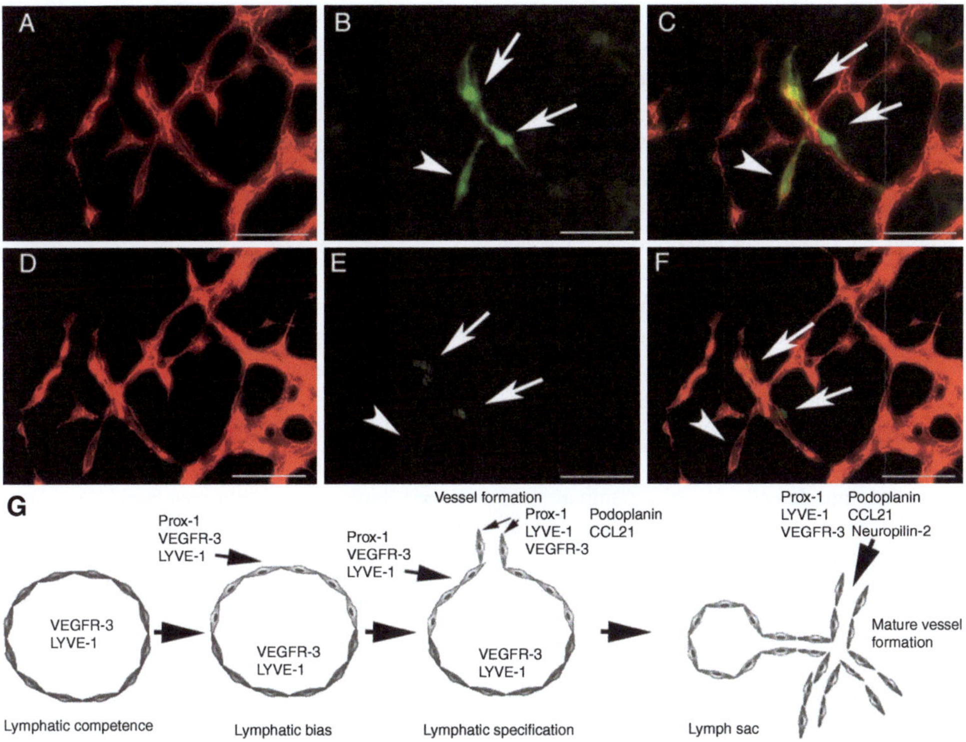

Fig. 8.1 Embryonic development of the lymph system. Lymphatic competence of vascular structures in embryoid bodies (EB) show differential expression of Lyve-1 and Prox-1. Double immunofluorescence stains of 21 days old EBs for CD31 (*red*; **a**, **d**) and Prox-1 (*green*, **e**) revealed CD31-positive blood vessels and CD31+/Prox-1+ (**e**; *arrow*) positive lymphatic vessels (f; merged image). Differential immunofluorescence stains for CD31 (**a**, **d**; *red*) and LYVE-1 (**b**; *green*) revealed that vascular structures are CD31+/Lyve-1 positive (b; *arrow/arrowhead*) with no expression of Prox-1 (e; *arrowhead*). (**c**, **f**) Merged images. Scale bars: 100 μm. (**g**) At early embryonic development endothelial cells of the cardinal vein express LYVE-1 and VEGFR-3 (lymphatic competence). Upon stimulation a subset of endothelial cells express the transcription factor Prox-1, a master regulator of lymphatic differentiation (lymphatic bias). These Prox-1 cells bud off and migrate out to form the primitive lymph sacs and then the mature lymphatic network. During this process, they upregulate the expression of additional lymphatic lineage markers

three-dimensional structures lymphatic endothelial cells (LEC) seem to develop not only from blood vessels. In agreement with earlier observation, LYVE-1/CD31 positive vessels develop much earlier than Prox-1 expression occurs. But Prox-1 was partially expressed not only in a subpopulation of LYVE-1/CD31 positive blood endothelial vessels (Fig. 8.1), but also in additional areas of newly formed lymphatic vessels not associated to any blood vessel.

In summary, until now published data suggest that the lymphatic vasculature is budding of from pre-existing veins, with a contribution from mesenchymal progenitors.

8.3 The Lymphatic Function

The lymphatic system consists of capillaries, collecting vessels, lymph nodes, trunks, and ducts. In the periphery, the blind-ended, finger shaped capillaries consist of a single layer of overlapping cells, connected to the surrounding tissue by fibrillin-containing anchoring filaments (Gerli et al. 2000). Due to an absent basal membrane, no smooth muscle cells, and lack of tight cell–cell junctions (Barsky et al. 1983; Leak and Burke 1968; Sauter et al. 1998), only these filaments stabilize the lymphatic capillaries and facilitate lymphatic flow and drainage (Leak and Burke 1966). Under physiological conditions, lymphatic capillaries remain collapsed, but especially in the case of increased interstitial pressure the anchoring filaments provide a better drainage by increasing their luminal volume. After the capillaries merge into collecting vessels, they consist of valves and are surrounded by smooth muscle cells. Intrinsic pump activity, nitric oxide–responsiveness (Shirasawa et al. 2000; von der Weid 2001), skeletal muscle action and valves regulate the unidirectional lymph flow (von der Weid 2001). Collecting vessels become the afferent lymphatics of lymph nodes, emptying into the subcapsular sinus. Lymph nodes are discrete structures surrounded by a capsule composed of connective tissue. Lymph nodes function as filters and reservoirs and exist for the activation of T-lymphocytes and B-lymphocytes. The capsule is perforated at various points by afferent lymphatics. Lymph fluid, macromolecules, and cells travel through the subcapsular, the trabecular, and marginal sinuses to reach the efferent lymphatic. The lining endothelium of the sinuses is lymphatic endothelium, expressing the typical lymphatic markers. Lymph node sinuses have an irregular surface with many reticular cells and fibers protruding into or crossing the lumen and, equivalent to the anchoring filaments of the peripheral capillaries, these fibers support the intranodal vessel lumen (Okada et al. 2002). Casts of these sinuses are connected with the surrounded nodal parenchyma and blood vessels by lymphaticovenous shunts (Okada et al. 2002). All collecting lymphatic vessels pass through lymph nodes, which are organized in clusters through the lymphatic systems. After leaving the lymph node, the efferent lymphatic vessels merge to thoracic ducts and drain the collected fluids, proteins, and cells back into the blood vascular circulation. Reflecting this specialized function in drainage, transport, and dissemination the lymphatic vasculature is crucially involved in the pathogenesis of various diseases or inflammatory conditions.

8.3.1 Molecular Players in the Regulation of Lymphangiogenesis

The lymphatic endothelium expresses most of the common endothelial cell markers and shares various biological similarities with the blood endothelium (Sauter et al. 1998; Wissmann and Detmar 2006). The main regulator of lymphatic differentiation is the homebox transcription factor *Prox-1* (Drosophila prospero related homeobox gene) (Alitalo and Carmeliet 2002; Wigle et al. 2002). Essential for lymph vessel growth are growth factors like *VEGF-C* and *VEGF-D* (Jeltsch et al. 1997; Oh et al. 1997; Veikkola et al. 2001). These were the first described stimulators of lymphangiogenesis (Fig. 8.2). Both are members of the VEGF-family, and they bind and activate the vascular endothelial growth factor receptor (VEGFR)-3 (Achen et al. 1998; Cao et al. 2004; Joukov et al. 1996; Lee et al. 1996; Makinen et al. 2001a; Veikkola et al. 2001), but after stepwise proteolytic processing by enzymes such as plasmin and proprotein convertases, they also bind VEGFR-2 (Joukov et al. 1997; Stacker et al. 1999) influencing angiogenesis as well (Cao et al. 1998; Marconcini et al. 1999; Witzenbichler et al. 1998). VEGFR-3, also known as FLT-4, was the first lymphangiogenic specific growth factor receptor (Kaipainen et al. 1995). It is expressed in early embryonic development in venous and lymphatic endothelium (Kaipainen et al. 1995) and synthesis is in parts controlled via activation of the p42/p44 MAPK signaling cascade, in protein C kinase dependent fashion, and via AKT phosphorylation (Makinen

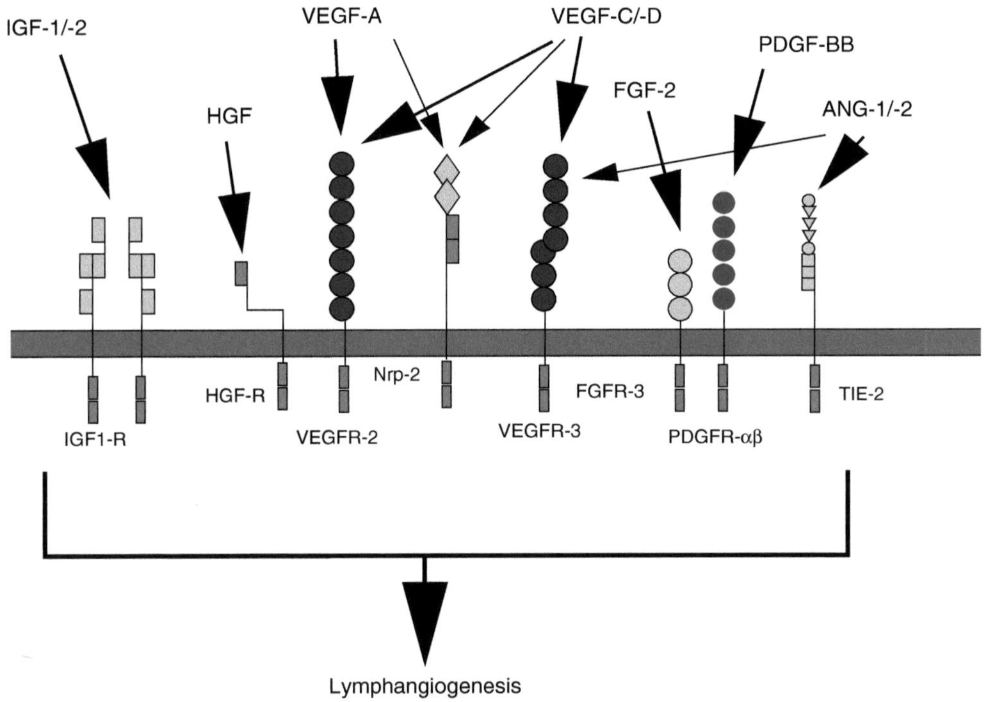

Fig. 8.2 Lymphangiogenic growth factors and their receptors. *VEGFR* vascular endothelial growth factor receptor; *HGFR* hepatocyte growth factor receptor; *IGFR* insulin-like growth factor receptor; *PDGFR* platelet derived growth factor receptor, *FGF* fibroblast growth factor, *TIE* Tyrosine kinase with immunoglobulin-like and EGF-like domains

et al. 2001b). However, in adults the expression of VEGFR-3 becomes confined to the lymphatic endothelium (Kaipainen et al. 1995), but in addition also monocytes, macrophages, dendritic cells, and fenestrated capillaries and veins express VEGFR-3 (Hamrah et al. 2003; Partanen et al. 2000; Schoppmann et al. 2002). Interestingly, VEGFR-3 is reexpressed on capillary endothelium in tumor tissue and is even involved in tumor-angiogenesis and tumor growth (Laakkonen et al. 2007). Signaling via VEGFR-3 is also important for the remodeling of primary vascular networks into larger blood vessels, a function essential for the development of the cardiovascular system in embryos (Dumont et al. 1998). Targeted inactivation of VEGFR-3 results in embryonic lethality as a result of failure to remodel the capillary network before the emergence of lymphatic vessels (Dumont et al. 1998). VEGF-C induces lymphangiogenesis both in embryos and tumors mainly by its interaction with VEGFR-3 (Jeltsch et al. 2003). VEGF-C knockouts fail to form initial lymphatic vessels indicating the pivotal role in embryogenesis (Karkkainen et al. 2004). In contrast, VEGF-D is not required for embryogenesis (Baldwin et al. 2005), but is the strongest inducer of lymphangiogenesis in the adult when given via adenoviral delivery (Rissanen et al. 2003). Exogenous VEGF-D can rescue the phenotype of VEGF-C deficient mice (Karkkainen et al. 2004). Recent studies revealed that VEGF-A also supports lymphangiogenesis through interaction with VEGFR-2, expressed on LEC (Fig. 8.2). VEGF-A induces proliferation of LEC and overexpression in vivo induces lymphangiogenesis in tissue repair and inflammation (Hong et al. 2004; Kunstfeld et al. 2004; Nagy et al. 2002). Even neutralizing anti-VEGF-A antibodies reduce both lymphatic vessel density (LVD) and lymph node metastasis in xenograft models (Whitehurst et al. 2007). Recently, it has been suggested that VEGF-A predominantly promotes lymphatic enlargement, but not the formation of lymphatic vessels (Wirzenius et al. 2007). However, whether the effect is mainly direct or indirect is still not well understood, because VEGF-A also might stimulate lymphangiogenesis indirectly by recruitment of VEGF-C/-D secreting mononuclear cells (Cursiefen et al. 2004b).

Podoplanin is a transmembrane sialomucoprotein expressed at high levels on lymphatic vessel endothelium (Breiteneder-Geleff et al. 1999). It appears to be important for their correct function and formation. In humans, podoplanin is also expressed in osteoblastic cells, kidney podocytes, and lung alveolar Type-I cells (Wetterwald et al. 1996). The precise function of podoplanin is unclear; however, mice with a targeted gene deletion were shown to have impaired lymphatic function and lymphedema (Schacht et al. 2003). Podoplanin knockout mice having defects in lymphatic, but not blood vessel patterning, show symptoms of lymphedema and die at birth due to respiratory failure (Schacht et al. 2003). Podoplanin is also able to aggregate platelets by interaction with the -C-type lectin-like receptor2 (CLEC-2), preventing leaks between the both vasculatures (Kato et al. 2003; Suzuki-Inoue et al. 2007). Interestingly, Wicki et al. (2006) recently published that podoplanin is upregulated in the invasive front of a number of human carcinomas and promotes tumor-cell invasion.

LYVE-1, the primary lymphatic endothelial receptor for hyaluronan has been shown to be a highly specific marker for lymphatic endothelium in a wide variety of different tissues, and to distinguish lymphatic from blood vascular endothelium in numerous human tumors (Banerji et al. 1999). The considerable structural similarity between LYVE-1 and the leukocyte inflammatory homing receptor CD44 suggests a potential role for LYVE-1 in lymphatic trafficking (Banerji et al. 1999). However, the precise function of LYVE-1 remains unknown, and LYVE-1 $^{-/-}$ mice display no obvious phenotype (Gale et al. 2007). Recently, Lyve-1 expression has also been reported to be absent in some tumor- and inflammation-associated lymphatic vessels (Rubbia-Brandt et al. 2004). It could be downregulated upon incubation of cultured LEC with tumor necrosis factor-alpha (Johnson et al. 2007).

Evidence is mounting concerning the role of *integrins* in lymphangiogenesis. Especially $\alpha9\beta1$ seems to have a crucial role in lymphangiogenesis. Mice deficient in the integrin $\alpha9$ subunit show edema, extra vascular lymphocytes surrounding lymphatic vessels, and die shortly after birth (Huang et al. 2000). Because integrin $\beta1$ can stimulate to some degree VEGFR-3, and VEGF-C and VEGF-D can bind $\alpha9\beta1$, the integrin-complex might be involved in lymphatic vessel formation and stabilization (Wang et al. 2001). Integrin $\alpha9\beta1$ has a role in growth factor induced lymphangiogenesis as Prox-1 upregulates the integrin and VEGFR-3 (Mishima et al. 2007). Antagonism of $\alpha9\beta1$ suppressed VEGF-C induced motility. Additional studies revealed that $\alpha1\beta1$ and $\alpha2\beta1$ are expressed on LEC in healing wounds, and antagonists could block lymphangiogenesis (Hong et al. 2004). Antagonists of $\alpha4\beta1$, which is expressed on tumor lymphatic endothelium, has been shown to block tumor metastasis as well as lymphangiogenesis (Garmy-Susini et al. 2007).

While Neuropilin-1 is mainly expressed on arterial endothelial cells, Neuropilin-2 is restricted to veins and lymphatics and is known to mediate axonal guidance during neuronal development. Neuropilin-2 is expressed by LEC and deficient mice develop a reduced small lymphatic endothelium (Yuan et al. 2002). It is also a receptor for VEGF-C and VEGF-D, raising the possibility that VEGF-C signaling is enhanced by Neuropilin, similar to Neuropilin-1 promotion of VEGF-A binding to VEGFR-2 (Karkkainen et al. 2001).

Subsequent studies have also identified *additional lymphangiogenic factors*, including fibroblast growth factor-2 (bFGF), platelet derived growth factor (PDGF-BB), HGF, insulin-like growth factor (IGF), and angiopoietins (Ang-1/-2). bFGF promotes lymphangiogensis in a mouse cornea assay, but it is more likely that this is due to an indirect effect by inducing VEGF-C production (Chang et al. 2004; Kubo et al. 2002). Recently, HGF was described as a novel lymphangiogenic growth factor. HGF promoted lymphangiogenesis and promoted peritumoral lymphangiogenesis (Kajiya et al. 2005). Of interest, HGF-receptor, also known as MET/c-met has been reported to correlate with metastatic spread of cancer (Danilkovitch-Miagkova and Zbar 2002). Studies also revealed that the insulin-like growth factor 1 and 2 (IGF-1/-2) induce lymphangiogenesis, but the effect could not be blocked by antagonist of VEGFR-3 (Bjorndahl et al. 2005), although IGF-receptors promoted expression of VEGF-C and lymph node metastasis in a Lewis lung carcinoma model (Tang et al. 2003). Whether IGF-1/-2 has a direct or indirect effect has to be further analyzed. In addition to Prox-1, VEGF-C, VEGF-D, and VEGFR-3, several molecules are known to be especially important for *later stages of lymphatic development*.

While *angiopoietin-2 (Ang-2)* is not required for the formation of lymphatics, it plays a key role in their subsequent remodeling and maturation. Mice lacking Ang-2 develop subcutaneous oedema and chylous ascites and die shortly after birth, due to impaired lymphatic vessel formation (Gale et al. 2002). Ang-1 can rescue these effects, although the abnormal angiogenesis also observed in Ang-2 $^{-/-}$ mice is not corrected (Gale et al. 2002). Interestingly, VEGF-C induces Ang-2 expression in cultured LEC through VEGFR-2, indicating a possible connection between the VEGF and angiopoietin families during lymphangiogenesis (Veikkola et al. 2003). However, so far there are no data published about the angiopoietins enhancing tumor-lymphangiogenesis and lymphatic metastasis, although a majority of tumors show an increased expression (for review (Tait and Jones 2004).

The *PDGF*-family (Platelet derived growth factor) includes at least four structurally related members, PDGF-AA, PDGF-BB, PDGF-CC, and PDGF-DD, that can form both homodimers and hetereodimers (Heldin and Westermark 1999). PDGF signaling is critical for proper embryonic development, whereas in the adult it plays a role in wound healing and in the control of interstitial fluid pressure. Besides stimulation of stromal cell recruitment, PDGF seems to be an important factor in regulating angiogenesis, pericyte recruitment, and tumor growth (Heldin and Westermark 1999; Ostman and Heldin 2007; Reinmuth et al. 2009). PDGF-BB plays a direct role in promoting lymphangiogenesis and metastasis. Expression of PDGF-BB in murine fibrosarcoma cells induce tumor lymphangiogenesis, leading to enhanced metastasis in lymph nodes (Cao et al. 2004). Cao et al. suggest that PDGF-BB acts as a survival factor for newly formed lymphatics through interaction with receptors PDGFR-alpha and -beta, both detected on isolated primary lymphatic endothelia cells. PDGFs may modulate the postnatal remodeling of lymphatic vessels, but not the development of rudimentary lymphatic vessels. This has to be validated in future.

Several other molecules were additionally found to be required for the development. The tyrosine kinase Syk and the adaptor protein SLP-76 were found to be involved in the separation of blood and lymph vessels (Abtahian et al. 2003). Deficiency resulted in arteriovenous shunting and connections between blood vessels and blood-filled lymph vessels. A similar role has been reported for Spred-1/Spred-2. In knockout mice, blood-filled lymphatic vessels have been reported indicating a possible role in vascular separation (Taniguchi et al. 2007) and angiopoietin-like protein-4 might be required for sustained separation of the two vasculatures (Backhed et al. 2007). Recently, two membrane proteins have been described specifically expressed in activated tumor-associated LEC. Applying double-staining techniques with established LEC markers, Fiedler et al. (2006) have screened endothelial cell differentiation antigens for their expression in LECs. Their experiments identified the sialomucin CD34 as being exclusively expressed by LECs in human tumors but not in corresponding normal tissues. LyP-1, a molecular marker of tumor lymphatics in the MDA-MB-435 breast carcinoma cell line, which was grown in nude mice, was identified by combining ex vivo screening of phage-displayed peptides and in vivo screening for tumor homing. LyP-1 does not appear in normal lymphatics, and it remains to be determined whether it is expressed in other tumor types (Laakkonen et al. 2002). Since LEC's can be successfully isolated by tissue micropreparation from lymphatic channels, embryonic stem cells, even when established in primary culture, provide a valuable opportunity to further explore molecular mechanisms of lymphangiogenesis and the biology of lymphatic metastasis (Hirakawa et al. 2003; Kono et al. 2006; Petrova et al. 2002; Podgrabinska et al. 2002; Wick et al. 2007). This may lead to the identification of endothelial lineage specific signatures.

8.4 Pathology of the Lymphatic Vasculature

Lymphatic vessels have multiple functions and play an important role in various diseases. Impaired function of lymphatic vessels results in lymphedema. Based on the cause, lymphedema occurs as a hereditary (primary) edema or acquired (secondary) edema, but share common features—the dysfunctional lymphatic vessel showing fibrosis and susceptibility to inflammation and infection. The secondary lymphedema is a frequent clinical finding in industrialized countries due to cancer treatment including surgery, radiotherapy, and chemotherapy.

8.4.1 Secondary Lymphedema

In the setting of *inflammation*, lymphatic vessels have multiple functions. In acute inflammation, edema is one typical sign and a significant feature. It results when the amount of inflamed tissue fluid exceeds the capacity of lymphatic vessel for drainage. Lymphatic vessels have the passive role to transport the interstitial fluid and cytokines to the sentinel lymph nodes. In addition, the lymphatic vessels actively participate in the inflammatory process and are responsible for the afferent immune response by enhancing the migration of dendritic cells, which could be induced in two different ways. One is the increasing level of markers such as the secondary lymphoid chemokine (CCL21) or by increased lymphangiogenesis, triggered by infiltrating immune cells. In the case of an inflammatory response, the infiltrating immune cells are a major source of growth factors and even stromal fibroblasts secrete chemokines and other cytokines such as VEGF-A, VEGF-C, and monocyte-colony stimulating factor (M-CSF). They are chemotactic for further monocytes and macrophages (Barleon et al. 1996; Melder et al. 1996). Macrophages, in particular, secrete many angiogenic and lymphangiogenic factors, including VEGF-C and VEGF-D (Schoppmann et al. 2002), and therefore trigger lymphangiogenesis. It has even been reported that macrophages contribute to lymphangiogenesis by incorporation into newly formed lymphatic vessels in the inflamed cornea (Kerjaschki et al. 2006). Thus, VEGFR-3 might have crucial roles in amplification of pathological lymphangiogenesis. Cornea inflammation increased the expression of VEGFR-3 and induced VEGF-C in dendritic cells, possibly by the secretion of proinflammatory cytokines (Hamrah et al. 2003).

It further induces pronounced recruitment of dendritic cells to lymph nodes and triggers graft-rejection. VEGF-C producing macrophages were also found to participate in lymphangiogenesis in human renal transplant rejection (Kerjaschki et al. 2004). Therefore, antilymphangiogenic strategies may improve transplant survival in the setting of transplantation (Cursiefen et al. 2004a, 2003).

In one setting of *lymphatic dysfunction*, the clinical finding of lymphedema is associated with a blockade of the lymphatic fluid uptake. Filiariasis, a parasitic worm infection (*Brugia malayi* or *Wuchereria bancrofti*), often causes massive fibrosis of the lymph nodes and lymph channels in the inguinal region. The resulting edema of the external genitalia and the lower limbs is so extreme that it is called elephantiasis. In Europe, one often finds edema resulting from trauma, surgery, tissue grafting, and congenital edema (Daroczy 1995; Gerber 1998; Mortimer 1998; Witte et al. 1998). Treatment of cancer by removal or irradiation of lymph nodes induces posttreatment lymphedema. Impaired lymphatic drainage produces swelling, scarring, and immundysregulatory disorders. Lymphedema can be a result of an induced imbalance between lymph formation and absorption. The induced fluid accumulation causes pain, chronic and disabling swelling, tissue fibrosis, adipose degeneration, poor immune function, and susceptibility to infections, as well as impaired wound healing (Rockson 2001). Recent studies of experimental lymphedema revealed that VEGF-C protein injection into the wounded area and virus-mediated VEGF-C gene therapy induce the growth of functional lymphatics (Karkkainen et al. 2001; Szuba et al. 2002). Furthermore, it has been shown that adenoviral delivery regenerated lymphatic vessels in mice (Tammela et al. 2007). Postsurgical lymphedemas might be a future indication for VEGF-C-based therapies; however, in the case of cancer treatment related lymphedema, future studies are warranted. VEGF-C might increase the risk of distant organ metastasis if not all tumor cells have been removed.

8.4.2 Primary Lymphedema

Primary lymphedemas are rare genetic developmental disorders which can manifest at birth (Milroy's disease) or at the onset of puberty (Meige's disease) (Witte et al. 1998). Milroy's disease is a congenital form of disease. It has been mapped to the telomeric part of chromosome 5q, in the region 5q34-q35 and Irrthum et al. (2000) have shown that this region includes a VEGFR-3 intragenic polymorphism. Several heterozygous VEGFR-3 missense mutations have been found in Milroy's disease, resulting in the expression of an inactive tyrosine kinase (Irrthum et al. 2003; Karkkainen et al. 2000). The effect of these mutations was the inhibition of autophosphorylation of the receptor causing this congenital hereditary lymphedema (Irrthum et al. 2000). In Milroy's disease, the superficial or subcutaneous lymphatic vessels are usually aplastic or hypoplastic, whereas in other lymphedema syndromes, such as in lymphedema distichiasis (LD), the microlymphatic network is normal or larger than in healthy controls (Bollinger et al. 1983). The inactivating mutation of the forkhead transcription factor FOXC2 in autosomal dominant LD syndrome relates to pubertal onset of lymphedema and double row of eyelashes (distichiasis) (Fang et al. 2000). FOXC2 is a member of the forkhead/winged helix family of transcription factors involved in developmental pathways. FOXC2 knockout mice display aortic arch and ventricular septal defects and also defective lymphatic valve formation and abnormal pericyte recruitment (Petrova et al. 2004). FOXC2 is necessary in lymphatic maturation and is expressed in the developing lymphatic vessels and lymphatic valves of adults (Dagenais et al. 2004; Petrova et al. 2004). Dysfunction of SOX18, a transcription factor of the SOX family, has been identified as a cause for hypotrichosis ly mphedema-teleangiectasia syndrome in humans (Irrthum et al. 2003), and is interestingly regulated by VEGFR-3 activation (Cermenati et al. 2008).

However, the detailed function is unclear. Reelin mutations, a gene coding for a protein guiding neuronal-cell migration, is accompanied with congenital lymphedema and chylous ascites (Hong et al. 2000).

In many lymphedema patients none of the aforementioned genetic defects are visible, indicating more relevant genes in human lymphatic development. Different familial lymphedema syndromes emphasize even bigger phenotypic and genotypic heterogeneity in inherited lymphedema angiodysplasia syndromes, where the mutated genes have not been characterized yet (Northup et al. 2003).

8.5 Role of Lymphangiogenesis in Cancer

The metastatic spread of tumor cells is responsible for the majority of cancer deaths, and with few exceptions, all cancers can metastasize. The lymphatic system is the primary pathway of metastasis for most human cancers. For migrating tumor cells, the lymphatic system has many advantages over the blood circulation. Even the smallest lymphatic vessels are larger than blood capillaries; flow velocities are lower and there is less interference with serum factors. High shear stress and mechanic deformation in the blood vascular system often kills metastatic cells (Liotta et al. 1991; Weiss 1992). Lymphatic vessels have no or a discontinuous basal membrane, intercellular gaps, and lymphatic capillaries are not surrounded by pericytes.

8.5.1 Lymphvascular Invasion

Lymphatic vessels in comparison to blood vessels are easier to invade and provide ideal conduits. In addition, LEC's secret chemotactic agents attract malignant tumor cells toward areas of high LVD (Shields et al. 2007). Tumor cells protrude and migrate between LEC, known as lymphovascular invasion (LVI), an important parameter in the prognosis of cancer patients associated with relapse-free and overall survival in various cancers (Lee et al. 2006, 2007; Lotan et al. 2005; May et al. 2007). Once tumor cells gain access to lymphatic vessels, they embolize as single cells or in clusters to the sentinel lymph node (SLN) (Yancopoulos et al. 2000). When tumor cells infiltrate, the SLN further metastasis to distant lymph nodes or distant organs occurs. Through lymphaticovenous connections cancer cells metastasize via blood vessels, although hematogenous metastasis could also occur without SLN metastasis (Fisher and Fisher 1966).

8.5.2 Tumor-Lymphangiogenesis

Lymphangiogenesis has been found in the tissue of many malignancies. Studies revealed that tumors can actively induce the formation of tumor lymphangiogenesis and promote metastasis (Mandriota et al. 2001; Skobe et al. 2001; Stacker et al. 2001). VEGF-C and VEGF-D induced lymphatic vessel proliferation intratumorally and peritumorally. Size of the peritumoral lymphatic vessel was observed to be a most reliable and significant predictor for cutaneous melanoma metastasis and survival (Dadras et al. 2003). There is still an ongoing controversy regarding the significance and functionality of intratumoral lymphatics or intratumoral lymphangiogenesis. Although there have been studies demonstrating that intratumoral lymphatics are nonfunctional for fluid drainage (Padera et al. 2002), others could describe the prognostic influence of intratumoral lymphatics in immunhistochemical analysis (Dadras et al. 2003). Tumor lymphangiogenesis predicts the presence of melanoma metastasis in sentinel lymph nodes at time of surgery (Dadras et al. 2003). In addition, several clinical studies have correlated intratumoral LVD with metastasis (reviewed by (Achen et al. 2005; Stacker et al. 2002), but nevertheless the importance of intratumoral lymphangiogenesis in regard to metastasis is debatable and may depend on the organ and/or experimental model used. This leads to the general problem that current methodology of lymphangiogenesis quantification is still characterized by high intra- and inter-observer variability. For using the amount of lymphatic vessels in a tumor as a clinically useful parameter, a reliable quantification technique needs to be developed.

8.5.3 Lymphatic Endothelial Cell Activation

Aside from peritumoral lymphangiogenesis, activation of lymphatic vessels has also been proposed as a way to enhance tumor cell infiltration and sentinel lymph node metastasis. He et al. (2005) recently noted that peritumoral LEC proximal to subcutaneous LNM35 lung tumors often displayed an activated phenotype – characterized by increased vessel sprouting, dilation, and permeability. VEGF-C may also activate lymphatics to promote tumor cell chemotaxis, lymphatic intravasation, blood vessel leakage with enhanced lymphatic vessel dilatation and hence tumor cell dissemination (Hoshida et al. 2006). Others have speculated that activated lymphatics might upregulate secretion of chemokines that could attract tumor cells (Alitalo et al. 2004). This activated phenotype can apparently be reversed by adenoviral delivery of soluble Flt-4 (He et al. 2005). Experimental evidence has been obtained suggesting that LEC's could attract tumor cells by secreting chemokines, and therefore actively promote lymphatic metastasis. One of the chemokines, named secondary lymphoid chemokine (SLC/CCL21), is highly expressed in lymph nodes, specifically in endothelial cells of high endothelial venules and T cell-rich areas, and also in the lymphatic endothelium of multiple organs (Gunn et al. 1998). CCL19 and CCL21, chemokines produced by LEC (Saeki et al. 1999), induce a biochemical change when bound to CCR7. Inactivation of CCR7 or CCL21 blocked dendritic cells to migrate from peripheral tissues to draining lymph nodes (Gunn et al. 1999). Recent reports have also shown that human (Takeuchi et al. 2004) and murine (Wiley et al. 2001) melanomas express CCR7, the receptor for CCL21 and CCL19 and that in gastric carcinoma, head/neck squamous cell carcinoma, nonsmall cell lung cancer, and breast cancer, these two factors are associated with lymph node metastasis (Mashino et al. 2002; Muller et al. 2001; Takanami 2003; Wang et al. 2004; Yan et al. 2004). It has been reported earlier that CCR7 and CXCR4, receptors for SLC/CCL21 and CXCL12, respectively, are significantly expressed in human breast cancer cells. Their ligands exhibit high levels of expression in regional lymph nodes, bone marrow, lung, and liver, which represent the first destinations of breast cancer metastasis (Muller et al. 2001). Inhibiting the interaction between this receptor–ligand pair in vivo reduced the ability of MDA-MB-231 breast cancer cells to metastasize to both lung and lymph nodes. These data suggest active interactions between tumor cells and endothelial cells. Furthermore, overexpression of CCR7 by B16 murine melanoma cells enhanced the incidence of lymph node but not lung metastasis when the tumor cells were implanted into the footpads of mice (Wiley et al. 2001). CCR7-mediated enhancement of lymphatic metastasis could be completely suppressed by treatment with neutralizing anti-SLC antibodies (Wiley et al. 2001). These data indicate that chemokines and their receptors play a critical role in determining the metastatic destination of tumor cells.

8.5.4 Lymph Node Lymphangiogenesis

Paget (1889) concluded that metastasis occurred only when certain favored tumor cells (the seed) had a special affinity for the growth milieu provided by certain specific organs (the soil). The

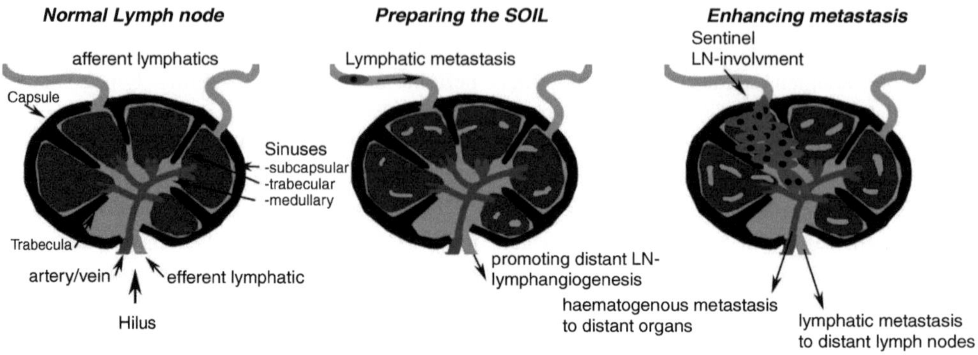

Fig. 8.3 Lymph node lymphangiogenesis. Cancer promotes tumor-associated lymphangiogenesis leading to enhanced metastasis to sentinel lymph nodes (SLN). Lymphangiogenic factors (VEGF-C or VEGF-A) are drained to the SLN where they induce expansion of the lymphatic network (lymph node lymphangiogenesis) preparing the lymph node for the later arrival of the metastatic cells. Metastatic cells then further stimulate sentinel lymph node lymphangiogenesis and distant lymph node lymphangiogenesis, enhancing cancer spread to distant lymph nodes and organs

concept of the *"Seed and soil hypothesis"* (Fig. 8.3) for tumor lymphangiogenesis has been recently described by Hirakawa et al. (2007, 2005). They describe an increased lymphangiogenesis in the sentinel lymph node, even prior to, and after metastatic colonization (Hirakawa et al. 2007, 2005) (Fig. 8.3). Similar observations have been also made in malignant melanoma experiments (Harrell et al. 2007) and in hematological malignancies such as lymphomas (Ruddell et al. 2003). Interestingly, these investigators also observed a 20-30-fold increase in lymph flow. Equivalent changes of lymph node lymphangiogenesis have been recently described in uninvolved axillary lymph nodes of human breast cancer patients (Qian et al. 2006), and lymph node lymphangiogenesis was even associated with nonsentinel lymph node metastasis (Van den Eynden et al. 2006, 2007). That lymph nodes respond to inflammation or neoplasia is a long-known fact. Activated lymph nodes can increase many-fold in size and weight (Cahill et al. 1976; Hall and Morris 1965; Hay and Hobbs 1977). This can be a morphological change known as reactive lymphadenopathy also observed during inflammatory processes. Although the exact mechanism underlying cancer-associated lymph node lymphangiogenesis remains unclear, it could be proposed as a possible way for tumors to disseminate faster throughout the lymphatic system and, subsequently, to distant sites.

8.6 Targeting Lymphangiogenesis

Dissemination of tumor cells is an early and common event and is associated with poorer prognosis for human cancer patients. Targeting lymphangiogenesis could prevent lymphatic metastasis and further dissemination to distant lymph nodes or even distant organs. In the setting of adjuvant tumor therapy, antilymphangiogenic treatment may be an interesting approach after the primary tumor has been surgically removed. Preventing the dissemination of micrometastasis and keeping the metastasis in a localized stage might increase the therapeutic opportunities and improve prognosis. Thus far, therapeutic agents include antibodies, soluble receptors, and tyrosine kinase inhibitors.

8.6.1 Antibodies

The most extensively targeted molecular system is the VEGFR-3/VEGF-C and VEGFR-3/VEGF-D system. Inhibition by neutralizing antibodies reduced lymphangiogenesis and prevented lymphatic metastasis in various animal models (He et al. 2002, 2005; Hoshida et al. 2006; Roberts et al. 2006; Stacker et al. 2001). Interestingly, neutralizing VEGFR-3 antibody blocked the formation of new lymphatics, while the preexisting lymphatics have not been affected (Pytowski et al. 2005). Of further importance is the expression of VEGFR-2 and the stimulation of LEC by VEGF-A and by proteolytically processed VEGF-C. Clinical studies inhibiting the activation of VEGFR-2 by the neutralizing VEGF-A antibody (bevacizumab) showed to be beneficial in human tumors (for review (Ferrara et al. 2004). An antilymphangiogenic effect of this antibody has never been evaluated systematically so far. Treatment of breast carcinoma in animal models with an anti-VEGF-A antibody revealed a reduced LVD and lymph node metastasis (Whitehurst et al. 2007). The effect might be more pronounced by a combined blockade of both VEGF-C and VEGF-A, leading to dual blocking of angiogenesis and lymphangiogenesis. Double blockade by an anti-receptor targeting may lead to enhanced antiangiogenic and antitumor effect (Tammela et al. 2008).

8.6.2 Soluble Receptors

Soluble receptors compete with membrane-bound receptors. They comprise their extracellular portions and retain the ability to bind their ligand. Even due to the binding of multiple soluble factors they might be very effective. Inhibition of VEGFR-3 signaling with a soluble receptor, VEGFR-3-Ig, suppressed tumor lymphangiogenesis and lymphatic metastasis in a breast and lung carcinoma model (He et al. 2002; Karpanen et al. 2001).

8.6.3 Small Molecule Inhibitor

A similar approach, but interacting intracellularly with the signal transduction are the receptor tyrosine kinase inhibitors such as sorafenib and sunitinib. Both interact with the VEGFR-2 and VEGFR-3 phosphorylation pockets and inhibit consecutive signaling pathways, but no studies have been published so far on their specific antilymphangiogenic effect. Cedarinib and vandetanib, which block VEGFR-2 and VEGFR-3 signaling, yielded no inhibition of lymphatic metastasis in animal models, suggesting that kinase inhibition of both receptors may not be enough (Padera et al. 2008). But further studies are warranted to determine the role of tyrosine kinase inhibitors in antilymphangiogenic treatment.

8.7 Conclusions

Lymphangiogenesis is currently receiving increasing scientific and clinical interest. The identification of novel mediators of lymphangiogenesis will likely lead to new advances in our understanding of the mechanisms underlying tumor metastasis. Comprehensive research strategies have revealed a number of novel targets supporting biologically based therapeutic studies. Novel lymphangiogenic targets for the treatment of cancers and inflammation support the future development of individualized therapies, possibly avoiding adverse side effects.

References

Abtahian F, Guerriero A, Sebzda E, Lu MM, Zhou R, Mocsai A, Myers EE, Huang B, Jackson DG, Ferrari VA, Tybulewicz V, Lowell CA, Lepore JJ,

8

Koretzky GA, Kahn ML (2003) Regulation of blood and lymphatic vascular separation by signaling proteins SLP-76 and Syk. Science 299: 247–251

Achen MG, Jeltsch M, Kukk E, Makinen T, Vitali A, Wilks AF, Alitalo K, Stacker SA (1998) Vascular endothelial growth factor D (VEGF-D) is a ligand for the tyrosine kinases VEGF receptor 2 (Flk1) and VEGF receptor 3 (Flt4). Proc Natl Acad Sci U S A 95:548–553

Achen MG, McColl BK, Stacker SA (2005) Focus on lymphangiogenesis in tumor metastasis. Cancer Cell 7:121–127

Alitalo K, Carmeliet P (2002) Molecular mechanisms of lymphangiogenesis in health and disease. Cancer Cell 1:219–227

Alitalo K, Mohla S, Ruoslahti E (2004) Lymphangiogenesis and cancer: meeting report. Cancer Res 64:9225–9229

Backhed F, Crawford PA, O'Donnell D, Gordon JI (2007) Postnatal lymphatic partitioning from the blood vasculature in the small intestine requires fasting-induced adipose factor. Proc Natl Acad Sci U S A 104:606–611

Baldwin ME, Halford MM, Roufail S, Williams RA, Hibbs ML, Grail D, Kubo H, Stacker SA, Achen MG (2005) Vascular endothelial growth factor D is dispensable for development of the lymphatic system. Mol Cell Biol 25:2441–2449

Banerji S, Ni J, Wang SX, Clasper S, Su J, Tammi R, Jones M, Jackson DG (1999) LYVE-1, a new homologue of the CD44 glycoprotein, is a lymph-specific receptor for hyaluronan. J Cell Biol 144:789–801

Barleon B, Sozzani S, Zhou D, Weich HA, Mantovani A, Marme D (1996) Migration of human monocytes in response to vascular endothelial growth factor (VEGF) is mediated via the VEGF receptor flt-1. Blood 87:3336–3343

Barsky SH, Baker A, Siegal GP, Togo S, Liotta LA (1983) Use of anti-basement membrane antibodies to distinguish blood vessel capillaries from lymphatic capillaries. Am J Surg Pathol 7: 667–677

Bjorndahl M, Cao R, Nissen LJ, Clasper S, Johnson LA, Xue Y, Zhou Z, Jackson D, Hansen AJ, Cao Y (2005) Insulin-like growth factors 1 and 2 induce lymphangiogenesis in vivo. Proc Natl Acad Sci U S A 102:15593–15598

Bollinger A, Isenring G, Franzeck UK, Brunner U (1983) Aplasia of superficial lymphatic capillaries in hereditary and connatal lymphedema (Milroy's disease). Lymphology 16:27–30

Breiteneder-Geleff S, Soleiman A, Horvat R, Amann G, Kowalski H, Kerjaschki D (1999) Podoplanin–a specific marker for lymphatic endothelium expressed in angiosarcoma. Verh Dtsch Ges Pathol 83:270–275

Cahill RN, Frost H, Trnka Z (1976) The effects of antigen on the migration of recirculating lymphocytes through single lymph nodes. J Exp Med 143:870–888

Cao Y, Linden P, Farnebo J, Cao R, Eriksson A, Kumar V, Qi JH, Claesson-Welsh L, Alitalo K (1998) Vascular endothelial growth factor C induces angiogenesis in vivo. Proc Natl Acad Sci U S A 95:14389–14394

Cao R, Bjorndahl MA, Religa P, Clasper S, Garvin S, Galter D, Meister B, Ikomi F, Tritsaris K, Dissing S, Ohhashi T, Jackson DG, Cao Y (2004) PDGF-BB induces intratumoral lymphangiogenesis and promotes lymphatic metastasis. Cancer Cell 6:333–345

Cermenati S, Moleri S, Cimbro S, Corti P, Del Giacco L, Amodeo R, Dejana E, Koopman P, Cotelli F, Beltrame M (2008) Sox18 and Sox7 play redundant roles in vascular development. Blood 111:2657–2666

Chang LK, Garcia-Cardena G, Farnebo F, Fannon M, Chen EJ, Butterfield C, Moses MA, Mulligan RC, Folkman J, Kaipainen A (2004) Dose-dependent response of FGF-2 for lymphangiogenesis. Proc Natl Acad Sci U S A 101:11658–11663

Cursiefen C, Chen L, Dana MR, Streilein JW (2003) Corneal lymphangiogenesis: evidence, mechanisms, and implications for corneal transplant immunology. Cornea 22:273–281

Cursiefen C, Cao J, Chen L, Liu Y, Maruyama K, Jackson D, Kruse FE, Wiegand SJ, Dana MR, Streilein JW (2004a) Inhibition of hemangiogenesis and lymphangiogenesis after normal-risk corneal transplantation by neutralizing VEGF promotes graft survival. Invest Ophthalmol Vis Sci 45:2666–2673

Cursiefen C, Chen L, Borges LP, Jackson D, Cao J, Radziejewski C, D'Amore PA, Dana MR, Wiegand SJ, Streilein JW (2004b) VEGF-A stimulates lymphangiogenesis and hemangiogenesis in inflammatory neovascularization via macrophage recruitment. J Clin Invest 113:1040–1050

Dadras SS, Paul T, Bertoncini J, Brown LF, Muzikansky A, Jackson DG, Ellwanger U, Garbe C, Mihm MC, Detmar M (2003) Tumor lymphangiogenesis: a novel prognostic indicator for cutaneous melanoma metastasis and survival. Am J Pathol 162:1951–1960

Dagenais SL, Hartsough RL, Erickson RP, Witte MH, Butler MG, Glover TW (2004) Foxc2 is expressed in developing lymphatic vessels and other tissues associated with lymphedema-distichiasis syndrome. Gene Expr Patterns 4:611–619

Danilkovitch-Miagkova A, Zbar B (2002) Dysregulation of Met receptor tyrosine kinase activity in invasive tumors. J Clin Invest 109:863–867

Daroczy J (1995) Pathology of lymphedema. Clin Dermatol 13:433–444

Dumont DJ, Jussila L, Taipale J, Lymboussaki A, Mustonen T, Pajusola K, Breitman M, Alitalo K (1998) Cardiovascular failure in mouse embryos deficient in VEGF receptor-3. Science 282: 946–949

Fang J, Dagenais SL, Erickson RP, Arlt MF, Glynn MW, Gorski JL, Seaver LH, Glover TW (2000) Mutations in FOXC2 (MFH-1), a forkhead family transcription factor, are responsible for the hereditary lymphedema-distichiasis syndrome. Am J Hum Genet 67:1382–1388

Ferrara N, Hillan KJ, Gerber HP, Novotny W (2004) Discovery and development of bevacizumab, an anti-VEGF antibody for treating cancer. Nat Rev Drug Discov 3:391–400

Fisher B, Fisher ER (1966) The interrelationship of hematogenous and lymphatic tumor cell dissemination. Surg Gynecol Obstet 122:791–798

Gale NW, Thurston G, Hackett SF, Renard R, Wang Q, McClain J, Martin C, Witte C, Witte MH, Jackson D, Suri C, Campochiaro PA, Wiegand SJ, Yancopoulos GD (2002) Angiopoietin-2 is required for postnatal angiogenesis and lymphatic patterning, and only the latter role is rescued by Angiopoietin-1. Dev Cell 3: 411–423

Gale NW, Prevo R, Espinosa J, Ferguson DJ, Dominguez MG, Yancopoulos GD, Thurston G, Jackson DG (2007) Normal lymphatic development and function in mice deficient for the lymphatic hyaluronan receptor LYVE-1. Mol Cell Biol 27:595–604

Garmy-Susini B, Makale M, Fuster M, Varner JA (2007) Methods to study lymphatic vessel integrins. Methods Enzymol 426:415–438

Gerber LH (1998) A review of measures of lymphedema. Cancer 83:2803–2804

Gerli R, Solito R, Weber E, Agliano M (2000) Specific adhesion molecules bind anchoring filaments and endothelial cells in human skin initial lymphatics. Lymphology 33:148–157

Gunn MD, Tangemann K, Tam C, Cyster JG, Rosen SD, Williams LT (1998) A chemokine expressed in lymphoid high endothelial venules promotes the adhesion and chemotaxis of naive T lymphocytes. Proc Natl Acad Sci U S A 95: 258–263

Gunn MD, Kyuwa S, Tam C, Kakiuchi T, Matsuzawa A, Williams LT, Nakano H (1999) Mice lacking expression of secondary lymphoid organ chemokine have defects in lymphocyte homing and dendritic cell localization. J Exp Med 189:451–460

Hall JG, Morris B (1965) The immediate effect of antigens on the cell output of a lymph node. Br J Exp Pathol 46:450–454

Hamrah P, Chen L, Zhang Q, Dana MR (2003) Novel expression of vascular endothelial growth factor receptor (VEGFR)-3 and VEGF-C on corneal dendritic cells. Am J Pathol 163:57–68

Harrell MI, Iritani BM, Ruddell A (2007) Tumor-induced sentinel lymph node lymphangiogenesis and increased lymph flow precede melanoma metastasis. Am J Pathol 170:774–786

Hay JB, Hobbs BB (1977) The flow of blood to lymph nodes and its relation to lymphocyte traffic and the immune response. J Exp Med 145:31–44

He Y, Kozaki K, Karpanen T, Koshikawa K, Yla-Herttuala S, Takahashi T, Alitalo K (2002) Suppression of tumor lymphangiogenesis and lymph node metastasis by blocking vascular endothelial growth factor receptor 3 signaling. J Natl Cancer Inst 94:819–825

He Y, Rajantie I, Pajusola K, Jeltsch M, Holopainen T, Yla-Herttuala S, Harding T, Jooss K, Takahashi T, Alitalo K (2005) Vascular endothelial cell growth factor receptor 3-mediated activation of lymphatic endothelium is crucial for tumor cell entry and spread via lymphatic vessels. Cancer Res 65:4739–4746

Heldin CH, Westermark B (1999) Mechanism of action and in vivo role of platelet-derived growth factor. Physiol Rev 79:1283–1316

Hirakawa S, Hong YK, Harvey N, Schacht V, Matsuda K, Libermann T, Detmar M (2003) Identification of vascular lineage-specific genes by transcriptional profiling of isolated blood vascular and lymphatic endothelial cells. Am J Pathol 162:575–586

Hirakawa S, Kodama S, Kunstfeld R, Kajiya K, Brown LF, Detmar M (2005) VEGF-A induces tumor and sentinel lymph node lymphangiogenesis and promotes lymphatic metastasis. J Exp Med 201:1089–1099

Hirakawa S, Brown LF, Kodama S, Paavonen K, Alitalo K, Detmar M (2007) VEGF-C-induced lymphangiogenesis in sentinel lymph nodes promotes tumor metastasis to distant sites. Blood 109: 1010–1017

Hong SE, Shugart YY, Huang DT, Shahwan SA, Grant PE, Hourihane JO, Martin ND, Walsh CA (2000) Autosomal recessive lissencephaly with cerebellar hypoplasia is associated with human RELN mutations. Nat Genet 26:93–96

Hong YK, Lange-Asschenfeldt B, Velasco P, Hirakawa S, Kunstfeld R, Brown LF, Bohlen P, Senger DR, Detmar M (2004) VEGF-A promotes tissue repair-associated lymphatic vessel formation via VEGFR-2 and the alpha1beta1 and alpha2beta1 integrins. FASEB J 18: 1111–1113

Hoshida T, Isaka N, Hagendoorn J, di Tomaso E, Chen YL, Pytowski B, Fukumura D, Padera TP, Jain RK (2006) Imaging steps of lymphatic metastasis reveals that vascular endothelial growth factor-C increases metastasis by increasing delivery of cancer cells to lymph nodes: therapeutic implications. Cancer Res 66:8065–8075

Huang XZ, Wu JF, Ferrando R, Lee JH, Wang YL, Farese RV Jr, Sheppard D (2000) Fatal bilateral chylothorax in mice lacking the integrin alpha-9beta1. Mol Cell Biol 20:5208–5215

Huntington G, McClure C (1910) The anatomy and development of the jugular lymph sac in the domestic cat (Felis domestica). Am J Anat 10: 177–311

Irrthum A, Karkkainen MJ, Devriendt K, Alitalo K, Vikkula M (2000) Congenital hereditary lymphedema caused by a mutation that inactivates VEGFR3 tyrosine kinase. Am J Hum Genet 67: 295–301

Irrthum A, Devriendt K, Chitayat D, Matthijs G, Glade C, Steijlen PM, Fryns JP, Van Steensel MA, Vikkula M (2003) Mutations in the transcription factor gene SOX18 underlie recessive and dominant forms of hypotrichosis-lymphedema-telangiectasia. Am J Hum Genet 72:1470–1478

Jeltsch M, Kaipainen A, Joukov V, Meng X, Lakso M, Rauvala H, Swartz M, Fukumura D, Jain RK, Alitalo K (1997) Hyperplasia of lymphatic vessels in VEGF-C transgenic mice. Science 276:1423–1425

Jeltsch M, Tammela T, Alitalo K, Wilting J (2003) Genesis and pathogenesis of lymphatic vessels. Cell Tissue Res 314:69–84

Johnson LA, Prevo R, Clasper S, Jackson DG (2007) Inflammation-induced uptake and degradation of the lymphatic endothelial hyaluronan receptor LYVE-1. J Biol Chem 282:33671–33680

Joukov V, Pajusola K, Kaipainen A, Chilov D, Lahtinen I, Kukk E, Saksela O, Kalkkinen N, Alitalo K (1996) A novel vascular endothelial growth factor, VEGF-C, is a ligand for the Flt4 (VEGFR-3) and KDR (VEGFR-2) receptor tyrosine kinases. EMBO J 15:1751

Joukov V, Sorsa T, Kumar V, Jeltsch M, Claesson-Welsh L, Cao Y, Saksela O, Kalkkinen N, Alitalo K (1997) Proteolytic processing regulates receptor specificity and activity of VEGF-C. EMBO J 16:3898–3911

Kaipainen A, Korhonen J, Mustonen T, van Hinsbergh VW, Fang GH, Dumont D, Breitman M, Alitalo K (1995) Expression of the fms-like tyrosine kinase 4 gene becomes restricted to lymphatic endothelium during development. Proc Natl Acad Sci U S A 92:3566–3570

Kajiya K, Hirakawa S, Ma B, Drinnenberg I, Detmar M (2005) Hepatocyte growth factor promotes lymphatic vessel formation and function. EMBO J 24:2885–2895

Karkkainen MJ, Ferrell RE, Lawrence EC, Kimak MA, Levinson KL, McTigue MA, Alitalo K, Finegold DN (2000) Missense mutations interfere with VEGFR-3 signalling in primary lymphoedema. Nat Genet 25:153–159

Karkkainen MJ, Saaristo A, Jussila L, Karila KA, Lawrence EC, Pajusola K, Bueler H, Eichmann A, Kauppinen R, Kettunen MI, Yla-Herttuala S, Finegold DN, Ferrell RE, Alitalo K (2001) A model for gene therapy of human hereditary lymphedema. Proc Natl Acad Sci U S A 98: 12677–12682

Karkkainen MJ, Haiko P, Sainio K, Partanen J, Taipale J, Petrova TV, Jeltsch M, Jackson DG, Talikka M, Rauvala H, Betsholtz C, Alitalo K (2004) Vascular endothelial growth factor C is required for sprouting of the first lymphatic vessels from embryonic veins. Nat Immunol 5:74–80

Karpanen T, Egeblad M, Karkkainen MJ, Kubo H, Yla-Herttuala S, Jaattela M, Alitalo K (2001) Vascular endothelial growth factor C promotes tumor lymphangiogenesis and intralymphatic tumor growth. Cancer Res 61:1786–1790

Kato Y, Fujita N, Kunita A, Sato S, Kaneko M, Osawa M, Tsuruo T (2003) Molecular identification of Aggrus/T1alpha as a platelet aggregation-inducing factor expressed in colorectal tumors. J Biol Chem 278:51599–51605

Kerjaschki D, Regele HM, Moosberger I, Nagy-Bojarski K, Watschinger B, Soleiman A, Birner P, Krieger S, Hovorka A, Silberhumer G,

Laakkonen P, Petrova T, Langer B, Raab I (2004) Lymphatic neoangiogenesis in human kidney transplants is associated with immunologically active lymphocytic infiltrates. J Am Soc Nephrol 15:603–612

Kerjaschki D, Huttary N, Raab I, Regele H, Bojarski-Nagy K, Bartel G, Krober SM, Greinix H, Rosenmaier A, Karlhofer F, Wick N, Mazal PR (2006) Lymphatic endothelial progenitor cells contribute to de novo lymphangiogenesis in human renal transplants. Nat Med 12: 230–234

Kono T, Kubo H, Shimazu C, Ueda Y, Takahashi M, Yanagi K, Fujita N, Tsuruo T, Wada H, Yamashita JK (2006) Differentiation of lymphatic endothelial cells from embryonic stem cells on OP9 stromal cells. Arterioscler Thromb Vasc Biol 26:2070–2076

Kreuger J, Nilsson I, Kerjaschki D, Petrova T, Alitalo K, Claesson-Welsh L (2006) Early lymph vessel development from embryonic stem cells. Arterioscler Thromb Vasc Biol 26:1073–1078

Kubo H, Cao R, Brakenhielm E, Makinen T, Cao Y, Alitalo K (2002) Blockade of vascular endothelial growth factor receptor-3 signaling inhibits fibroblast growth factor-2-induced lymphangiogenesis in mouse cornea. Proc Natl Acad Sci U S A 99:8868–8873

Kunstfeld R, Hirakawa S, Hong YK, Schacht V, Lange-Asschenfeldt B, Velasco P, Lin C, Fiebiger E, Wei X, Wu Y, Hicklin D, Bohlen P, Detmar M (2004) Induction of cutaneous delayed-type hypersensitivity reactions in VEGF-A transgenic mice results in chronic skin inflammation associated with persistent lymphatic hyperplasia. Blood 104:1048–1057

Laakkonen P, Porkka K, Hoffman JA, Ruoslahti E (2002) A tumor-homing peptide with a targeting specificity related to lymphatic vessels. Nat Med 8:751–755

Laakkonen P, Waltari M, Holopainen T, Takahashi T, Pytowski B, Steiner P, Hicklin D, Persaud K, Tonra JR, Witte L, Alitalo K (2007) Vascular endothelial growth factor receptor 3 is involved in tumor angiogenesis and growth. Cancer Res 67:593–599

Leak LV, Burke JF (1966) Fine structure of the lymphatic capillary and the adjoining connective tissue area. Am J Anat 118:785–809

Leak LV, Burke JF (1968) Electron microscopic study of lymphatic capillaries in the removal of connective tissue fluids and particulate substances. Lymphology 1:39–52

Lee J, Gray A, Yuan J, Luoh SM, Avraham H, Wood WI (1996) Vascular endothelial growth factor-related protein: a ligand and specific activator of the tyrosine kinase receptor Flt4. Proc Natl Acad Sci U S A 93:1988–1992

Lee AH, Pinder SE, Macmillan RD, Mitchell M, Ellis IO, Elston CW, Blamey RW (2006) Prognostic value of lymphovascular invasion in women with lymph node negative invasive breast carcinoma. Eur J Cancer 42:357–362

Lee CC, Wu CW, Lo SS, Chen JH, Li AF, Hsieh MC, Shen KH, Lui WY (2007) Survival predictors in patients with node-negative gastric carcinoma. J Gastroenterol Hepatol 22:1014–1018

Liersch R, Nay F, Lu L, Detmar M (2006) Induction of lymphatic endothelial cell differentiation in embryoid bodies. Blood 107:1214–1216

Liotta LA, Stetler-Stevenson WG, Steeg PS (1991) Cancer invasion and metastasis: positive and negative regulatory elements. Cancer Invest 9: 543–551

Lotan Y, Gupta A, Shariat SF, Palapattu GS, Vazina A, Karakiewicz PI, Bastian PJ, Rogers CG, Amiel G, Perotte P, Schoenberg MP, Lerner SP, Sagalowsky AI (2005) Lymphovascular invasion is independently associated with overall survival, cause-specific survival, and local and distant recurrence in patients with negative lymph nodes at radical cystectomy. J Clin Oncol 23:6533–6539

Makinen T, Jussila L, Veikkola T, Karpanen T, Kettunen MI, Pulkkanen KJ, Kauppinen R, Jackson DG, Kubo H, Nishikawa S, Yla-Herttuala S, Alitalo K (2001a) Inhibition of lymphangiogenesis with resulting lymphedema in transgenic mice expressing soluble VEGF receptor-3. Nat Med 7:199–205

Makinen T, Veikkola T, Mustjoki S, Karpanen T, Catimel B, Nice EC, Wise L, Mercer A, Kowalski H, Kerjaschki D, Stacker SA, Achen MG, Alitalo K (2001b) Isolated lymphatic endothelial cells transduce growth, survival and migratory signals via the VEGF-C/D receptor VEGFR-3. EMBO J 20:4762–4773

Mandriota SJ, Jussila L, Jeltsch M, Compagni A, Baetens D, Prevo R, Banerji S, Huarte J, Montesano R, Jackson DG, Orci L, Alitalo K, Christofori G, Pepper MS (2001) Vascular endothelial growth factor-C-mediated lymphangiogenesis promotes tumour metastasis. EMBO J 20:672–682

Marconcini L, Marchio S, Morbidelli L, Cartocci E, Albini A, Ziche M, Bussolino F, Oliviero S (1999) c-fos-induced growth factor/vascular endothelial growth factor D induces angiogenesis in vivo and in vitro. Proc Natl Acad Sci U S A 96:9671–9676

Mashino K, Sadanaga N, Yamaguchi H, Tanaka F, Ohta M, Shibuta K, Inoue H, Mori M (2002) Expression of chemokine receptor CCR7 is associated with lymph node metastasis of gastric carcinoma. Cancer Res 62:2937–2941

May M, Kaufmann O, Hammermann F, Loy V, Siegsmund M (2007) Prognostic impact of lymphovascular invasion in radical prostatectomy specimens. BJU Int 99:539–544

Melder RJ, Koenig GC, Witwer BP, Safabakhsh N, Munn LL, Jain RK (1996) During angiogenesis, vascular endothelial growth factor and basic fibroblast growth factor regulate natural killer cell adhesion to tumor endothelium. Nat Med 2:992–997

Mishima K, Watabe T, Saito A, Yoshimatsu Y, Imaizumi N, Masui S, Hirashima M, Morisada T, Oike Y, Araie M, Niwa H, Kubo H, Suda T, Miyazono K (2007) Prox1 induces lymphatic endothelial differentiation via integrin alpha9 and other signaling cascades. Mol Biol Cell 18: 1421–1429

Mortimer PS (1998) The pathophysiology of lymphedema. Cancer 83:2798–2802

Muller A, Homey B, Soto H, Ge N, Catron D, Buchanan ME, McClanahan T, Murphy E, Yuan W, Wagner SN, Barrera JL, Mohar A, Verastegui E, Zlotnik A (2001) Involvement of chemokine receptors in breast cancer metastasis. Nature 410:50–56

Nagy JA, Vasile E, Feng D, Sundberg C, Brown LF, Detmar MJ, Lawitts JA, Benjamin L, Tan X, Manseau EJ, Dvorak AM, Dvorak HF (2002) Vascular permeability factor/vascular endothelial growth factor induces lymphangiogenesis as well as angiogenesis. J Exp Med 196:1497–1506

Northup KA, Witte MH, Witte CL (2003) Syndromic classification of hereditary lymphedema. Lymphology 36:162–189

Ny A, Koch M, Schneider M, Neven E, Tong RT, Maity S, Fischer C, Plaisance S, Lambrechts D, Heligon C, Terclavers S, Ciesiolka M, Kalin R, Man WY, Senn I, Wyns S, Lupu F, Brandli A, Vleminckx K, Collen D, Dewerchin M, Conway EM, Moons L, Jain RK, Carmeliet P (2005) A genetic *Xenopus laevis* tadpole model to study lymphangiogenesis. Nat Med 11:998–1004

Oh SJ, Jeltsch MM, Birkenhager R, McCarthy JE, Weich HA, Christ B, Alitalo K, Wilting J (1997) VEGF and VEGF-C: specific induction of angiogenesis and lymphangiogenesis in the differentiated avian chorioallantoic membrane. Dev Biol 188:96–109

Okada S, Albrecht RM, Aharinejad S, Schraufnagel DE (2002) Structural aspects of the lymphocyte traffic in rat submandibular lymph node. Microsc Microanal 8:116–133

Ostman A, Heldin CH (2007) PDGF receptors as targets in tumor treatment. Adv Cancer Res 97:247–274

Padera TP, Kadambi A, di Tomaso E, Carreira CM, Brown EB, Boucher Y, Choi NC, Mathisen D, Wain J, Mark EJ, Munn LL, Jain RK (2002) Lymphatic metastasis in the absence of functional intratumor lymphatics. Science 296:1883–1886

Padera TP, Kuo AH, Hoshida T, Liao S, Lobo J, Kozak KR, Fukumura D, Jain RK (2008) Differential response of primary tumor versus lymphatic metastasis to VEGFR-2 and VEGFR-3 kinase inhibitors cediranib and vandetanib. Mol Cancer Ther 7:2272–2279

Paget S. The distribution of secondary growths in cancer of the breast. *Lancet.* 1889;1:571–573.

Partanen TA, Arola J, Saaristo A, Jussila L, Ora A, Miettinen M, Stacker SA, Achen MG, Alitalo K (2000) VEGF-C and VEGF-D expression in neuroendocrine cells and their receptor, VEGFR-3, in fenestrated blood vessels in human tissues. FASEB J 14:2087–2096

Petrova TV, Makinen T, Makela TP, Saarela J, Virtanen I, Ferrell RE, Finegold DN, Kerjaschki D, Yla-Herttuala S, Alitalo K (2002) Lymphatic endothelial reprogramming of vascular endothelial cells by the Prox-1 homeobox transcription factor. EMBO J 21:4593–4599

Petrova TV, Karpanen T, Norrmen C, Mellor R, Tamakoshi T, Finegold D, Ferrell R, Kerjaschki D, Mortimer P, Yla-Herttuala S, Miura N, Alitalo K (2004) Defective valves and abnormal mural cell recruitment underlie lymphatic vascular failure in lymphedema distichiasis. Nat Med 10:974–981

Podgrabinska S, Braun P, Velasco P, Kloos B, Pepper MS, Skobe M (2002) Molecular characterization of lymphatic endothelial cells. Proc Natl Acad Sci U S A 99:16069–16074

Pytowski B, Goldman J, Persaud K, Wu Y, Witte L, Hicklin DJ, Skobe M, Boardman KC, Swartz MA (2005) Complete and specific inhibition of adult

lymphatic regeneration by a novel VEGFR-3 neutralizing antibody. J Natl Cancer Inst 97:14–21
Qian CN, Berghuis B, Tsarfaty G, Bruch M, Kort EJ, Ditlev J, Tsarfaty I, Hudson E, Jackson DG, Petillo D, Chen J, Resau JH, Teh BT (2006) Preparing the "soil": the primary tumor induces vasculature reorganization in the sentinel lymph node before the arrival of metastatic cancer cells. Cancer Res 66:10365–10376
Reinmuth N, Liersch R, Raedel M, Fehrmann F, Fehrmann N, Bayer M, Schwoeppe C, Kessler T, Berdel W, Thomas M, Mesters RM (2009) Combined anti-PDGFRalpha and PDGFRbeta targeting in non-small cell lung cancer. Int J Cancer 124(7):1535–1544
Rissanen TT, Markkanen JE, Gruchala M, Heikura T, Puranen A, Kettunen MI, Kholova I, Kauppinen RA, Achen MG, Stacker SA, Alitalo K, Yla-Herttuala S (2003) VEGF-D is the strongest angiogenic and lymphangiogenic effector among VEGFs delivered into skeletal muscle via adenoviruses. Circ Res 92:1098–1106
Roberts N, Kloos B, Cassella M, Podgrabinska S, Persaud K, Wu Y, Pytowski B, Skobe M (2006) Inhibition of VEGFR-3 activation with the antagonistic antibody more potently suppresses lymph node and distant metastases than inactivation of VEGFR-2. Cancer Res 66:2650–2657
Rockson SG (2001) Lymphedema. Am J Med 110: 288–295
Rubbia-Brandt L, Terris B, Giostra E, Dousset B, Morel P, Pepper MS (2004) Lymphatic vessel density and vascular endothelial growth factor-C expression correlate with malignant behavior in human pancreatic endocrine tumors. Clin Cancer Res 10:6919–6928
Ruddell A, Mezquita P, Brandvold KA, Farr A, Iritani BM (2003) B lymphocyte-specific c-Myc expression stimulates early and functional expansion of the vasculature and lymphatics during lymphomagenesis. Am J Pathol 163:2233–2245
Sabin F (1902) On the origin of the lymphatics system from the veins and the development of the lymph hearts and thorarcic duct in the pig. Am J Anat 1:367–391
Sabin F (1904) On the development of the superficial lymphatics in the skin of the pig. Am J Anat 3:183–195
Saeki H, Moore AM, Brown MJ, Hwang ST (1999) Cutting edge: secondary lymphoid-tissue chemokine (SLC) and CC chemokine receptor 7 (CCR7) participate in the emigration pathway of mature dendritic cells from the skin to regional lymph nodes. J Immunol 162:2472–2475
Sauter B, Foedinger D, Sterniczky B, Wolff K, Rappersberger K (1998) Immunoelectron microscopic characterization of human dermal lymphatic microvascular endothelial cells. Differential expression of CD31, CD34, and type IV collagen with lymphatic endothelial cells vs blood capillary endothelial cells in normal human skin, lymphangioma, and hemangioma in situ. J Histochem Cytochem 46: 165–176
Schacht V, Ramirez MI, Hong YK, Hirakawa S, Feng D, Harvey N, Williams M, Dvorak AM, Dvorak HF, Oliver G, Detmar M (2003) T1alpha/podoplanin deficiency disrupts normal lymphatic vasculature formation and causes lymphedema. EMBO J 22:3546–3556
Schneider M, Othman-Hassan K, Christ B, Wilting J (1999) Lymphangioblasts in the avian wing bud. Dev Dyn 216:311–319
Schoppmann SF, Birner P, Stockl J, Kalt R, Ullrich R, Caucig C, Kriehuber E, Nagy K, Alitalo K, Kerjaschki D (2002) Tumor-associated macrophages express lymphatic endothelial growth factors and are related to peritumoral lymphangiogenesis. Am J Pathol 161:947–956
Shields JD, Emmett MS, Dunn DB, Joory KD, Sage LM, Rigby H, Mortimer PS, Orlando A, Levick JR, Bates DO (2007) Chemokine-mediated migration of melanoma cells towards lymphatics–a mechanism contributing to metastasis. Oncogene 26:2997–3005
Shirasawa Y, Ikomi F, Ohhashi T (2000) Physiological roles of endogenous nitric oxide in lymphatic pump activity of rat mesentery in vivo. Am J Physiol Gastrointest Liver Physiol 278:G551–G556
Skobe M, Hawighorst T, Jackson DG, Prevo R, Janes L, Velasco P, Riccardi L, Alitalo K, Claffey K, Detmar M (2001) Induction of tumor lymphangiogenesis by VEGF-C promotes breast cancer metastasis. Nat Med 7:192–198
Stacker SA, Stenvers K, Caesar C, Vitali A, Domagala T, Nice E, Roufail S, Simpson RJ, Moritz R, Karpanen T, Alitalo K, Achen MG (1999) Biosynthesis of vascular endothelial growth factor-D involves proteolytic processing which generates non-covalent homodimers. J Biol Chem 274:32127–32136
Stacker SA, Caesar C, Baldwin ME, Thornton GE, Williams RA, Prevo R, Jackson DG, Nishikawa S,

Kubo H, Achen MG (2001) VEGF-D promotes the metastatic spread of tumor cells via the lymphatics. Nat Med 7:186–191

Stacker SA, Achen MG, Jussila L, Baldwin ME, Alitalo K (2002) Lymphangiogenesis and cancer metastasis. Nat Rev Cancer 2:573–583

Suzuki-Inoue K, Kato Y, Inoue O, Kaneko MK, Mishima K, Yatomi Y, Yamazaki Y, Narimatsu H, Ozaki Y (2007) Involvement of the snake toxin receptor CLEC-2, in podoplanin-mediated platelet activation, by cancer cells. J Biol Chem 282: 25993–26001

Szuba A, Skobe M, Karkkainen MJ, Shin WS, Beynet DP, Rockson NB, Dakhil N, Spilman S, Goris ML, Strauss HW, Quertermous T, Alitalo K, Rockson SG (2002) Therapeutic lymphangiogenesis with human recombinant VEGF-C. FASEB J 16:1985–1987

Tait CR, Jones PF (2004) Angiopoietins in tumours: the angiogenic switch. J Pathol 204:1–10

Takanami I (2003) Overexpression of CCR7 mRNA in nonsmall cell lung cancer: correlation with lymph node metastasis. Int J Cancer 105:186–189

Takeuchi H, Fujimoto A, Tanaka M, Yamano T, Hsueh E, Hoon DS (2004) CCL21 chemokine regulates chemokine receptor CCR7 bearing malignant melanoma cells. Clin Cancer Res 10:2351–2358

Tammela T, Saaristo A, Holopainen T, Lyytikka J, Kotronen A, Pitkonen M, Abo-Ramadan U, Yla-Herttuala S, Petrova TV, Alitalo K (2007) Therapeutic differentiation and maturation of lymphatic vessels after lymph node dissection and transplantation. Nat Med 13:1458–1466

Tammela T, Zarkada G, Wallgard E, Murtomaki A, Suchting S, Wirzenius M, Waltari M, Hellstrom M, Schomber T, Peltonen R, Freitas C, Duarte A, Isoniemi H, Laakkonen P, Christofori G, Yla-Herttuala S, Shibuya M, Pytowski B, Eichmann A, Betsholtz C, Alitalo K (2008) Blocking VEGFR-3 suppresses angiogenic sprouting and vascular network formation. Nature 454:656–660

Tang Y, Zhang D, Fallavollita L, Brodt P (2003) Vascular endothelial growth factor C expression and lymph node metastasis are regulated by the type I insulin-like growth factor receptor. Cancer Res 63:1166–1171

Taniguchi K, Kohno R, Ayada T, Kato R, Ichiyama K, Morisada T, Oike Y, Yonemitsu Y, Maehara Y, Yoshimura A (2007) Spreds are essential for embryonic lymphangiogenesis by regulating vascular endothelial growth factor receptor 3 signaling. Mol Cell Biol 27:4541–4550

Van den Eynden GG, Van der Auwera I, Van Laere SJ, Huygelen V, Colpaert CG, van Dam P, Dirix LY, Vermeulen PB, Van Marck EA (2006) Induction of lymphangiogenesis in and around axillary lymph node metastases of patients with breast cancer. Br J Cancer 95:1362–1366

Van den Eynden GG, Vandenberghe MK, van Dam PJ, Colpaert CG, van Dam P, Dirix LY, Vermeulen PB, Van Marck EA (2007) Increased sentinel lymph node lymphangiogenesis is associated with nonsentinel axillary lymph node involvement in breast cancer patients with a positive sentinel node. Clin Cancer Res 13:5391–5397

Veikkola T, Jussila L, Makinen T, Karpanen T, Jeltsch M, Petrova TV, Kubo H, Thurston G, McDonald DM, Achen MG, Stacker SA, Alitalo K (2001) Signalling via vascular endothelial growth factor receptor-3 is sufficient for lymphangiogenesis in transgenic mice. EMBO J 20:1223–1231

Veikkola T, Lohela M, Ikenberg K, Makinen T, Korff T, Saaristo A, Petrova T, Jeltsch M, Augustin HG, Alitalo K (2003) Intrinsic versus microenvironmental regulation of lymphatic endothelial cell phenotype and function. FASEB J 17:2006–2013

von der Weid PY (2001) Lymphatic vessel pumping and inflammation–the role of spontaneous constrictions and underlying electrical pacemaker potentials. Aliment Pharmacol Ther 15:1115–1129

Wang JF, Zhang XF, Groopman JE (2001) Stimulation of beta 1 integrin induces tyrosine phosphorylation of vascular endothelial growth factor receptor-3 and modulates cell migration. J Biol Chem 276:41950–41957

Wang J, Xi L, Hunt JL, Gooding W, Whiteside TL, Chen Z, Godfrey TE, Ferris RL (2004) Expression pattern of chemokine receptor 6 (CCR6) and CCR7 in squamous cell carcinoma of the head and neck identifies a novel metastatic phenotype. Cancer Res 64:1861–1866

Weiss L (1992) Biomechanical interactions of cancer cells with the microvasculature during hematogenous metastasis. Cancer Metastasis Rev 11: 227–235

Wetterwald A, Hoffstetter W, Cecchini MG, Lanske B, Wagner C, Fleisch H, Atkinson M (1996) Characterization and cloning of the E11 antigen, a marker expressed by rat osteoblasts and osteocytes. Bone 18:125–132

Whitehurst B, Flister MJ, Bagaitkar J, Volk L, Bivens CM, Pickett B, Castro-Rivera E, Brekken RA, Gerard RD, Ran S (2007) Anti-VEGF-A therapy reduces lymphatic vessel density and expression of VEGFR-3 in an orthotopic breast tumor model. Int J Cancer 121:2181–2191

Wick N, Saharinen P, Saharinen J, Gurnhofer E, Steiner CW, Raab I, Stokic D, Giovanoli P, Buchsbaum S, Burchard A, Thurner S, Alitalo K, Kerjaschki D (2007) Transcriptomal comparison of human dermal lymphatic endothelial cells ex vivo and in vitro. Physiol Genomics 28:179–192

Wicki A, Lehembre F, Wick N, Hantusch B, Kerjaschki D, Christofori G (2006) Tumor invasion in the absence of epithelial-mesenchymal transition: podoplanin-mediated remodeling of the actin cytoskeleton. Cancer Cell 9:261–272

Wigle JT, Oliver G (1999) Prox1 function is required for the development of the murine lymphatic system. Cell 98:769–778

Wigle JT, Harvey N, Detmar M, Lagutina I, Grosveld G, Gunn MD, Jackson DG, Oliver G (2002) An essential role for Prox1 in the induction of the lymphatic endothelial cell phenotype. EMBO J 21:1505–1513

Wiley HE, Gonzalez EB, Maki W, Wu MT, Hwang ST (2001) Expression of CC chemokine receptor-7 and regional lymph node metastasis of B16 murine melanoma. J Natl Cancer Inst 93:1638–1643

Wilting J, Neeff H, Christ B (1999) Embryonic lymphangiogenesis. Cell Tissue Res 297:1–11

Wirzenius M, Tammela T, Uutela M, He Y, Odorisio T, Zambruno G, Nagy JA, Dvorak HF, Yla-Herttuala S, Shibuya M, Alitalo K (2007) Distinct vascular endothelial growth factor signals for lymphatic vessel enlargement and sprouting. J Exp Med 204:1431–1440

Wissmann C, Detmar M (2006) Pathways targeting tumor lymphangiogenesis. Clin Cancer Res 12:6865–6868

Witte MH, Erickson R, Bernas M, Andrade M, Reiser F, Conlon W, Hoyme HE, Witte CL (1998) Phenotypic and genotypic heterogeneity in familial Milroy lymphedema. Lymphology 31:145–155

Witzenbichler B, Asahara T, Murohara T, Silver M, Spyridopoulos I, Magner M, Principe N, Kearney M, Hu JS, Isner JM (1998) Vascular endothelial growth factor-C (VEGF-C/VEGF-2) promotes angiogenesis in the setting of tissue ischemia. Am J Pathol 153:381–394

Yan C, Zhu ZG, Yu YY, Ji J, Zhang Y, Ji YB, Yan M, Chen J, Liu BY, Yin HR, Lin YZ (2004) Expression of vascular endothelial growth factor C and chemokine receptor CCR7 in gastric carcinoma and their values in predicting lymph node metastasis. World J Gastroenterol 10: 783–790

Yancopoulos GD, Davis S, Gale NW, Rudge JS, Wiegand SJ, Holash J (2000) Vascular-specific growth factors and blood vessel formation. Nature 407:242–248

Yuan L, Moyon D, Pardanaud L, Breant C, Karkkainen MJ, Alitalo K, Eichmann A (2002) Abnormal lymphatic vessel development in Neuropilin-2 mutant mice. Development 129: 4797–4806

Compounds in Clinical Phase III and Beyond

9

Torsten Kessler, Michael Bayer, Christian Schwöppe,
Rüdiger Liersch, Rolf M. Mesters, and Wolfgang E. Berdel

Abstract Targeted therapies against cancer have become more and more important. In particular, the inhibition of tumor angiogenesis and vascular targeting have been the focus of new treatment strategies. Numerous new substances were developed as angiogenesis inhibitors and evaluated in clinical trials for safety, tolerance, and efficacy. With positive study results, some of these molecules have already been approved for clinical use. For example, this is true for the vascular endothelial growth factor neutralizing antibody bevacizumab (BEV) in metastatic colorectal cancer, nonsmall cell lung cancer, renal cancer, and breast cancer. The tyrosine kinase (TK) inhibitors sorafenib and sunitinib have been approved for metastatic renal cancer as well as for hepatocellular carcinoma, and sunitinib has also been approved for gastrointestinal stroma tumors. In this chapter we try to give an overview of the substances currently investigated in Phase III studies and beyond with regard to antiangiogenesis in cancer therapy.

T. Kessler (✉)
Department of Medicine,
Hematology and Oncology, University of Münster,
Albert-Schweitzer-Strasse, 33, 48129,
Münster, Germany
e-mail: torstenkessler@uni-muenster.de

9.1 Introduction

Besides surgery and radiation, chemotherapy has been the cornerstone of cancer treatment for decades. Over the past ten years, a new generation of substances has come into focus targeting molecular pathways in the malignant cell itself or in cells supporting tumor growth, more specifically. For example, strategies aiming at tumor angiogenesis have been extensively studied, following observations that the growth and metastasis of tumors depend on the development of vascular supply. This research led to the isolation of an array of mediators that are capable of inhibiting tumor angiogenesis. Possibly the most pivotal positive regulator of angiogenesis is vascular endothelial growth factor (VEGF). Strategies to either block binding of VEGF to its receptors or to block intracellular signaling events in the downstream cascade represent the basis of many new developments in antiangiogenic cancer therapy (Ferrara et al. 2003).

During the 1990s, the first angiogenesis inhibitors entered clinical trials for cancer therapy. The first drug in this class that was granted approval by the Food and Drug Administration (FDA) in the United States was the anti-VEGF antibody BEV in 2004 (Ferrara et al. 2004). Soon, broad-spectrum receptor tyrosine kinase

R. Liersch et al. (eds.), *Angiogenesis Inhibition,* Recent Results in Cancer Research,
DOI: 10.1007/978-3-540-78281-0_9, © Springer Verlag Berlin Heidelberg 2010

9

(TK) inhibitors (RTKI) targeting the VEGF/VEGFR pathway followed in clinical development. The idea behind the development of these compounds was partly based on the rather modest activity of the BEV when used as monotherapy, giving a rationale for higher efficacy when aiming at more than one target. In fact, most agents currently investigated in clinical studies work by mechanisms illustrated in Fig. 9.1. By now at least the RTKIs sorafenib and sunitinib are also approved for treatment of certain cancers, and more than 40 other drugs that were preclinically screened and selected for their anti-angiogenic activity are listed in clinical trials of the National Cancer Institute's (NCI) database.

This chapter summarizes some of the substances currently approved or investigated as antiangiogenic cancer drugs in Phase III studies and beyond.

9.1.1 Anti-VEGF Antibody (Bevacizumab, Avastin™)

The humanized monoclonal anti-VEGF antibody BEV is the first VEGF targeting drug which has been officially approved for cancer therapy (Ferrara et al. 2004). In particular, BEV is approved, in combination with intravenous 5-fluorouracil-based (5-FU) chemotherapy, for

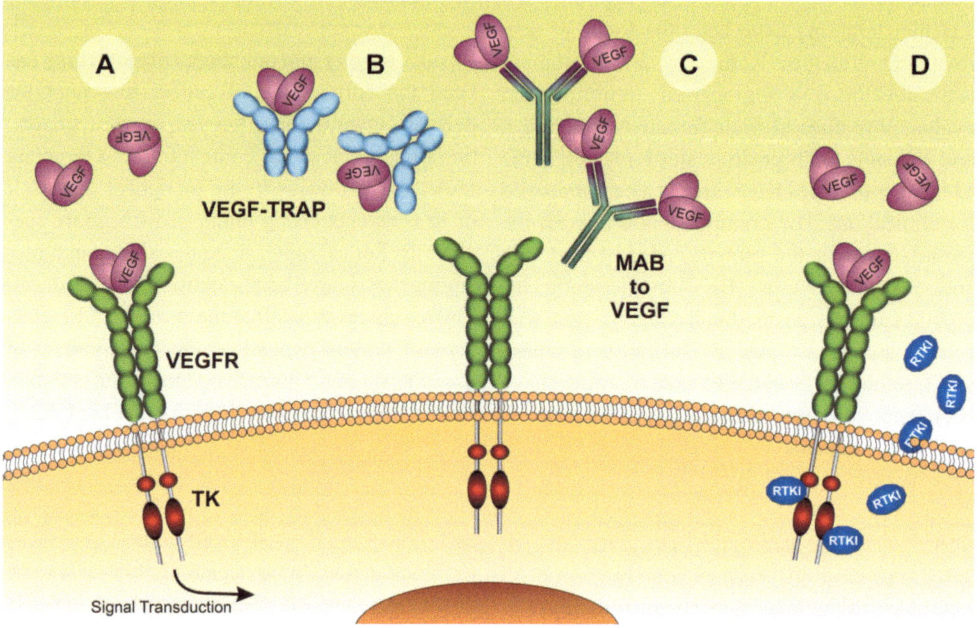

Fig. 9.1 *Therapeutic strategies to target the VEGF/VEGF receptor (VEGFR) system.* (**a**) Tumors secrete VEGF in response to hypoxia, VEGF binds to VEGFR-2 on endothelial cells, thereby switching on the intracellular tyrosine kinase (TK) activity. Subsequent signal transduction steps promote proliferation, migration, invasion and tumor angiogenesis. Downregulation of VEGF secretion on the tumor side can be achieved by antagonists of the Epidermal Growth Factor Receptor (EGFR) and other "accidental" antiangiogenic drugs. (**b**) VEGF-TRAP (Aflibercept), fusion protein of the second IgG domain of VEGFR-1, the third IgG domain of VEGFR-2 and the Fc region of human IgG functions as decoy receptor. (**c**) Mab against VEGF (bevacizumab; Avastin™) prevents binding to VEGFR. (**d**) Small molecule Receptor tyrosine kinase inhibitors (RTKI) suppress kinase activity of VEGFR after VEGF binding; e.g., sorafenib, sunitinib, axitinib, vatalanib, vandetanib, cediranib

first- or second-line treatment of patients with metastatic carcinoma of the colon or rectum and in combination with carboplatin and paclitaxel for the first-line treatment of patients with unresectable, locally advanced, recurrent, or metastatic nonsquamous nonsmall cell lung cancer (NSCLC). Furthermore, it has been approved in combination with paclitaxel for first-line treatment of patients with metastatic breast cancer and in combination with interferon α-2a for first-line treatment of patients with advanced and/or metastatic renal cell cancer (RCC). The original FDA approval for BEV in 2004 was based on data from a large, placebo-controlled, randomized study demonstrating prolongation in the median survival of patients with metastatic colorectal cancer (CRC) treated with BEV in addition to a combination chemotherapy regimen containing 5-FU, Leucovorin, and Irinotecan (IFL) by approximately five months, compared to patients treated with the IFL chemotherapy regimen alone (20.3 vs. 15.6 months). At that time, this study represented one of the largest improvements in survival ever reported in a randomized, Phase III study of patients with metastatic CRC (Hurwitz et al. 2004). The following approval for second-line therapy was based on results of a randomized, controlled, multicenter Phase III trial (E3200) of 829 patients with advanced or metastatic CRC who had received previous treatment with irinotecan and 5-FU as initial therapy for metastatic disease or as adjuvant therapy (Giantonio et al. 2007). In detail, it could be shown that patients who received BEV plus the 5-FU-based chemotherapy regimen known as FOLFOX4 (oxaliplatin/5-FU/leucovorin) had a 33% improvement in overall survival (OS), compared to patients who received FOLFOX4 alone (hazard ratio (HR) 0.75). Median OS for patients receiving BEV plus FOLFOX4 was 13.0 months, compared to 10.8 months for those receiving FOLFOX4 alone. The third approval and first in another cancer type was based on results from E4599, a randomized, controlled, multicenter trial that enrolled 878 patients with unresectable, locally advanced, recurrent, or metastatic nonsquamous NSCLC (Sandler et al. 2006). Results showed that patients receiving BEV plus paclitaxel and carboplatin chemotherapies had a 25% improvement in OS, the trial's primary end point, compared to patients who received chemotherapy alone (hazard ratio (HR) 0.80). One-year survival was 51% in the BEV arm vs. 44% in the chemotherapy-alone arm. Median OS of patients treated with BEV plus chemotherapy was 12.5 months, compared to 10.2 months for patients treated with chemotherapy alone. Notably, a pilot study including NSCLC patients with squamous histology prior to E4599 showed an increased death rate in the BEV arm due to fatal pulmonal hemorrhages, leading to exclusion of this subtype for further studies (Johnson et al. 2004). Subsequently, BEV has been approved in first-line therapy of metastatic breast cancer, which was based on an improvement in progression-free survival (PFS) only. In this study 722 patients who had not received chemotherapy for locally recurrent or metastatic breast cancer were randomized to receive either paclitaxel alone or in combination with BEV (Miller et al. 2007). The addition of BEV to paclitaxel resulted in an improvement in PFS (11.3 vs. 5.8 months; $p<0.0001$) with no significant improvement in OS (26.5 vs. 24.8 months; $p=0.14$). Partial response (PR) rates in patients with measurable disease were higher with BEV plus paclitaxel, but no complete responses (CR) were observed. This has led to a limited approval of BEV not including patients with breast cancer that has progressed following anthracycline and taxane chemotherapy administered for metastatic disease. The most recent approval for BEV has been granted for the combination with interferon-α (IFN-α) as first-line treatment of patients with advanced and/or metastatic clear RCC. This was based on a multicentre, randomized, Phase III study, randomizing 649 patients with previously untreated metastatic RCC to receive IFN-α plus BEV or placebo (Escudier et al. 2007a). Median duration of PFS was significantly longer in the BEV plus IFN-α group than it was in the control group (10.2 vs. 5.4 months; $p<0.0001$). With regard to OS, only a trend in favor of the BEV group could be observed.

Currently, BEV is listed in 47 clinical phase III trials, mostly evaluating new combinations for approved indications such as breast cancer, CRC, and NSCLC, but also for other entities such as lymphoma or osteosarcoma (see Table 9.1).

9.1.2 Aflibercept (VEGF – Trap)

Another approach to target the VEGF/VEGF receptor system is to deliver a soluble decoy for VEGF. To this end, a recombinant fusion protein was constructed from the second Ig domain of VEGFR-1 and the third Ig domain of VEGFR-2, fused to the Fc region of human IgG (Aflibercept; VEGF – trap, Regeneron in cooperation with Sanofi-Aventis). The resulting decoy receptor possesses an affinity for all VEGF isoforms that is significantly higher than that of the monoclonal antibody. In addition, aflibercept binds Placental Growth Factor (PLGF), which has also been implicated in tumor angiogenesis. Numerous preclinical models demonstrated significant inhibition of angiogenesis and tumor growth (Holash et al. 2002; Kim et al. 2002a). The first clinical Phase II study published is an open-label, multicenter, two-stage trial in patients with metastatic CRC with at least one prior systemic therapy and good performance status (Tang et al. 2008). Prior treatment with a VEGF or VEGFR inhibitor other than BEV was not allowed. Aflibercept (4 mg/kg) was administered every 2 weeks intravenously. In total, 51 patients were included (BEV naive=24 patients; prior BEV=27; median age=59). During 287 therapy cycles, most common adverse events (AE) of any grade were fatigue (n=40), hypertension (n=28), proteinuria (n=25), headache (n=22), voice alteration (n=16), anorexia (n=12), and joint pain (n=9). Serious AE (Grade 3/4) consisted of hypertension (n=4), proteinuria (n=4), fatigue (n=3), headache (n=3). One patient died during treatment due to progressive disease (PD). In the BEV naïve group (n=24), disease control rate defined as either PR or stable disease (SD) for at least 16 weeks was 29% (95% Confidence Interval (CI) 13–51%), and median PFS was 2.0 months (95% CI 1.7 – not reached). In the group with prior BEV treatment (n=27), disease control rate was 30% (95% CI 14–50%) and median PFS was 3.4 months (95% CI 1.9 – not reached). The authors concluded that aflibercept is well tolerated in pretreated patients with CRC and shows single agent activity (Tang et al. 2008). Based on the study results, aflibercept is now tested in a randomized Phase III study in combination with irinotecan based second-line chemotherapy for patients with CRC. Other currently listed Phase III studies for aflibercept evaluate its efficacy in prostate cancer, NSCLC, advanced ovarian and pancreatic cancer (see Table 9.1).

9.1.2.1 Sorafenib (Nexavar™)

Sorafenib (Nexavar™; Bayer Pharmaceuticals) represents the class of small-molecule compounds with activity against a broad spectrum of receptor tyrosine kinases. Originally developed as RAF-1 inhibitor in a high-throughput screening program, sorafenib later was found to be active against VEGFR-1/-2/-3; platelet derived growth factor (PDGF) -β receptor; Fms-like tyrosine kinase-3 (FLT-3); c-Kit protein and RET receptor tyrosine kinases (Adnane et al. 2006). Thereby, sorafenib inhibits tumor growth by targeting the endothelial cell as well as the tumor cell and was shown to inhibit proliferation, promote apoptosis, and disrupt angiogenesis. In preclinical mechanism of action studies, sorafenib demonstrated a potent antiangiogenic effect in nearly all models tested, resulting in significant reduction of micro-vessel density (Strumberg 2005; Wilhelm et al. 2006). It also showed promising activity in tumor xenograft models in nude mice in combination with

Table 9.1 Inhibitors of angiogenesis currently approved and investigated in clinical phase III studies (Numbers in brackets according to the U.S. National Cancer Institute Clinical Trial Identifier Code)

Drug	Approved	Phase III
Bevacizumab (Avastin™) Monoclonal antibody that binds and inactivates VEGF	First approval 2004: in combination with chemotherapy for metastatic CRC (first and second line), unresectable NSCLC (2006), metastatic breast cancer (2007), in combination with IFN-α for RCC	Forty-seven active phase III trials: evaluating further combinations for approved entities but also new indications such as mesothelioma (NCT00651456), ovarian cancer (NCT00262847), GIST (NCT00324987), lymphoma (NCT00486759), gastric cancer (NCT00548548), carcinoid (NCT00569127), head-and-neck cancer (NCT00588770), osteosarcoma (NCT00667342), and cervix carcinoma (NCT00803062)
Aflibercept (VEGF-trap) binds and neutralizes VEGF as decoy receptor		Four active phase III trials: with docetaxel in metastatic HRPC (NCT00519285), with docetaxel as second-line therapy in metastatic NSCLC (NCT00532155), with irinotecan and 5-FU for metastatic CRC as second line after oxaliplation failure (NCT00561470), with gemcitabine for first-line therapy of metastatic pancreatic cancer (NCT00574275)
Sorafenib (Nexavar™) RTKI active against VEGFRs, PDGFR, c-Kit, FLT-3, RET, RAF-1	First approval 2005: advanced RCC after failure of cytokine therapy or patients unsuitable for such therapy. Advanced HCC as first-line therapy (2008)	Ten active phase III trials: further combinations for approved entities, new indications include unresectable stage III and IV melanoma (NCT00111007) and in combination with gemcitabine for advanced pancreatic cancer (NCT00541021)
Sunitinib (Sutent™) RTKI active against VEGFRs, PDGFR, c-Kit, FLT-3	First approval 2006: advanced RCC as first-line therapy. Advanced GIST after imatinib failure	Twenty active phase III trials: further combinations for approved entities, new indications include the combination with paclitaxel in breast cancer (NCT00373256), with capecitabine in breast cancer (NCT00373113), for pancreatic islet tumors (NCT00428597), with erlotinib in NSCLC (NCT00457392), with FOLFIRI in mCRC (NCT00457691), after failure of docetaxel in HRPC (NCT00676650). Head-to-head study against sorafenib for advanced HCC first line therapy (NCT00699374)
Axitinib (AG-013736) RTKI active against VEGFRs, PDGFR, c-Kit		Two active phase III trials: in combination with gemcitabine for advanced pancreatic cancer (NCT00471146), as second-line therapy for metastatic RCC (NCT00678392)

(*continued*)

Table 9.1 (continued)

Drug	Approved	Phase III
Cediranib (AZD2171; Recentin™) RTKI active against VEGFRs, PDGFR, c-Kit, EGFR		Five active phase III trials: in combination with FOLFOX or XELOX for first-line therapy of mCRC (NCT00384176, NCT00399035), with platinum based chemotherapy for ovarian epithelial, fallopian tube or primary peritoneal carcinoma (NCT00544973), with lomustin in recurrent glioblastoma (NCT00777153), with carboplatin/paclitaxel in stage IIIb/IV NSCLC (NCT00795340)
Vandetanib (ZD6474; Zactima™) RTKI active against VEGFR-2 and -3, RET and EGFR		Four recently completed phase III trials: vs. erlotinib in second line therapy of NSCLC (NCT00364351), after EGFR-antagonist failure as monotherapy (NCT00404924), in combination with pemetrexed in second-line therapy of NSCLC (NCT00418886), combined with docetaxel in second-line therapy of NSCLC (NCT00312377). Significant improvement in PFS for vandetanib (press release)
Vatalanib (PTK787/ ZK222584) RTKI active against VEGFRs, c-KIT and PDGFR		Two completed phase III trials: in combination with FOLFOX in first-line (NCT00056459) and second-line therapy of mCRC (NCT00068679). Clinical benefits in LDH high patients
rh-Endostatin (YH-16, Endostar™) endogenous angiogenesis inhibitor	First approval in 2005 (China): in combination with chemotherapy as first-line therapy of NSCLC	Two active phase III trials (China): in combination with Cisplatin and Vinorelbine as adjuvant therapy in stage IB-IIIA NSCLC after complete resection (NCT00576914). Combined with chemotherapy in metastatic NSCLC (biomarker analysis; NCT00657423)
Thalidomide not fully clarified mechanism: postulated direct apoptotic effect on endothelial cells via downregulation of angiogenic growth factors	First approval 1998: treatment of erythema nodosum leprosum (ENL). in combination with Dexamethason as first-line therapy of multiple myeloma (MM) (2003)	Twenty active phase III trials: new indications in MM, e.g., maintenance therapy after autologous stem cell transplantation (NCT00049673), in advanced HCC with poor liver reserve (NCT00225290), with transarterial chemoembolization in advanced HCC (NCT00522405)
Combretastatin-A4 (Zybrestat™) VDA with direct disrupting effect on the endothelial cytoskeleton	"Fast-track" status for anaplastic thyroid cancer	One active phase III trial: in combination with paclitaxel/carboplatin in the treatment of anaplastic thyroid cancer (NCT00507429)
DMXAA (ASA404) VDA with direct disrupting effect on the endothelial cytoskeleton and cytokine induction		Two active phase III trials: in combination with paclitaxel/carboplatin as first line therapy of stage IIIB/IV NSCLC (NCT00662597). In combination with docetaxel in second-line therapy of stage IIIB/IV NSCLC (NCT00738387)

chemotherapy. The first clinical entity in which sorafenib was tested again was clear-cell RCC (Kane et al. 2006). This cancer is special due to its loss of the von Hippel-Lindau tumor suppressor gene, which results in overexpression of hypoxia inducible factors (HIF) – 1 and – 2, subsequently upregulating pro-angiogenic factors (e.g., VEGF). The tumors are usually hypervascularized and increased RAF-1 activity also is found. All these pathways are within the target range for sorafenib providing a strong rationale for testing it in RCC.

In a number of Phase I/II trials, the optimal dose was determined to be 400 mg twice daily (b.i.d.) with dose-limiting toxicities (DLT) such as fatigue, skin rash, hand-foot syndrome, and diarrhea (Richly et al. 2006; Siu et al. 2006; Strumberg et al. 2006). Also, the postulated antiangiogenic effect was confirmed by diminished blood flow in dynamic contrast-enhanced magnetic resonance imaging (Flaherty et al. 2008). The most promising result was the significant increase in PFS in RCC patients treated with sorafenib (24 weeks) vs. placebo (6 weeks; $p=0.0087$) (Ratain et al. 2006).

This prompted the Phase III treatment approach in RCC global evaluation trial (TARGET), which represents the biggest randomized treatment trial for this disease so far (Escudier et al. 2007b). From November 2003 to March 2005, the participating 117 centers in 19 countries randomized 903 patients with advanced or metastatic RCC who failed standard therapy to receive either continuous treatment with oral sorafenib (at a dose of 400 mg b.i.d.) or placebo; resulting in 451 patients who received sorafenib and 452 who received placebo. A single planned analysis of PFS in January 2005 already demonstrated a statistically significant benefit of sorafenib over placebo. Regarding this result, patients who were on placebo were allowed to crossover to the sorafenib arm later that year. In detail, the PFS was 5.5 months in the sorafenib group and 2.8 months in the placebo group (HR for disease progression in the sorafenib group=0.44; 95% CI 0.35–0.55; $p<0.01$). The first interim analysis of the primary end point OS in May 2005 indicated that sorafenib reduced the risk of death, as compared with placebo (HR=0.72; 95% CI 0.54–0.94; $p=0.02$). However, this survival benefit did not meet the previously specified criteria for statistical significance. Only in a preplanned placebo-censored analysis, excluding patients who crossed over to sorafenib, results showed a significant survival advantage (17.8 months median OS vs. 14.3 months; HR=0.78; 95% CI 0.62–0.97; $p=0.0287$) (Bukowski et al. 2007). Partial responses were reported as the best response in 10% of patients receiving sorafenib and in 2% of those receiving placebo ($p<0.001$). Again, diarrhea, rash, fatigue, and hand-foot skin reactions were the most common AE associated with sorafenib. Hypertension and cardiac ischemia were more common in patients receiving sorafenib than in those receiving placebo. At the time of publication, the authors concluded that sorafenib prolongs PFS as compared with placebo in patients with advanced clear-cell RCC in whom previous therapy has failed. However, sorafenib therapy was associated with increased toxicities (Escudier et al. 2007b). In a concomitant quality of life (QOL) analysis it was shown that sorafenib had a positive effect on cancer-related symptoms and did not negatively impact QOL (Cella et al. 2006).

This result led to the approval of sorafenib for the treatment of patients with advanced RCC who have failed prior IFN-α or interleukin-2-based therapy, or are considered unsuitable for such therapy.

Apart from RCC, hepatocellular carcinoma (HCC) also represents a rather chemoresistant, but highly vascularized tumor with vast expression of VEGF. Furthermore, Raf-1 is constitutely overexpressed in HCC offering a rationale for treatment with sorafenib. A number of Phase I and II trials showed promising results for sorafenib either as monotherapy or in combination with doxorubicin (Abou-Alfa et al. 2006; Furuse et al. 2008; Gollob et al. 2007;

Richly et al. 2008). This prompted a randomized Phase III trial for patients with advanced or metastatic HCC in which sorafenib was compared with placebo (SHARP-trial). Patients with advanced measurable HCC in good performance status and Child-Pugh status A were treated with either sorafenib 400 mg b.i.d. or placebo. Overall, 602 patients were randomized leaving 299 in the sorafenib arm and 303 in the placebo arm. Baseline characteristics were similar for both arms. Based on 321 deaths (Sorafenib $n=143$; Placebo $n=178$), the HR for OS was 0.69 (95% CI 0.55–0.87; $p=0.0006$), representing a 44% improvement. This met early stopping criteria and median OS was 10.7 months for sorafenib vs. 7.9 for placebo. There was no accumulation of serious AE in the sorafenib arm. The most frequent grade 3/4 AE for sorafenib vs. placebo were diarrhea (11 vs. 2%), hand-foot skin reaction (8 vs. 1%), fatigue (10 vs. 15%), and bleeding (6 vs. 9%). At the time of presentation at the annual meeting of the American Society of Clinical Oncology (ASCO) in 2007, the authors concluded that sorafenib is the first drug to demonstrate a statistically significant improvement in OS for patients with advanced HCC (Llovet et al. 2007). Again, these findings led to the approval of sorafenib for this indication.

Currently, sorafenib is listed in ten active Phase III studies for treatment of RCC, HCC, NSCLC, unresectable melanoma and adenocarcinoma of the pancreas (see Table 9.1).

9.1.3 Sunitinib Malate (SU11248; Sutent™)

Sunitinib (SU11248; Sutent™; Pfizer Oncology) is a broad-spectrum orally available TK inhibitor of VEGFR, PDGFR, c-kit, and Flt-3 kinase activity. Just like sorafenib, it emerged from a drug-discovery program that was initiated to identify compounds with activity against selected receptor tyrosine kinases involved in tumor angiogenesis (Atkins et al. 2006; Roskoski 2007). Again, the highly vascularized clear cell RCC was one of the first diseases in which sunitinib was tested. After the promising Phase I and II results, a large multicentered, international randomized Phase III trial was started (Motzer et al. 2007). Single-agent sunitinib was compared with IFN-α in patients with treatment-naive advanced or metastatic RCC. Altogether, 750 patients were randomized (1:1) to receive either 50 mg sunitinib once daily in 6-week cycles (4 weeks on treatment, 2 weeks off) or to receive IFN-α administered subcutaneously at nine million units 3 times a week until disease progression or withdrawal from the trial.

Median duration of treatment was 11 months for sunitinib vs. 4 months for IFN-α. The 2008-updated response rate was 47% (95% CI 42–52%) for sunitinib vs. 12% (95% CI 9–16%) for IFN-α ($p<0.000001$), including 11 CR for sunitinib and four for IFN-α (Figlin et al. 2008). Median PFS was significantly higher in the sunitinib arm (11 months vs. 5 months; $p<0.000001$). Also the median OS was significantly longer for sunitinib (26.4 months; 95% CI 23.0–32.9) vs. IFN-α (21.8 months; 95% CI 17.9–26.9), which results in a HR of 0.821 (95% CI 0.673–1.001; $p=0.051$). The most common grade 3/4 treatment-related AEs for the sunitinib group were hypertension (12%), fatigue (11%), diarrhea and hand-foot syndrome (both 8%), and for IFN-α fatigue (13%) and anorexia (2%).

These results led to the approval of sunitinib in patients with advanced or metastatic RCC as first-line therapy and based on two other Phase II studies also as second-line therapy after cytokine or interferon failure (Motzer et al. 2006a, b).

Another malignant disease for which sunitinib has been approved is the gastrointestinal stroma tumor (GIST). Based on its strong activity against the GIST driving c-kit receptor, there was an imminent rationale for the therapy with sunitinib. Also, in cases of advanced, unresectable, or metastatic disease, the other TK inhibitor imatinib was already established as standard first-line therapy for this indication. However, after failure of imatinib, there was no accepted standard therapy available in unresectable GIST tumors (Faivre et al. 2007; Heinrich et al. 2008; Liegl et al. 2008).

Sunitinib was first tested in a population of GIST patients in two multicenter randomized studies. The first one represented a two-sided, randomized, double-blind, placebo-controlled trial of sunitinib in patients with GIST who had disease progression during prior imatinib treatment or who were intolerant of imatinib. Altogether, 312 patients were randomized (2:1) to receive either 50 mg sunitinib ($n=207$) or placebo orally ($n=105$), once daily, on the same 4 weeks on and 2 weeks off schedule until disease progression or withdrawal from the study for another reason. Patients randomized to placebo were then offered to crossover to open-label sunitinib (Demetri et al. 2006).

Demographics were comparable between the sunitinib and placebo groups with regard to age (69 vs. 72% younger than 65 years for sunitinib vs. placebo, respectively), gender (male: 64 vs. 61%), performance status (ECOG 0: 44 vs. 46%, ECOG 1: 55 vs. 52% and ECOG 2: 1 vs. 2%). Prior treatment included surgery (94 vs. 93%) and radiotherapy (8 vs. 15%). Reasons for imatinib failure were also comparably balanced between both arms; being intolerance (4 vs. 4%), progression within 6 months of starting treatment (17 vs. 16%), or progression beyond 6 months (78 vs. 80%).

The trial was unblinded early after the preplanned interim analysis including the first 149 cases of disease progression or death revealed significantly longer time to tumor progression (TTP) in patients initially treated with sunitinib than in those who started with placebo. In detail, the primary study endpoint, median TTP, was more than 4 times as long with sunitinib (27.3 weeks; 95% CI 16.0–32.1) as with placebo treatment (6.4 weeks; 95% CI 4.4–10.0; HR 0.33, 95% CI 0.23–0.47; $p<0{\cdot}0001$). All other efficacy analyzes were uniformly statistically and clinically significant and confirmed the findings of the primary endpoint data. The median PFS was similar to TPP (24.1 weeks; 95% CI 11.1–28.3 for sunitinib; 6.0 weeks for placebo, respectively; HR 0.33; 95% CI 0.24–0.47; $p<0{\cdot}0001$). Moreover, 16% (33) of patients in the sunitinib group were progression-free for at least 26 weeks, compared with 1% (one) in the placebo group. As more than half the patients in the initial sunitinib group were still alive at the time of the interim analysis, OS data were not mature at the time of publication and a median OS was not calculated. However, there was a gain in OS in patients treated initially with sunitinib compared to those who started on placebo despite the availability of the crossover option (HR 0.49, 95% CI 0.29–0.83; $p=0.007$). Later on, an update presented at the ASCO 2008 conventional analysis showed that OS converged in the two treatment groups (Sunitinib median 74.7 weeks; 95% CI 61.4–85.7; placebo 64.9 weeks, 45.7–98.4; HR 0.82, $p=0.128$) as expected for the crossover design (Demetri et al. 2008). However, rank-preserving structural failure time analysis yielded an estimated median OS for placebo of 36.0 weeks (95% CI 25.9–51.0), revealing a significant sunitinib treatment effect (HR 0.46, $p<0.0001$) comparable to that of the blinded phase. The most common treatment-related AEs throughout the entire study were fatigue, diarrhea, nausea, and skin discoloration, mainly grade 1/2; incidences increased slightly with extended duration of sunitinib treatment. In terms of best overall objective tumor response, 7% (14) of patients in the sunitinib group showed PR as the best response, 58% (120) had SD, and 19% (39) had PD, compared with rates of 0 48 (50), and 37% (39), respectively, for placebo. Six of fifty-nine patients who crossed over to sunitinib from the placebo group also had confirmed PR (10.2%, 95% CI 3.8–20.8). Four patients (7% overall) who crossed over to sunitinib from placebo had SD for at least 26 weeks after crossover. Based on these results, sunitinib is now approved for the therapy of GIST patients with advanced or unresectable disease after imatinib failure or intolerance (Goodman et al. 2007).

Currently, sunitinib is listed for 20 Phase III studies involving the approved indications RCC and GIST, as well as NSCLC, breast cancer, CRC, and pancreatic islet cell tumors (see Table 9.1).

9.1.4 Axitinib (AG-013736)

Axitinib (AG-013736; Pfizer Oncology) represents a potent small molecule TK inhibitor of all known VEGFRs at subnanomolar concentrations and PDGFR-ß and c-Kit in low nanomolar concentrations. Structurally, it is a substituted indazole derivative discovered by using a structure-based drug design. In vitro, axitinib selectively blocks VEGF stimulated receptor autophosphorylation leading to inhibition of endothelial cell proliferation and survival. In numerous preclinical models, axitinib inhibited tumor angiogenesis and the growth of human colorectal and murine lung tumors. In a transgenic mouse model of spontaneous islet cell tumors, axitinib eliminated suppressed vascular sprouting within 24 h. At 7 days, vascular density decreased more than 70%, and significant tumor shrinkage was seen at 21 days (Inai et al. 2004).

The first-in-human Phase I trial was conducted to test axitinib in patients with advanced solid malignancies in order to determine DLTs and the maximum-tolerated dose (MTD). Altogether, 36 patients received axtinib at doses ranging from 5 to 30 mg orally b.i.d. (Rugo et al. 2005). Similar to other TK inhibitors, observed DLTs included hypertension, hemoptysis, and stomatitis primarily seen at higher dose levels. All toxicities were manageable with medication or drug holidays. The MTD and recommended Phase II dose of AG-013736 was specified for 5 mg b.i.d. The trial demonstrated three confirmed partial responses and other evidence of clinical activity (Rugo et al. 2005). Subsequently, axitinib was tested in advanced or metastatic RCC in a multicenter, open-label, Phase II study (Dutcher et al. 2008). Altogether, 58 patients with sorafenib or sunitinib-refractory (progression or unacceptable toxicity) metastatic RCC, and measurable disease, regardless of additional prior therapies, were enrolled. All patients received a starting dose of axitinib 5 mg orally b.i.d., which was titrated to 7 mg b.i.d. and then to 10 mg b.i.d. according to tolerance. Stratification was performed by prior therapy into three groups: 14 patients were refractory to sunitinib and sorafenib (Group 1), 29 patients were refractory to cytokines and sorafenib (Group 2), and 15 patients were refractory to sorafenib alone (Group 3). With a median follow-up of 10.3 months, the overall response rate (ORR) was 7, 28, and 27% and the median PFS was 7.1, 9.0, and 7.7 months for groups 1, 2, and 3, respectively. Overall, grade 3/4 treatment-related AEs included fatigue (13%), hypertension (11%), hand-foot syndrome (11%), diarrhea (5%), and dyspnea (5%). The authors concluded, that axitinib appears to have antitumor activity in metastatic RCC refractory to sunitinib and sorafenib (Dutcher et al. 2008). To this end, a randomized Phase III trial is currently recruiting patients. The Axis-trial is a head-to-head comparison of axitinib (5 mg b.i.d.) and sorafenib (400 mg b.i.d.) for second-line therapy of metastatic RCC and is designed to enroll 540 patients until 2010 (NCT00678392).

The other malignant disease in which axitinib is currently evaluated in a Phase III trial is pancreatic cancer (see Table 9.1). So far, standard of care for patients with advanced pancreatic cancer is gemcitabine-based chemotherapy. Therefore, axitinib was tested in a Phase I/II trial in combination with gemcitabine in patients with pancreatic cancer (Spano et al. 2008). In detail, eight patients were treated on the Phase I part and 103 for the Phase II part of the trial. Prior gemcitabine or VEGF/VEGFR inhibitors were not allowed. The randomization took place between standard dose gemcitabine (1,000 mg/ m^2 over 30 min on days 1, 8, 15) plus axitinib (5 mg b.i.d.) or placebo. The median number of days on axitinib was 158 days (range: 57–330 days). The most commonly reported AEs were anemia (48%), alkaline phosphatase elevations (48%), leukopenia (45%), and thrombocytopenia (27%). The most common nonhematologic AEs were nausea (24%), vomiting (20%), fatigue (19%), diarrhea (18%), anorexia (18%), constipation (13%), dyspnea (12%), and fever (12%). In the axitinib group 66% of patients ($n=45$) reached at least disease stabilization, including 7% PRs compared to 59% SD ($n=20$) and no PR for gemcitabine plus placebo. This yielded a median OS of 210 days in the axitinib group in comparison to 169 days for gemcitabine plus placebo (HR 0.74; 95% CI 0.427–1.284) for the whole study group. For the subpopulation in very good performance status (ECOG PS 0/1), the calculated death risk reduction for axitinib was even bigger with 33% (HR 0.67; 95% CI 0.372–1.196). These results prompted the currently recruiting randomized, double-blind Phase III study of gemcitabine plus axitinib vs. gemcitabine plus placebo for the first-line treatment of patients in good performance status with locally advanced, unresectable, or metastatic pancreatic cancer. The trial is estimated to enroll more than 500 patients until planned completion date in September 2009 (NCT00471146).

9.1.5 Cediranib (AZD2171; Recentin™)

Another broad-spectrum kinase inhibitor is cediranib (AZD2171; Recentin™; AstraZeneca). Its predominant effect is directed against VEGFR-2 with additional potent inhibition of VEGFR-1 and -3, c-Kit, Flt-3 and to a lesser extent against epidermal growth factor receptor (EGFR). This broad activity range was determined in a wide range of cell lines (Wedge et al. 2005). Cediranib significantly inhibits VEGF driven vascular sprouting and demonstrated potent antitumor effects in a number of preclinical studies. It is orally bioavailable and was preclinically tested at a dose range of 1.5–6 mg/kg bodyweight per day. Based on these observations, a range of clinical Phase I studies were performed, the first being a dose-finding trial with 83 patients suffering of different solid tumors. In this study, cediranib was generally well tolerated at doses not higher than 45 mg/day and gave encouraging antitumor activity. Pharmacokinetic data revealed a half-life of approximately 20 h and the optimal dosing was determined to be 20–30 mg once daily (Drevs et al. 2007).

The next step was the initiation of Phase I/II study in conjunction with standard doses of carboplatin (AUC 6) and paclitaxel (200 mg/m^2) in order to assess the tolerability, safety, and antitumor activity of this combination in patients with stage IIIB / IV NSCLC of any histology in first-line therapy (Laurie et al. 2006; Laurie et al. 2008). Cediranib was started on Day 2 of the first cycle at a dose of 30 mg p.o. daily. Of the 20 enrolled patients, nine received cediranib at 30 mg/day, 11 at 45 mg/day. Again, most common grade 3/4 toxicity was hypertension, other common toxicities were: fatigue, anorexia, mucositis, and diarrhea. Hematologic toxicity was not greater than that expected with chemotherapy alone. At time of presentation, 15 patients were evaluable for response, with 6 PR, 8 SD, and 1 PD. The authors concluded that, full single-agent dose of cediranib may be administered with standard chemotherapy. However, the subsequent started randomized Phase II/III trial CTG BR.24 comparing carboplatin/paclitaxel plus cediranib (30 mg/day) vs. this chemotherapy combination plus placebo did not reach Phase III. The National Cancer Institute of Canada Clinical Trials Group (NCIC-CTG) decided in 2008 that the BR.24 study should not continue into Phase III following the planned end of

Phase II efficacy and tolerability analysis by the study's data safety monitoring committee, mostly because of an imbalance in toxicity. Although cediranib gave evidence of clinical activity, the study did not meet the predefined criteria for automatic continuation into Phase III (Laurie et al. 2008). Instead, NCIC-CTG agreed to start a new randomized Phase III study evaluating this combination in advanced or metastatic NSCLC with a lower dose of cediranib (20 mg/day); this BR.29 trial is expected to enroll the first patients in 2009.

Another step in the clinical development of cediranib was the initiation of a two-stage, multicenter Phase II clinical trial in patients with recurrent ovarian, peritoneal, or fallopian tube cancer (Hirte et al. 2008). Of the 60 patients who were enrolled; 49 had ovarian, 8 peritoneal, and 3 fallopian tube cancer; follow up was available for 154 cycles of treatment given to 46 patients. As in other Phase I studies with cediranib, the most frequent AEs were fatigue (85%), diarrhea (80%), hypertension (72%), anorexia (57%). Hypertension (33%) and fatigue (20%) were the most frequent grade 3/4 AEs. The median TTP and median OS for all patients was 4.1 months (95% CI 3.4–7.6) and 11.9 months (95% CI 9.9-not reached). This prompted a randomized Phase III study evaluating the combination of carboplatin/paclitaxel with or without cediranib in treating women with relapsed ovarian epithelial cancer, fallopian tube cancer, or primary peritoneal cancer.

Altogether, cediranib is currently listed in five active Phase III studies, such as the HORIZON II Phase II/III study of chemotherapy with cediranib vs. placebo in first-line metastatic CRC and HORIZON III, which represents a head-to-head comparison with bevacizumab (Avastin™) for this indication. Both studies completed recruitment by the end of 2008 and results are eagerly awaited. Also, the Phase III REGAL trial, in recurrent glioblastoma comparing cediranib monotherapy vs. lomustine±cediranib began enrolling patients in late 2008 (see Table 9.1).

9.1.6 Vandetanib (ZD6474; Zactima®)

Vandetanib (ZD6474; Zactima™; AstraZeneca), an orally bioavailable 4-anilinoquinazoline derivate, acts as selective and reversible inhibitor of ATP binding to TK receptors VEGFR-2, -3, RET, and EGFR. In comparison to other kinase inhibitors, vandetanib is somehow more selective, which is demonstrated by a lack of effect against structurally related receptors such as PDGFR or c-Kit. Its antiangiogenic and antitumor activity has been shown in a wide range of preclinical animal models (Herbst et al. 2007). The potent anti-EGFR activity gave a reasonable rationale for testing vandetanib in cancers in which EGFR antagonists have been proven effective.

The clinical development so far was focused on NSCLC. First, the antitumor activity of vandetanib monotherapy or vandetanib with paclitaxel and carboplatin was compared with paclitaxel and carboplatin in previously untreated patients with NSCLC in a partially blinded, placebo-controlled, randomized Phase II study (Heymach et al. 2008). Patients were randomly assigned 2:1:1 to receive vandetanib alone, vandetanib plus chemotherapy, or chemotherapy alone. Interestingly, the risk of progression was reduced for patients receiving vandetanib plus chemotherapy ($n=56$) vs. chemotherapy alone ($n=52$; HR=0.76; $p=0.098$); but median PFS differed only by 1 week (24 vs. 23 weeks). The vandetanib monotherapy arm ($n=73$) was discontinued after a planned interim PFS analysis met the criterion for discontinuation. Also, the OS was not significantly different between groups. Rash, diarrhea, and hypertension were common adverse events. The authors concluded, that vandetanib could be safely administered to patients with NSCLC, including those with squamous cell histology and treated brain metastases. The slightly longer PFS for vandetanib met the prespecified study end point, but was not significant (Heymach et al. 2008).

The next set of studies focused on vandetanib in second-line therapy of NSCLC. Eligible patients had locally advanced or metastatic (stage IIIB/IV) NSCLC after failure of first-line platinum-based chemotherapy (Heymach et al. 2007). First, a randomized Phase II study was initiated comparing vandetanib (100 or 300 mg/day) plus docetaxel (75 mg/m^2 intravenous infusion every 21 days) vs. placebo plus docetaxel. After including 127 patients, median PFS was 18.7 weeks for vandetanib 100 mg plus docetaxel ($n=42$; HR=0.64; $p=0.037$); 17.0 weeks for vandetanib 300 mg plus docetaxel ($n=44$; HR=0.83; $p=0.231$); and 12 weeks for docetaxel ($n=41$). There was no statistically significant difference in OS among the three treatment arms. Common AEs included diarrhea, rash, and asymptomatic prolongation of corrected QT (QT_C) interval. At the time of publication, the authors concluded that the primary objective was achieved, with vandetanib 100 mg plus docetaxel demonstrating a significant prolongation of PFS compared with docetaxel in relation to the prespecified significance level. On the basis of these encouraging data, Phase III evaluation of vandetanib 100 mg plus docetaxel in second-line NSCLC (ZODIAC trial) was initiated in 2006. Until completion in September 2008, the study enrolled 1,391 patients previously treated with one prior anticancer therapy for advanced NSCLC. Median duration of follow-up was 12.8 months, with 87% patients progressed and 59% dead. Addition of vandetanib to docetaxel showed a statistically significant improvement in PFS versus docetaxel (HR 0.79, 97.58% CI 0.70-0.90; P<0.001). Significant advantages for vandetanib plus docetaxel were also seen for ORR (17% vs 10%, P<0.001). Overall survival showed a positive trend for vandetanib plus docetaxel that was not statistically significant (HR 0.91, 97.52% CI 0.78-1.07; P=0.196). The adverse event profile was consistent with that previously observed for vandetanib in NSCLC. Common AEs occurring more frequently in the vandetanib arm included diarrhea (42% vs 33%), rash (42% vs 24%) and neutropenia (32% vs 27%). (see Table 9.1).

Three other Phase III trials with vandetanib in second- and third-line therapy of NSCLC recently stopped recruiting patients and will complete data collection in 2009. The so-called ZEAL trial is a randomized, double-blind, placebo-controlled Phase III study evaluating the combination of vandetanib 100 mg with pemetrexed vs. pemetrexed alone. This study enrolled 534 patients previously treated with one prior anticancer therapy for advanced NSCLC. There were positive trends seen for vandetanib plus pemetrexed for both PFS (HR 0.86, 97.58% CI 0.69 -1.06; P=0.108) and OS (HR 0.86, 97.54% CI 0.65 -1.13; P=0.219). There was a statistically significant advantage for ORR (19.1% vs 7.9%, P<0.001) in the combination arm. The ZEST study also is a randomized, double-blind, Phase III study evaluating the efficacy of vandetanib 300 mg vs. erlotinib 150 mg, which enrolled 1,240 patients with locally advanced or metastatic NSCLC after failure of at least one prior anticancer therapy. There was no difference in PFS for patients treated with vandetanib versus erlotinib (HR 0.98, 95.22% CI 0.87 -1.10; P=0.721), and no difference in the secondary endpoints of OS (HR 1.01, 95.08% CI 0.89 -1.16; P=0.830) and ORR (both 12%). Finally, the ZEPHYR trial is a randomized Phase III study to assess the efficacy of vandetanib vs. best supportive care in patients with NSCLC (Stage IIIB-IV) after therapy with an EGFR inhibitor. This study is expected to enroll over 900 patients and data collection will be completed by April 2009.

At the time of writing this review, there was no active Phase III trial listed in the NCI's database, but 26 Phase II and 17 Phase I studies, including trials on medullary thyroid carcinoma, breast cancer, and glioma, were ongoing.

9.1.7 Vatalanib (PTK787/ZK222584)

Vatalanib (PTK787/ZK222584; Bayer Schering Pharma AG, Berlin; Novartis, East Hanover, NJ) is an oral multitargeted kinase inhibitor that acts on VEGFR-1, -2, -3, c-KIT, and PDGFR (Wood et al. 2000). After oral administration, vatalanib reaches peak concentration in 1.0–2.5 h and has a half-life of 4.5 h, with no evidence of accumulation at steady state following once-daily dosing. Vatalanib demonstrated clinical activity in patients with several types of human cancer (Drevs et al. 2000; Roboz et al. 2006; Sharma et al. 2009; Thomas et al. 2005; Thomas et al. 2007). For further clinical development, vatalanib was investigated in two multinational randomized phase III studies in first- (CONFIRM-1) and second-line (CONFIRM-2) metastatic CRC. In CONFIRM-2, 855 patients were randomized to FOLFOX4 chemotherapy plus vatalanib (1,250 mg/day) or placebo (Kohne et al. 2007). Eligibility included histologically documented metastatic CRC, pretreatment for metastatic disease with irinotecan-/fluoropyrimidine- based therapy, measurable disease by Response Evaluation Criteria In Solid Tumors (RECIST), good performance status, and adequate organ function. In both trials, toxicities were similar. In detail, for the CONFIRM-2 trial, grade 3–4 AEs were hypertension (21% for vatalanib vs. 5% for placebo), diarrhea (16 vs. 8%), fatigue (15 vs. 7%), nausea (11 vs. 5%), vomiting (9 vs. 5%), and dizziness (9 vs. 1%). Thrombotic and embolic events of all grades occurred in 6% of the vatalanib treated patients vs. 1% of the placebo group. At the time of interim analysis in July 2005, OS was 12.1 months in the vatalanib and 11.8 months in the placebo group (HR 0.94; $p=0.511$). PFS was significantly longer in the vatalanib arm (5.5 vs. 4.1 months; HR 0.83; $p=0.026$). Interestingly, Lactat dehydrogenase (LDH), a rather unspecific marker related to poor prognosis in CRC, was predictive for the outcome in the vatalanib group. Especially patients with high LDH gained improvement in PFS when treated with vatalanib (5.6 vs. 3.8 months; HR 0.63; $p<0.001$) and in OS (9.6 vs. 7.5 months; HR 0.78; $p=0.10$). For CONFIRM-1, 1,168 patients were randomized to receive FOLFOX-4 plus vatalanib (1250 mg/day) or FOLFOX-4 plus placebo. The addition of vatalanib did not result in differences in the response rate (42% for FOLFOX-4 plus vatalanib vs. 46% for FOLFOX-4 plus placebo) or PFS time (7.7 months for FOLFOX-4 plus vatalanib vs. 7.6 months for FOLFOX-4 plus placebo). Thus, it was concluded that significant clinical benefits for vatalanib treatment in CRC seems to be limited to LDH-high patients, the reason for this remains unclear (Hecht et al. 2005; Kohne et al. 2007).

Currently, no active Phase III studies with vatalanib are listed, but six Phase II and four Phase I studies for therapy of glioma, multiple myeloma, pancreatic cancer, and melanoma are active.

9.1.8 Endostatin (rh-Endostatin, YH-16, Endostar™)

Endostatin, a 20-kiloDalton (kDa) fragment of collagen XVIII, is a group member of endogenous antiangiogenic proteins activated by proteolytic processing (Ferreras et al. 2000). Endostatin was shown to inhibit endothelial cell proliferation, migration, invasion, and vascular sprouting (O'Reilly et al. 1997). The reduction in endothelial cell survival induced by endostatin has been proposed to involve binding to the fibronectin receptor $\alpha_5\beta_1$ (Sudhakar et al. 2003), interference with VEGF/VEGFR signaling (Hajitou et al. 2002; Kim et al. 2002b), inhibition of matrix metalloproteinases (MMP), e.g., MMP-2 (Kim et al. 2000), and downregulation of c-myc and cyclin-D1 (Hanai et al. 2002; Shichiri and Hirata 2001). Also, endostatin seems to downregulate a number of proteins essential to angiogenesis such as the Id1 and -3, HIF1-α and Ephrin B1 and B2 (Shichiri and Hirata 2001). Despite initial high hopes, the clinical development of endostatin came close to an unsuccessful end after treatment of about 160 cancer patients in Phase I and II studies when the sole manufacturer (EntreMed, Rockville, USA) announced the cease of production in 2003 due to lack of efficacy, difficult application scheme, and concerns about its production in yeast. Some years later, the Chinese protein chemist Luo may have solved the folding problem by adding nine amino acids to the endostatin molecule (Fu et al. 2008). This reformulation apparently made it possible to manufacture a soluble rh-endostatin (Endostar™, Simcere Pharmaceutical Co., Nanjing, China) using not yeast but bacteria and providing higher in vivo stability, now eligible for daily application once rather than twice. Phase I/II studies revealed that rh-endostatin was effective as single agent with good tolerance in clinical use. The first randomized study presented was designed to compare the response rate, median TTP, clinical benefit, and safety in patients with advanced NSCLC, treated with rh-endostatin (7.5 mg/m^2 on days 1–14) plus standard dose vinorelbine (25 mg/m^2 on day 1 and 5) and cisplatin (30 mg/m^2 on Days 2–4), or placebo plus chemotherapy (Sun et al. 2005). Altogether, 493 NSCLC patients in good performance status were recruited for this double-blind study (326 in the rh-endostatin group, 167 as control). Of the 486 assessable patients, overall response rates were 35.4% for rh-endostatin and 19.5% in the control group (p=0.0003). The median TTP were 6.3 and 3.6 months for rh-endostatin vs. control (p<0.001), yielding a clinical benefit rate of 73.3 vs. 64.0% respectively (p=0.035). Grade 3/4 neutropenia, anemia, nausea/vomiting were comparable in both arms. There was no data on OS reported. The authors concluded that the addition of rh-endostatin to standard chemotherapy resulted in significant improvement in response rate, median TTP, and clinical benefit rate compared with chemotherapy alone in advanced NSCLC patients (Sun et al. 2005). Subsequently, the national Food and Drug Administration of China approved Endostar™ for this setting. The currently listed Phase III studies involving rh-endostatin exclusively originate in China and enroll only NSCLC patients testing different combinations with chemotherapy or application in the adjuvant setting (see Table 9.1).

9.1.9 Thalidomide

One drug that exhibits an antiangiogenic effect by still not fully clarified mechanisms is thalidomide (D'Amato et al. 1994). Originally introduced as sedative and withdrawn due to deleterious side effects, today there is increasing evidence for the efficacy of thalidomide in cancer therapy. Thalidomide was developed in the 1950s and chiefly sold from 1957 to 1961 in almost 50 countries under at least 40 names to pregnant women, as an antiemetic to combat morning sickness and sleeping problems. Later, the teratogenic effects of thalidomide became clear when approximately 10,000 children mainly in Africa and Europe were born with severe malformations, including phocomelia in the late 1950s and early 1960s (Lenz 1967; Lenz and Knapp 1962). However, it was soon found that the teratogenicity caused by thalidomide was only associated with one particular optical isomer. Research continued, although the drug was not prescribed for decades, and finally the US FDA granted approval for treatment of erythema nodosum leprosum (ENL) in 1998. One year later, the first report was presented demonstrating activity of thalidomide in multiple myeloma (MM) tested in 180 patients with advanced disease (Singhal et al. 1999). Clinical development continued under strict regulations regarding the pregnancy status of patients and even their partners and finally the US FDA granted accelerated approval for thalidomide in combination with dexamethasone for the treatment of newly diagnosed MM in 2006. Since then, thalidomide was shown to be useful in a variety of tumors. Its mechanism of action in cancer is attributed to multiple, including direct cytotoxic, antiangiogenic, and antiinflammatory effects (Kumar 2006). The combination of temozolomide and thalidomide has shown promising activity in metastatic melanoma (Hwu et al. 2003), metastatic neuroendocrine tumors (Kulke et al. 2006), and unresectable or metastatic leiomyosarcoma (Boyar et al. 2008). Recently, the surprising effects of thalidomide have led to the development of a series of immunomodulatory drugs (IMiDs) and selective cytokine inhibitory drugs (SELCIDs) with even higher antiangiogenic potency (Dredge et al. 2005; List et al. 2005). The modulation of the immune system consists of stimulation of T – cells and NK – cells (Chang et al. 2006). In our own studies, thalidomide demonstrated biological and clinical activity in myelodysplastic syndrome (MDS) and acute myeloid leukemia (AML) with ORR up to 56 and 25%, respectively (Steins et al. 2003; Steins et al. 2002). Responding patients experienced hematologic improvements including an increase in hemoglobin values and platelet counts. In four of 20 AML patients, a bone marrow blast clearance of at least 50% was achieved after treatment with thalidomide for at least 1 month (PR). Furthermore, we observed a long-term response in one AML patient of more than 20 months, subsequently meeting the criteria of complete remission. Interestingly, the decrease in leukemic blast infiltration in the bone marrow of responders was accompanied by a significant reduction of MVD. While it still remains unclear how exactly thalidomide inhibits angiogenesis, some data suggests a downregulation of VEGF as one possible mode of action (Komorowski et al. 2006; Li et al. 2003).

Currently, thalidomide and the subsequently developed IMiDs Revlimid™ (lenalidomide, CC-5013) and Actimid™ (CC-4047) are listed in 27 active Phase III trials in the NCI database. Apart from hematological malignancies, these substances are tested for treatment of poor liver function HCC and RCC (see Table 9.1).

9.1.10 Vascular Disrupting Agents

While classic inhibitors of tumor angiogenesis mostly compromise the formation of new blood vessels, occlusion of the existing tumor vasculature by inducing thrombosis or extensive endothelial damage leading to severe hemorrhagic necrosis is the main goal of the substances referred to as vascular disrupting agents (VDA). The largest group of VDAs already in clinical stage of development is the family of combretastatins, which act as microtubulin destabilizing drugs, and the structurally distinct flavonoid 5,6-dimethylxanthenone-4-acetic acid (DMXAA).

The first agent extensively studied was Combretastatin-4 (CA-4), which demonstrated rapid and extensive vascular disruption concomitant with hemorrhagic necrosis within the first hour of treatment in preclinical models (Dark et al. 1997). The fast onset of action is attributed to cytoskeletal shift changes including contraction of actinomyosin and the malformed assembly of stress fibers (see Fig. 9.2). Subsequently, this leads to disruption of the endothelial monolayer with increased permeability for macromolecules and shear-stress activation of platelets with intravascular thrombosis (Galbraith et al. 2001; Kanthou and Tozer 2002; Tozer et al. 1999). Finally, this endothelial disruption and platelet aggregation results in rapid almost complete vascular obstruction and tumor necrosis.

For the clinical setting, Combretastatin-A4P is developed by OXiGENE (Waltham, MA, USA) as Zybrestat™. In July 2007, the company initiated a 180-patient pivotal registration study with Zybrestat™ for the treatment of anaplastic thyroid cancer, under a Special Protocol Assessment (SPA) agreement with the US FDA. For this study, the FDA granted Zybrestat™ "Fast-Track" status as potential cancer therapy. This is a randomized open-label Phase II/III study in which the experimental drug is tested in combination with conventional chemotherapeutics carboplatin and paclitaxel (NCT00507429).

In a previous Phase II study with 18 patients suffering of advanced anaplastic thyroid cancer Zybrestat™ as monotherapy achieved a median

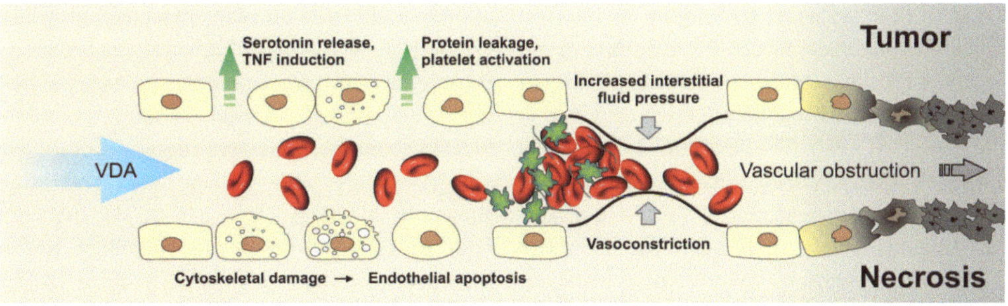

Fig. 9.2 *Proposed mechanism of vascular disrupting agents.* The lead compounds of this class, Combretastatin A-4 (Zybrestat™) or 5,6-dimethylxantheonone-4-acetic acid (DMXAA; ASA404) induce rapid vascular obstruction within the tumor by acting on the endothelial cytoskeleton. In detail, shape changes and intracellular damage is seen leading to subsequent disruption of the endothelial monolayer. Increased vascular permeability and high interstitial fluid pressure in the tumor adds up to vascular collapse and obstruction. Due to direct exposure of the basement membrane to blood cells, platelets and plasmatic coagulation are activated leading to rapid tumor vessel thrombosis within minutes of exposure

PFS of 7.4 weeks (range 2–84 weeks); with five patients remaining progression-free for more than 3 months (Cooney et al. 2006). The median OS in this study was approximately 20 weeks. Zybrestat™ also demonstrated activity in other Phase I studies for treatment of advanced solid neoplasms, such as NSCLC and ovarian cancer (Anderson et al. 2003; Bilenker et al. 2005; Dowlati et al. 2002; Rustin et al. 2003a; Stevenson et al. 2003). It is also the first VDA that has been clinically tested in combination with classic antiangiogenic drugs such as bevacizumab (Avastin™) (Nathan et al. 2008). In this study, 9 of 14 patients with advanced solid tumors experienced disease stabilization for more than 12 weeks. Three patients experienced SD for more than 24 weeks. Besides, DCE-MRI demonstrated statistically significant reductions in tumor perfusion. This effect rapidly reversed after Zybrestat™ alone, but was sustained following the combination of Zybrestat™ and BEV (Nathan et al. 2008). This observation and other preclinical evidence have prompted another randomized Phase II study in which the combination of carboplatin, paclitaxel, and BEV is evaluated with and without Zybrestat™ for patients with advanced NSCLC (Stadium IIIb and IV) as first-line therapy. Like in other studies involving antiangiogenic drugs, patients with predominant squamous cell histology are excluded. This study started in March 2008 and is aimed for enrollment of 60 patients until 2010 (NCT00653939).

The current lead compound of the structurally and mechanistically distinct flavonoids is DMXAA (AS1404, Antisoma Research Limited, London, UK) (Rewcastle et al. 1991). In contrast to combretastatins, cytoskeletal effects of DMXAA seem to be confined to actin assembly leaving interphase microtubules unharmed. In experimental models, DMXAA has been shown to enhance antitumor effects of melphalan and other cytotoxic agents as well as hyperthermia and radiation (Murata et al. 2001; Pruijn et al. 1997; Siim et al. 2003).

The first clinical Phase I study was presented in 2003 (Rustin et al. 2003b). DMXAA was applied to 46 patients for a total of 247 infusions of over 15 dose levels ranging from 6 to 4,900 mg/m^2. The MTD was reached at 3,700 mg/m^2 with DLTs observed in form of urinary incontinence, visual disturbance, and anxiety at the highest dose level (4,900 mg/m^2). Dose-dependent increases in the serotonin metabolite 5-hydroxyindoleacetic acid were found at dose levels of 650 mg/m^2 and above. There was one unconfirmed PR at 1,300 mg/m^2.

Phase II studies have been published for ovarian cancer, NSCLC, and hormone refractory prostate cancer (HRPC). The first randomized study evaluated DMXAA in combination with carboplatin (AUC 6) and paclitaxel (175 mg/m^2) in NSCLC with histologically confirmed stage IIIb or IV NSCLC previously untreated with chemotherapy (McKeage 2006). Until 2006, 77 patients were randomized to receive up to six cycles of carboplatin/paclitaxel with or without DMXAA (1,200 or 1,800 mg/m^2). Thirty-five patients received chemotherapy alone, 36 chemotherapy plus 1,200 mg/m^2 DMXAA and 6 plus 1,800 mg/m^2 DMXAA. The safety profile in the control arm and DMXAA arm was comparable. Twenty-three of thirty patients in the control arm achieved disease control and seven progressed, for the 1,200 mg/m^2 DMXAA arm 28 of 33 patients reached disease control and five progressed. Finally, all six patients receiving 1,800 mg/m^2 DMXAA achieved disease control, with three confirmed PRs. The encouraging updated survival data was presented in 2008 (McKeage and Jameson 2008); median OS for chemotherapy alone being 8.8 months ($n=36$), 14.0 months for chemotherapy plus 1,200 mg/m^2 DMXAA ($n=34$) and 14.9 months for the 1,800 mg/m^2 DMXAA group ($n=30$). It is noteworthy that in this trial, patients with squamous NSCLC were also benefited.

These data prompted the currently recruiting international multicenter, randomized Phase III trial ATTRACT-1 (Antivascular Targeted Therapy Researching ASA404 in Cancer Treatment; NCT00662597). Previously untreated patients with advanced NSCLC (St. IIIb or IV) are randomized to receive standard chemotherapy carboplatin/paclitaxel in combination with 1,800 mg/m^2 DMXAA (AS1404, now licensed to Novartis, Basel, Switzerland) or placebo. It is planned to recruit 1,200 patients with comparison of OS as primary objective. Safety data from the previous studies described earlier indicates a different toxicity profile in contrast to other antiangiogenic drugs. Typical vascular effects such as proteinuria, arterial hypertension and thrombosis, pulmonary hemorrhage, wound healing or other bleeding complications were almost not observed with DMXAA both in squamous and non-squamous histology. This allows also patients with predominant squamous histology to be recruited, a group that is usually ruled out in other trials involving most other antiangiogenic agents. Also, a second randomized Phase III study (ATTRACT-2) evaluating the efficacy of DMXAA in second-line therapy of NSCLC was initiated in late 2008 (see Table 9.1).

9.1.11 Accidental Antiangiogenesis Agents

Apart from the aforementioned agents, some already FDA-approved anticancer drugs were later to be shown to have antiangiogenic activity as well. For example, the FDA-approved EGFR antibodies cetuximab (Erbitux™; Merck) and panitumumab (Vectibix™; Amgen) as well as the EGFR antagonists erlotinib (Tarceva™; Genentech, OSI Pharmaceuticals in collaboration with Genentech and Roche) and gefitinib (ZD1839; Iressa™; AstraZeneca) were shown to inhibit tumor angiogenesis by partly blocking the VEGF receptor and downregulation of various pro-angiogenic factors such as VEGF (Ciardiello et al. 2001; Hoffmann et al. 2007; Huang et al. 2002; Perrotte et al. 1999; Pore et al. 2006), basic fibroblast growth factor (bFGF) (Albanell et al. 2001), HIF1-α (Li et al. 2008) and transforming growth factor- (TGF) (Pino et al. 2006). Also, the proteasome inhibitor bortezomib (Velcade™; Millennium Pharmaceuticals), approved for multiple myeloma, demonstrated potent antiangiogenic activity in clinical and preclinical models (Galimberti et al. 2008; Nawrocki et al. 2002; Williams et al. 2003). Even drugs like celecoxib (Celebrex™; Pfizer Inc.) originally approved not for therapy of malignant disease but for treatment of rheumatoid arthritis have been shown to increase production of endogenous angiogenesis inhibitors like endostatin and demonstrated clinical anticancer activity as well. Celecoxib is currently listed in four randomized Phase III trials for therapy of metastatic CRC, NSCLC, pancreatic, and prostate cancer (NCT00268476, NCT00295035, NCT00300729, NCT00486460). Also, the concept of metronomic chemotherapy was introduced meaning the inhibition of tumor angiogenesis by simply changing the dose and frequency of a cytotoxic chemotherapeutic agent like cyclophosphamide (Browder et al. 2000; Hanahan et al. 2000). Vice versa to these "accidental" antiangiogenic drugs, it became clear that "classic" antiangiogenic drugs affect not only endothelial but also tumor cells directly (Beaudry et al. 2008). Especially pancreatic and breast cancer cells were shown to express VEGFR-2 offering the possibility to directly target them with VEGF/VEGFR antagonists (Higgins et al. 2006a; Higgins et al. 2006b).

9.1.12 Conclusions and Future Perspectives

Taken together, the classic concept in cancer therapy that a drug is either directed exclusively against the tumor cell or against the vascular cell in tumor angiogenesis has been replaced by a far more complex model of tumor-stroma interactions. Thus, (multi-)targeted therapies against cancer have become more and more important. Up to date, numerous new substances were developed as angiogenesis inhibitors and evaluated in clinical trials for safety, tolerance, and efficacy. Yielding positive study results, some of these molecules have already been approved for clinical use as described earlier. Although the clinical benefit for patient groups studied is only in the range of few months, the benefit for single patients can be considerably more long-lasting. Treatment results begin to change even in diseases where no therapeutic advances could be made for decades. Today, the wide array of available agents offers the clinician multiple treatment choices.

However, the question of the optimal antiangiogenic approach is still an open debate and subject to a number of clinical studies described in this chapter; for example, which combinations for what tumors, treatment in early stage vs. advanced stage or maintenance?

In particular, the concept of tumor dormancy induced or maintained by angiogenesis inhibitors is widely discussed in the expert field. One intriguing observation for this model is the vast difference between the prevalence of clinically presenting cancer and unapparent malignant tumors found in autopsy studies. Besides, tumor dormancy may be a clinically relevant phenomenon in patients who have been treated for primary cancer and relapse after a long disease-free period (Demicheli et al. 2005; Uhr et al. 1997). Hypothetically, a small number of remaining malignant cells are able to re-activate their tumorigenic potential even years later. Most often, this phenomenon has been explained as consequence of a complex and poorly understood shift in the balance between host and tumor, the angiogenic switch. Historically, the failure to induce the angiogenic switch has been proposed as one of the mechanisms that may be responsible for tumor dormancy (Brem and Folkman 1975; Folkman and Kalluri 2004; Hanahan and Folkman 1996).

However, it is not clear whether a sustained production of angiogenic factors is required to finally break the balance or a short-term angiogenic burst may suffice to break dormancy. To this end, it is absolute speculative that the lower incidence of clinically apparent breast cancer in women with Down syndrome might be due to constant elevated serum values of endogenous angiogenesis inhibitor endostatin regulated on chromosome 21 (Retsky et al. 2009; Zorick et al. 2001). So far, it is still just an outlook into the future when hopefully our diagnostic tools are sensitive enough to detect recurrent disease before it leaves the dormant state and becomes

9

symptomatic again or even better it might be possible to actively halt the tumor dormancy by antiangiogenic maintenance. However, the challenge for both basic researchers and clinicians will remain to integrate these numerous novel treatment approaches into existing protocols to eventually improve individual patient outcome.

Acknowledgment Supported by a grant of the Deutsche Forschungsgemeinschaft (SPP1190) and the Institute for Innovative Medical Research (IMF KE 110715; IMF LI 110633)

References

Abou-Alfa GK, Schwartz L, Ricci S, Amadori D, Santoro A, Figer A, De Greve J, Douillard JY, Lathia C, Schwartz B, Taylor I, Moscovici M, Saltz LB (2006) Phase II study of sorafenib in patients with advanced hepatocellular carcinoma. J Clin Oncol 24:4293–4300

Adnane L, Trail PA, Taylor I, Wilhelm SM (2006) Sorafenib (BAY 43–9006, Nexavar), a dual-action inhibitor that targets RAF/MEK/ERK pathway in tumor cells and tyrosine kinases VEGFR/PDGFR in tumor vasculature. Methods Enzymol 407:597–612

Albanell J, Codony-Servat J, Rojo F, Del Campo JM, Sauleda S, Anido J, Raspall G, Giralt J, Rosello J, Nicholson RI, Mendelsohn J, Baselga J (2001) Activated extracellular signal-regulated kinases: association with epidermal growth factor receptor/transforming growth factor alpha expression in head and neck squamous carcinoma and inhibition by anti-epidermal growth factor receptor trea. Cancer Res 61:6500–6510

Anderson HL, Yap JT, Miller MP, Robbins A, Jones T, Price PM (2003) Assessment of pharmacodynamic vascular response in a phase I trial of combretastatin A4 phosphate. J Clin Oncol 21: 2823–2830

Atkins M, Jones CA, Kirkpatrick P (2006) Sunitinib maleate. Nat Rev Drug Discov 5:279–280

Beaudry P, Nilsson M, Rioth M, Prox D, Poon D, Xu L, Zweidler-Mckay P, Ryan A, Folkman J, Ryeom S, Heymach J (2008) Potent antitumor effects of ZD6474 on neuroblastoma via dual targeting of tumor cells and tumor endothelium. Mol Cancer Ther 7:418–424

Bilenker JH, Flaherty KT, Rosen M, Davis L, Gallagher M, Stevenson JP, Sun W, Vaughn D, Giantonio B, Zimmer R, Schnall M, O'Dwyer PJ (2005) Phase I trial of combretastatin a-4 phosphate with carboplatin. Clin Cancer Res 11: 1527–1533

Boyar MS, Hesdorffer M, Keohan ML, Jin Z, Taub RN (2008) Phase II study of temozolomide and thalidomide in patients with unresectable or metastatic leiomyosarcoma. Sarcoma 2008:412503

Brem H, Folkman J (1975) Inhibition of tumor angiogenesis mediated by cartilage. J Exp Med 141:427–439

Browder T, Butterfield CE, Kraling BM, Shi B, Marshall B, O'Reilly MS, Folkman J (2000) Antiangiogenic scheduling of chemotherapy improves efficacy against experimental drug-resistant cancer. Cancer Res 60:1878–1886

Bukowski RM, Eisen T, Szczylik C, Stadler WM, Simantov R, Shan M, Elting J, Pena C, Escudier B (2007) Final results of the randomized phase III trial of sorafenib in advanced renal cell carcinoma: survival and biomarker analysis. J Clin Oncol 25(Suppl):5023 (abstract)

Cella D, Yount S, Du H, Dhanda R, Gondek K, Langefeld K, George J, Bro WP, Kelly C, Bukowski R (2006) Development and validation of the functional assessment of cancer therapy-kidney symptom index (FKSI). J Support Oncol 4:191–199

Chang DH, Liu N, Klimek V, Hassoun H, Mazumder A, Nimer SD, Jagannath S, Dhodapkar MV (2006) Enhancement of ligand-dependent activation of human natural killer T cells by lenalidomide: therapeutic implications. Blood 108:618–621

Ciardiello F, Caputo R, Bianco R, Damiano V, Fontanini G, Cuccato S, De Placido S, Bianco AR, Tortora G (2001) Inhibition of growth factor production and angiogenesis in human cancer cells by ZD1839 (Iressa), a selective epidermal growth factor receptor tyrosine kinase inhibitor. Clin Cancer Res 7:1459–1465

Cooney MM, Savvides P, Agarwala S, Wang D, Flick S, Bergant S, Bhakta S, Lavertu P, Ortiz J, Remick SC (2006) Phase II study of combretastatin A4 phosphate (CA4P) in patients with advanced anaplastic thyroid carcinoma (ATC). J Clin Oncol 24(Suppl):5580 (abstract)

D'Amato RJ, Loughnan MS, Flynn E, Folkman J (1994) Thalidomide is an inhibitor of angiogenesis. Proc Natl Acad Sci USA 91:4082–4085

Dark GG, Hill SA, Prise VE, Tozer GM, Pettit GR, Chaplin DJ (1997) Combretastatin A-4, an agent that displays potent and selective toxicity toward tumor vasculature. Cancer Res 57:1829–1834

Demetri GD, Huang X, Garrett CR, Schoeffski P, Blackstein ME, Shah MH, Verweij J, Tassell V, Baum CM, Casali PG (2008) Novel statistical analysis of long-term survival to account for cross-over in a phase III trial of sunitinib (SU) vs. placebo (PL) in advanced GIST after imatinib (IM) failure. J Clin Oncol 26(Suppl):10524 (abstract)

De Boer R, Arrieta O, Gottfried M, Blackhall FH, Raats J, Yang CH, Langmuir P, Milenkova T, Read J, Vansteenkiste J (2009) Vandetanib plus pemetrexed versus pemetrexed as second-line therapy in patients with advanced non-small cell lung cancer (NSCLC): A randomized, double-blind phase III trial (ZEAL). J Clin Oncol 27: 8010

Demetri GD, van Oosterom AT, Garrett CR, Blackstein ME, Shah MH, Verweij J, McArthur G, Judson IR, Heinrich MC, Morgan JA, Desai J, Fletcher CD, George S, Bello CL, Huang X, Baum CM, Casali PG (2006) Efficacy and safety of sunitinib in patients with advanced gastrointestinal stromal tumour after failure of imatinib: a randomised controlled trial. Lancet 368: 1329–1338

Demicheli R, Miceli R, Moliterni A, Zambetti M, Hrushesky WJ, Retsky MW, Valagussa P, Bonadonna G (2005) Breast cancer recurrence dynamics following adjuvant CMF is consistent with tumor dormancy and mastectomy-driven acceleration of the metastatic process. Ann Oncol 16:1449–1457

Dowlati A, Robertson K, Cooney M, Petros WP, Stratford M, Jesberger J, Rafie N, Overmoyer B, Makkar V, Stambler B, Taylor A, Waas J, Lewin JS, McCrae KR, Remick SC (2002) A phase I pharmacokinetic and translational study of the novel vascular targeting agent combretastatin a-4 phosphate on a single-dose intravenous schedule in patients with advanced cancer. Cancer Res 62: 3408–3416

Dredge K, Horsfall R, Robinson SP, Zhang LH, Lu L, Tang Y, Shirley MA, Muller G, Schafer P, Stirling D, Dalgleish AG, Bartlett JB (2005) Orally administered lenalidomide (CC-5013) is anti-angiogenic in vivo and inhibits endothelial cell migration and Akt phosphorylation in vitro. Microvasc Res 69:56–63

Drevs J, Hofmann I, Hugenschmidt H, Wittig C, Madjar H, Muller M, Wood J, Martiny-Baron G, Unger C, Marme D (2000) Effects of PTK787/ZK 222584, a specific inhibitor of vascular endothelial growth factor receptor tyrosine kinases, on primary tumor, metastasis, vessel density, and blood flow in a murine renal cell carcinoma model. Cancer Res 60:4819–4824

Drevs J, Siegert P, Medinger M, Mross K, Strecker R, Zirrgiebel U, Harder J, Blum H, Robertson J, Jurgensmeier JM, Puchalski TA, Young H, Saunders O, Unger C (2007) Phase I clinical study of AZD2171, an oral vascular endothelial growth factor signaling inhibitor, in patients with advanced solid tumors. J Clin Oncol 25:3045–3054

Dutcher JP, Wilding G, Hudes GR, Stadler WM, Kim S, Tarazi JC, Rosbrook B, Rini BI (2008) Sequential axitinib (AG-013736) therapy of patients (pts) with metastatic clear cell renal cell cancer (RCC) refractory to sunitinib and sorafenib, cytokines and sorafenib, or sorafenib alone. J Clin Oncol 26(Suppl):5127 (abstract)

Escudier B, Pluzanska A, Koralewski P, Ravaud A, Bracarda S, Szczylik C, Chevreau C, Filipek M, Melichar B, Bajetta E, Gorbunova V, Bay JO, Bodrogi I, Jagiello-Gruszfeld A, Moore N (2007a) Bevacizumab plus interferon alfa-2a for treatment of metastatic renal cell carcinoma: a randomised, double-blind phase III trial. Lancet 370: 2103–2111

Escudier B, Eisen T, Stadler WM, Szczylik C, Oudard S, Siebels M, Negrier S, Chevreau C, Solska E, Desai AA, Rolland F, Demkow T, Hutson TE, Gore M, Freeman S, Schwartz B, Shan M, Simantov R, Bukowski RM (2007b) Sorafenib in advanced clear-cell renal-cell carcinoma. N Engl J Med 356:125–134

Faivre S, Demetri G, Sargent W, Raymond E (2007) Molecular basis for sunitinib efficacy and future clinical development. Nat Rev Drug Discov 6:734–745

Ferrara N, Gerber HP, LeCouter J (2003) The biology of VEGF and its receptors. Nat Med 9:669–676

Ferrara N, Hillan KJ, Gerber HP, Novotny W (2004) Discovery and development of bevacizumab, an anti-VEGF antibody for treating cancer. Nat Rev Drug Discov 3:391–400

Ferreras M, Felbor U, Lenhard T, Olsen BR, Delaisse J (2000) Generation and degradation of human endostatin proteins by various proteinases. FEBS Lett 486:247–251

Figlin RA, Hutson TE, Tomczak P, Michaelson MD, Bukowski RM, Negrier S, Huang J, Kim ST, Chen I, Motzer RJ (2008) Overall survival with sunitinib versus interferon (IFN)-alfa as first-line

9

treatment of metastatic renal cell carcinoma (mRCC). J Clin Oncol 26(Suppl):5024 (abstract)
Flaherty KT, Rosen MA, Heitjan DF, Gallagher ML, Schwartz B, Schnall MD, O'Dwyer PJ (2008) Pilot study of DCE-MRI to predict progression-free survival with sorafenib therapy in renal cell carcinoma. Cancer Biol Ther 7:496–501
Folkman J, Kalluri R (2004) Cancer without disease. Nature 427:787
Fu Y, Wu X, Han Q, Liang Y, He Y, Luo Y (2008) Sulfate stabilizes the folding intermediate more than the native structure of endostatin. Arch Biochem Biophys 471:232–239
Furuse J, Ishii H, Nakachi K, Suzuki E, Shimizu S, Nakajima K (2008) Phase I study of sorafenib in Japanese patients with hepatocellular carcinoma. Cancer Sci 99:159–165
Galbraith SM, Chaplin DJ, Lee F, Stratford MR, Locke RJ, Vojnovic B, Tozer GM (2001) Effects of combretastatin A4 phosphate on endothelial cell morphology in vitro and relationship to tumour vascular targeting activity in vivo. Anticancer Res 21:93–102
Galimberti S, Canestaro M, Ciancia E, Fazzi R, Marasca R, Petrini M (2008) Bortezomib is able to reduce angiogenesis in half of patients affected by idiopathic myelofibrosis: an ex vivo study. Leuk Res 32:1324–1325
Giantonio BJ, Catalano PJ, Meropol NJ, O'Dwyer PJ, Mitchell EP, Alberts SR, Schwartz MA, Benson AB 3rd (2007) Bevacizumab in combination with oxaliplatin, fluorouracil, and leucovorin (FOLFOX4) for previously treated metastatic colorectal cancer: results from the Eastern Cooperative Oncology Group Study E3200. J Clin Oncol 25:1539–1544
Gollob JA, Rathmell WK, Richmond TM, Marino CB, Miller EK, Grigson G, Watkins C, Gu L, Peterson BL, Wright JJ (2007) Phase II trial of sorafenib plus interferon alfa-2b as first- or second-line therapy in patients with metastatic renal cell cancer. J Clin Oncol 25:3288–3295
Goodman VL, Rock EP, Dagher R, Ramchandani RP, Abraham S, Gobburu JV, Booth BP, Verbois SL, Morse DE, Liang CY, Chidambaram N, Jiang JX, Tang S, Mahjoob K, Justice R, Pazdur R (2007) Approval summary: sunitinib for the treatment of imatinib refractory or intolerant gastrointestinal stromal tumors and advanced renal cell carcinoma. Clin Cancer Res 13: 1367–1373
Hajitou A, Grignet C, Devy L, Berndt S, Blacher S, Deroanne CF, Bajou K, Fong T, Chiang Y, Foidart JM, Noel A (2002) The antitumoral effect of endostatin and angiostatin is associated with a down-regulation of vascular endothelial growth factor expression in tumor cells. FASEB J 16:1802–1804
Hanahan D, Folkman J (1996) Patterns and emerging mechanisms of the angiogenic switch during tumorigenesis. Cell 86:353–364
Hanahan D, Bergers G, Bergsland E (2000) Less is more, regularly: metronomic dosing of cytotoxic drugs can target tumor angiogenesis in mice. J Clin Invest 105:1045–1047
Hanai J, Dhanabal M, Karumanchi SA, Albanese C, Waterman M, Chan B, Ramchandran R, Pestell R, and Sukhatme VP (2002) Endostatin causes G1 arrest of endothelial cells through inhibition of cyclin D1. J Biol Chem 277: 16464–16469
Hecht JR, Trarbach T, Jaeger E, Hainsworth J, Wolff R, Lloyd K, Bodoky G, Borner M, Laurent D, Jacques C (2005) A randomized, double-blind, placebo-controlled, phase III study in patients (Pts) with metastatic adenocarcinoma of the colon or rectum receiving first-line chemotherapy with oxaliplatin/5-fluorouracil/leucovorin and PTK787/ZK 222584 or placebo (CONFIRM-1). J Clin Oncol 23(Suppl):3 (abstract)
Heinrich MC, Maki RG, Corless CL, Antonescu CR, Harlow A, Griffith D, Town A, McKinley A, Ou WB, Fletcher JA, Fletcher CD, Huang X, Cohen DP, Baum CM, Demetri GD (2008) Primary and secondary kinase genotypes correlate with the biological and clinical activity of sunitinib in imatinib-resistant gastrointestinal stromal tumor. J Clin Oncol 26:5352–5359
Herbst RS, Heymach JV, O'Reilly MS, Onn A, Ryan AJ (2007) Vandetanib (ZD6474): an orally available receptor tyrosine kinase inhibitor that selectively targets pathways critical for tumor growth and angiogenesis. Expert Opin Investig Drugs 16:239–249
Herbst RS, Sun Y, Korfee S, Germonpre P, Saijo N, Zhou C, Wang J, Langmuir P, Kennedy SJ, Johnson BE (2009) Vandetanib plus docetaxel versus docetaxel as second-line treatment for patients with advanced non-small cell lung cancer (NSCLC): A randomized, double-blind phase III trial (ZODIAC). J Clin Oncol 27: CRA8003
Heymach JV, Johnson BE, Prager D, Csada E, Roubec J, Pesek M, Spasova I, Belani CP, Bodrogi I, Gadgeel S, Kennedy SJ, Hou J, Herbst RS (2007) Randomized, placebo-controlled phase II study of vandetanib plus

docetaxel in previously treated non small-cell lung cancer. J Clin Oncol 25:4270–4277

Heymach JV, Paz-Ares L, De Braud F, Sebastian M, Stewart DJ, Eberhardt WE, Ranade AA, Cohen G, Trigo JM, Sandler AB, Bonomi PD, Herbst RS, Krebs AD, Vasselli J, Johnson BE (2008) Randomized phase II study of vandetanib alone or with paclitaxel and carboplatin as first-line treatment for advanced non-small-cell lung cancer. J Clin Oncol 26:5407–5415

Higgins KJ, Abdelrahim M, Liu S, Yoon K, Safe S (2006a) Regulation of vascular endothelial growth factor receptor-2 expression in pancreatic cancer cells by Sp proteins. Biochem Biophys Res Commun 345:292–301

Higgins KJ, Liu S, Abdelrahim M, Yoon K, Vanderlaag K, Porter W, Metz RP, Safe S (2006b) Vascular endothelial growth factor receptor-2 expression is induced by 17beta-estradiol in ZR-75 breast cancer cells by estrogen receptor alpha/Sp proteins. Endocrinology 147:3285–3295

Hirte HW, Vidal L, Fleming GF, Sugimoto AK, Morgan RJ, Biagi JJ, Wang L, McGill S, Ivy SP, Oza AM (2008) A phase II study of cediranib (AZD2171) in recurrent or persistent ovarian, peritoneal or fallopian tube cancer: final results of a PMH, Chicago and California consortia trial. J Clin Oncol 26:5521 (abstract)

Hoffmann S, Burchert A, Wunderlich A, Wang Y, Lingelbach S, Hofbauer LC, Rothmund M, Zielke A (2007) Differential effects of cetuximab and AEE 788 on epidermal growth factor receptor (EGF-R) and vascular endothelial growth factor receptor (VEGF-R) in thyroid cancer cell lines. Endocrine 31:105–113

Holash J, Davis S, Papadopoulos N, Croll SD, Ho L, Russell M, Boland P, Leidich R, Hylton D, Burova E, Ioffe E, Huang T, Radziejewski C, Bailey K, Fandl JP, Daly T, Wiegand SJ, Yancopoulos GD, Rudge JS (2002) VEGF-Trap: a VEGF blocker with potent antitumor effects. Proc Natl Acad Sci USA 99:11393–11398

Huang SM, Li J, Armstrong EA, Harari PM (2002) Modulation of radiation response and tumor-induced angiogenesis after epidermal growth factor receptor inhibition by ZD1839 (Iressa). Cancer Res 62:4300–4306

Hurwitz H, Fehrenbacher L, Novotny W, Cartwright T, Hainsworth J, Heim W, Berlin J, Baron A, Griffing S, Holmgren E, Ferrara N, Fyfe G, Rogers B, Ross R, Kabbinavar F (2004) Bevacizumab plus irinotecan, fluorouracil, and leucovorin for metastatic colorectal cancer. N Engl J Med 350:2335–2342

Hwu WJ, Krown SE, Menell JH, Panageas KS, Merrell J, Lamb LA, Williams LJ, Quinn CJ, Foster T, Chapman PB, Livingston PO, Wolchok JD, Houghton AN (2003) Phase II study of temozolomide plus thalidomide for the treatment of metastatic melanoma. J Clin Oncol 21: 3351–3356

Inai T, Mancuso M, Hashizume H, Baffert F, Haskell A, Baluk P, Hu-Lowe DD, Shalinsky DR, Thurston G, Yancopoulos GD, McDonald DM (2004) Inhibition of vascular endothelial growth factor (VEGF) signaling in cancer causes loss of endothelial fenestrations, regression of tumor vessels, and appearance of basement membrane ghosts. Am J Pathol 165:35–52

Johnson DH, Fehrenbacher L, Novotny WF, Herbst RS, Nemunaitis JJ, Jablons DM, Langer CJ, DeVore RF 3rd, Gaudreault J, Damico LA, Holmgren E, Kabbinavar F (2004) Randomized phase II trial comparing bevacizumab plus carboplatin and paclitaxel with carboplatin and paclitaxel alone in previously untreated locally advanced or metastatic non-small-cell lung cancer. J Clin Oncol 22:2184–2191

Kane RC, Farrell AT, Saber H, Tang S, Williams G, Jee JM, Liang C, Booth B, Chidambaram N, Morse D, Sridhara R, Garvey P, Justice R, Pazdur R (2006) Sorafenib for the treatment of advanced renal cell carcinoma. Clin Cancer Res 12:7271–7278

Kanthou C, Tozer GM (2002) The tumor vascular targeting agent combretastatin A-4-phosphate induces reorganization of the actin cytoskeleton and early membrane blebbing in human endothelial cells. Blood 99:2060–2069

Kim ES, Serur A, Huang J, Manley CA, McCrudden KW, Frischer JS, Soffer SZ, Ring L, New T, Zabski S, Rudge JS, Holash J, Yancopoulos GD, Kandel JJ, Yamashiro DJ (2002a) Potent VEGF blockade causes regression of coopted vessels in a model of neuroblastoma. Proc Natl Acad Sci USA 99:11399–11404

Kim YM, Hwang S, Pyun BJ, Kim TY, Lee ST, Gho YS, Kwon YG (2002b) Endostatin blocks vascular endothelial growth factor-mediated signaling via direct interaction with KDR/Flk-1. J Biol Chem 277:27872–27879

Kim YM, Jang JW, Lee OH, Yeon J, Choi EY, Kim KW, Lee ST, Kwon YG (2000) Endostatin inhibits endothelial and tumor cellular invasion by blocking the activation and catalytic activity of matrix metalloproteinase. Cancer Res 60: 5410–5413

Kohne C, Bajetta E, Lin E, Valle JW, Van Cutsem E, Hecht JR, Moore MJ, Germond CJ, Meinhardt G, Jacques C (2007) Final results of CONFIRM 2: a multinational, randomized, double-blind, phase III study in 2nd line patients (pts) with metastatic colorectal cancer (mCRC) receiving FOLFOX4 and PTK787/ZK 222584 (PTK/ZK) or placebo. J Clin Oncol 25(Suppl):4033 (abstract)

Komorowski J, Jerczynska H, Siejka A, Baranska P, Lawnicka H, Pawlowska Z, Stepien H (2006) Effect of thalidomide affecting VEGF secretion, cell migration, adhesion and capillary tube formation of human endothelial EA.hy 926 cells. Life Sci 78:2558–2563

Kulke MH, Stuart K, Enzinger PC, Ryan DP, Clark JW, Muzikansky A, Vincitore M, Michelini A, Fuchs CS (2006) Phase II study of temozolomide and thalidomide in patients with metastatic neuroendocrine tumors. J Clin Oncol 24:401–406

Kumar S (2006) Progress in the treatment of multiple myeloma. Lancet 367:791–792

Laurie SA, Arnold A, Gauthier I, Chen E, Goss G, Ellis PM, Shepherd FA, Matthews S, Robertson J, Seymour L (2006) Final results of a phase I study of daily oral AZD2171, an inhibitor of vascular endothelial growth factor receptors (VEGFR), in combination with carboplatin (C)+paclitaxel (T) in patients with advanced non-small cell lung cancer (NSCLC): a study of the National Cancer Institute of Canada Clinical Trials Group (NCIC CTG). J Clin Oncol 24:3054 (abstract)

Laurie SA, Gauthier I, Arnold A, Shepherd FA, Ellis PM, Chen E, Goss G, Powers J, Walsh W, Tu D, Robertson J, Puchalski TA, Seymour L (2008) Phase I and pharmacokinetic study of daily oral AZD2171, an inhibitor of vascular endothelial growth factor tyrosine kinases, in combination with carboplatin and paclitaxel in patients with advanced non-small-cell lung cancer: the National Cancer Institute of Canada clinical trials group. J Clin Oncol 26:1871–1878

Lenz W (1967) Perthes-like changes in thalidomide children. Lancet 2:562

Lenz W, Knapp K (1962) Thalidomide embryopathy. Arch Environ Health 5:100–105

Li X, Lu Y, Liang K, Pan T, Mendelsohn J, Fan Z (2008) Requirement of hypoxia-inducible factor-1alpha down-regulation in mediating the antitumor activity of the anti-epidermal growth factor receptor monoclonal antibody cetuximab. Mol Cancer Ther 7:1207–1217

Li X, Liu X, Wang J, Wang Z, Jiang W, Reed E, Zhang Y, Liu Y, Li QQ (2003) Thalidomide down-regulates the expression of VEGF and bFGF in cisplatin-resistant human lung carcinoma cells. Anticancer Res 23:2481–2487

Liegl B, Kepten I, Le C, Zhu M, Demetri GD, Heinrich MC, Fletcher CD, Corless CL, Fletcher JA (2008) Heterogeneity of kinase inhibitor resistance mechanisms in GIST. J Pathol 216:64–74

List A, Kurtin S, Roe DJ, Buresh A, Mahadevan D, Fuchs D, Rimsza L, Heaton R, Knight R, Zeldis JB (2005) Efficacy of lenalidomide in myelodysplastic syndromes. N Engl J Med 352:549–557

Llovet J, Ricci S, Mazzaferro V, Hilgard P, Raoul J, Zeuzem S, Poulin-Costello M, Moscovici M, Voliotis D, Bruix J (2007) Sorafenib improves survival in advanced hepatocellular carcinoma (HCC): results of a phase III randomized placebo-controlled trial (SHARP trial). J Clin Oncol 25(18 S):LBA1 (abstract)

McKeage M (2006) Phase Ib/II study of DMXAA combined with carboplatin and paclitaxel in non-small cell lung cancer (NSCLC). J Clin Oncol 24(suppl):7102 (abstract)

McKeage MJ, and Jameson MB (2008) Comparison of safety and efficacy between squamous and non-squamous non-small cell lung cancer (NSCLC) patients in phase II studies of DMXAA (ASA404). J Clin Oncol 26(suppl):8072 (abstract)

Miller K, Wang M, Gralow J, Dickler M, Cobleigh M, Perez EA, Shenkier T, Cella D, Davidson NE (2007) Paclitaxel plus bevacizumab versus paclitaxel alone for metastatic breast cancer. N Engl J Med 357:2666–2676

Motzer RJ, Hutson TE, Tomczak P, Michaelson MD, Bukowski RM, Rixe O, Oudard S, Negrier S, Szczylik C, Kim ST, Chen I, Bycott PW, Baum CM, Figlin RA (2007) Sunitinib versus interferon alfa in metastatic renal-cell carcinoma. N Engl J Med 356:115–124

Motzer RJ, Rini BI, Bukowski RM, Curti BD, George DJ, Hudes GR, Redman BG, Margolin KA, Merchan JR, Wilding G, Ginsberg MS, Bacik J, Kim ST, Baum CM, Michaelson MD (2006a) Sunitinib in patients with metastatic renal cell carcinoma. JAMA 295:2516–2524

Motzer RJ, Michaelson MD, Redman BG, Hudes GR, Wilding G, Figlin RA, Ginsberg MS, Kim ST,

Baum CM, DePrimo SE, Li JZ, Bello CL, Theuer CP, George DJ, Rini BI (2006b) Activity of SU11248, a multitargeted inhibitor of vascular endothelial growth factor receptor and platelet-derived growth factor receptor, in patients with metastatic renal cell carcinoma. J Clin Oncol 24: 16–24

Murata R, Siemann DW, Overgaard J, Horsman MR (2001) Improved tumor response by combining radiation and the vascular-damaging drug 5, 6-dimethylxanthenone-4-acetic acid. Radiat Res 156:503–509

Natale RB, Thongprasert S, Greco FA, Thomas M, Tsai CM, Sunpaweravong P, Ferry D, Langmuir P, Rowbottom JA, Goss GD (2009) Vandetanib versus erlotinib in patients with advanced non-small cell lung cancer (NSCLC) after failure of at least one prior cytotoxic chemotherapy: A randomized, double-blind phase III trial (ZEST). J Clin Oncol 27: 8009

Nathan PD, Judson I, Padhani AR, Harris A, Carden CP, Smythe J, Collins D, Leach M, Walicke P, Rustin GJ (2008) A phase I study of combretastatin A4 phosphate (CA4P) and bevacizumab in subjects with advanced solid tumors. J Clin Oncol 26(Suppl):3550 (abstract)

Nawrocki ST, Bruns CJ, Harbison MT, Bold RJ, Gotsch BS, Abbruzzese JL, Elliott P, Adams J, McConkey DJ (2002) Effects of the proteasome inhibitor PS-341 on apoptosis and angiogenesis in orthotopic human pancreatic tumor xenografts. Mol Cancer Ther 1:1243–1253

O'Reilly MS, Boehm T, Shing Y, Fukai N, Vasios G, Lane WS, Flynn E, Birkhead JR, Olsen BR, Folkman J (1997) Endostatin: an endogenous inhibitor of angiogenesis and tumor growth. Cell 88:277–285

Perrotte P, Matsumoto T, Inoue K, Kuniyasu H, Eve BY, Hicklin DJ, Radinsky R, Dinney CP (1999) Anti-epidermal growth factor receptor antibody C225 inhibits angiogenesis in human transitional cell carcinoma growing orthotopically in nude mice. Clin Cancer Res 5:257–265

Pino MS, Shrader M, Baker CH, Cognetti F, Xiong HQ, Abbruzzese JL, McConkey DJ (2006) Transforming growth factor alpha expression drives constitutive epidermal growth factor receptor pathway activation and sensitivity to gefitinib (Iressa) in human pancreatic cancer cell lines. Cancer Res 66:3802–3812

Pore N, Jiang Z, Gupta A, Cerniglia G, Kao GD, Maity A (2006) EGFR tyrosine kinase inhibitors decrease VEGF expression by both hypoxia-inducible factor (HIF)-1-independent and HIF-1-dependent mechanisms. Cancer Res 66:3197–3204

Pruijn FB, van Daalen M, Holford NH, Wilson WR (1997) Mechanisms of enhancement of the antitumour activity of melphalan by the tumour-blood-flow inhibitor 5, 6-dimethylxanthenone-4-acetic acid. Cancer Chemother Pharmacol 39:541–546

Ratain MJ, Eisen T, Stadler WM, Flaherty KT, Kaye SB, Rosner GL, Gore M, Desai AA, Patnaik A, Xiong HQ, Rowinsky E, Abbruzzese JL, Xia C, Simantov R, Schwartz B, O'Dwyer PJ (2006) Phase II placebo-controlled randomized discontinuation trial of sorafenib in patients with metastatic renal cell carcinoma. J Clin Oncol 24: 2505–2512

Retsky MW, Hrushesky WJ, Gukas ID (2009) Hypothesis: primary antiangiogenic method proposed to treat early stage breast cancer. BMC Cancer 9:7

Rewcastle GW, Atwell GJ, Li ZA, Baguley BC, Denny WA (1991) Potential antitumor agents. 61. Structure-activity relationships for in vivo colon 38 activity among disubstituted 9-oxo-9H-xanthene-4-acetic acids. J Med Chem 34: 217–222

Richly H, Schultheis B, Adamietz IA, Kupsch P, Grubert M, Hilger RA, Ludwig M, Brendel E, Christensen O, Strumberg D (2009) Combination of sorafenib and doxorubicin in patients with advanced hepatocellular carcinoma: results from a phase I extension trial. Eur J Cancer 45(4): 579–587

Richly H, Henning BF, Kupsch P, Passarge K, Grubert M, Hilger RA, Christensen O, Brendel E, Schwartz B, Ludwig M, Flashar C, Voigtmann R, Scheulen ME, Seeber S, Strumberg D (2006) Results of a phase I trial of sorafenib (BAY 43–9006) in combination with doxorubicin in patients with refractory solid tumors. Ann Oncol 17:866–873

Roboz GJ, Giles FJ, List AF, Cortes JE, Carlin R, Kowalski M, Bilic S, Masson E, Rosamilia M, Schuster MW, Laurent D, Feldman EJ (2006) Phase 1 study of PTK787/ZK 222584, a small molecule tyrosine kinase receptor inhibitor, for the treatment of acute myeloid leukemia and myelodysplastic syndrome. Leukemia 20:952–957

Roskoski R Jr (2007) Sunitinib: a VEGF and PDGF receptor protein kinase and angiogenesis inhibitor. Biochem Biophys Res Commun 356:323–328

Rugo HS, Herbst RS, Liu G, Park JW, Kies MS, Steinfeldt HM, Pithavala YK, Reich SD,

9

Freddo JL, Wilding G (2005) Phase I trial of the oral antiangiogenesis agent AG-013736 in patients with advanced solid tumors: pharmacokinetic and clinical results. J Clin Oncol 23: 5474–5483
Rustin GJ, Galbraith SM, Anderson H, Stratford M, Folkes LK, Sena L, Gumbrell L, Price PM (2003a) Phase I clinical trial of weekly combretastatin A4 phosphate: clinical and pharmacokinetic results. J Clin Oncol 21:2815–2822
Rustin GJ, Bradley C, Galbraith S, Stratford M, Loadman P, Waller S, Bellenger K, Gumbrell L, Folkes L, Halbert G, PIITCoCR UK (2003b) 5, 6-dimethylxanthenone-4-acetic acid (DMXAA), a novel antivascular agent: phase I clinical and pharmacokinetic study. Br J Cancer 88:1160–1167
Sandler A, Gray R, Perry MC, Brahmer J, Schiller JH, Dowlati A, Lilenbaum R, Johnson DH (2006) Paclitaxel-carboplatin alone or with bevacizumab for non-small-cell lung cancer. N Engl J Med 355:2542–2550
Sharma S, Freeman B, Turner J, Symanowski J, Manno P, Berg W, Vogelzang N (2009) A phase I trial of PTK787/ZK222584 in combination with pemetrexed and cisplatin in patients with advanced solid tumors. Invest New Drugs 27:63–65
Shichiri M, Hirata Y (2001) Antiangiogenesis signals by endostatin. FASEB J 15:1044–1053
Siim BG, Lee AE, Shalal-Zwain S, Pruijn FB, McKeage MJ, Wilson WR (2003) Marked potentiation of the antitumour activity of chemotherapeutic drugs by the antivascular agent 5, 6-dimethylxanthenone-4-acetic acid (DMXAA). Cancer Chemother Pharmacol 51:43–52
Singhal S, Mehta J, Desikan R, Ayers D, Roberson P, Eddlemon P, Munshi N, Anaissie E, Wilson C, Dhodapkar M, Zeddis J, Barlogie B (1999) Antitumor activity of thalidomide in refractory multiple myeloma. N Engl J Med 341:1565–1571
Siu LL, Awada A, Takimoto CH, Piccart M, Schwartz B, Giannaris T, Lathia C, Petrenciuc O, Moore MJ (2006) Phase I trial of sorafenib and gemcitabine in advanced solid tumors with an expanded cohort in advanced pancreatic cancer. Clin Cancer Res 12:144–151
Spano J, Chodkiewicz C, Maurel J, Wong RP, Wasan HS, Pithavala YK, Bycott PW, Liau KF, Kim S, Rixe O (2008) A randomized phase II study of axitinib (AG-013736) and gemcitabine versus gemcitabine in advanced pancreatic cancer, preceded by a phase I component. J Clin Oncol 25:4551 (abstract)
Steins MB, Bieker R, Padro T, Kessler T, Kienast J, Berdel WE, Mesters RM (2003) Thalidomide for the treatment of acute myeloid leukemia. Leuk Lymphoma 44:1489–1493
Steins MB, Padro T, Bieker R, Ruiz S, Kropff M, Kienast J, Kessler T, Buechner T, Berdel WE, Mesters RM (2002) Efficacy and safety of thalidomide in patients with acute myeloid leukemia. Blood 99:834–839
Stevenson JP, Rosen M, Sun W, Gallagher M, Haller DG, Vaughn D, Giantonio B, Zimmer R, Petros WP, Stratford M, Chaplin D, Young SL, Schnall M, O'Dwyer PJ (2003) Phase I trial of the antivascular agent combretastatin A4 phosphate on a 5-day schedule to patients with cancer: magnetic resonance imaging evidence for altered tumor blood flow. J Clin Oncol 21:4428–4438
Strumberg D (2005) Preclinical and clinical development of the oral multikinase inhibitor sorafenib in cancer treatment. Drugs Today (Barc) 41: 773–784
Strumberg D, Awada A, Hirte H, Clark JW, Seeber S, Piccart P, Hofstra E, Voliotis D, Christensen O, Brueckner A, Schwartz B (2006) Pooled safety analysis of BAY 43–9006 (sorafenib) monotherapy in patients with advanced solid tumours: is rash associated with treatment outcome? Eur J Cancer 42:548–556
Sudhakar A, Sugimoto H, Yang C, Lively J, Zeisberg M, Kalluri R (2003) Human tumstatin and human endostatin exhibit distinct antiangiogenic activities mediated by alpha v beta 3 and alpha 5 beta 1 integrins. Proc Natl Acad Sci USA 100:4766–4771
Sun Y, Wang J, Liu Y, Song X, Zhang Y, Li K, Zhu Y, Zhou Q, You L, Yao C (2005) Results of phase III trial of endostarTM (rh-endostatin, YH-16) in advanced non-small cell lung cancer (NSCLC) patients. J Clin Oncol 23:7138 (abstract)
Tang P, Cohen SJ, Bjarnason GA, Kollmannsberger C, Virik K, MacKenzie MJ, Brown J, Wang L, Chen AP, Moore MJ (2008) Phase II trial of aflibercept (VEGF Trap) in previously treated patients with metastatic colorectal cancer (MCRC): a PMH phase II consortium trial. J Clin Oncol 26: 4027 (abstract)
Thomas AL, Morgan B, Horsfield MA, Higginson A, Kay A, Lee L, Masson E, Puccio-Pick M, Laurent D, Steward WP (2005) Phase I study of the safety, tolerability, pharmacokinetics, and pharmacodynamics of PTK787/ZK 222584

administered twice daily in patients with advanced cancer. J Clin Oncol 23:4162–4171

Thomas AL, Trarbach T, Bartel C, Laurent D, Henry A, Poethig M, Wang J, Masson E, Steward W, Vanhoefer U, Wiedenmann B (2007) A phase IB, open-label dose-escalating study of the oral angiogenesis inhibitor PTK787/ZK 222584 (PTK/ZK), in combination with FOLFOX4 chemotherapy in patients with advanced colorectal cancer. Ann Oncol 18:782–788

Tozer GM, Prise VE, Wilson J, Locke RJ, Vojnovic B, Stratford MR, Dennis MF, Chaplin DJ (1999) Combretastatin A-4 phosphate as a tumor vascular-targeting agent: early effects in tumors and normal tissues. Cancer Res 59:1626–1634

Uhr JW, Scheuermann RH, Street NE, Vitetta ES (1997) Cancer dormancy: opportunities for new therapeutic approaches. Nat Med 3:505–509

Wedge SR, Kendrew J, Hennequin LF, Valentine PJ, Barry ST, Brave SR, Smith NR, James NH, Dukes M, Curwen JO, Chester R, Jackson JA, Boffey SJ, Kilburn LL, Barnett S, Richmond GH, Wadsworth PF, Walker M, Bigley AL, Taylor ST, Cooper L, Beck S, Jurgensmeier JM, Ogilvie DJ (2005) AZD2171: a highly potent, orally bioavailable, vascular endothelial growth factor receptor-2 tyrosine kinase inhibitor for the treatment of cancer. Cancer Res 65:4389–4400

Wilhelm S, Carter C, Lynch M, Lowinger T, Dumas J, Smith RA, Schwartz B, Simantov R, Kelley S (2006) Discovery and development of sorafenib: a multikinase inhibitor for treating cancer. Nat Rev Drug Discov 5:835–844

Williams S, Pettaway C, Song R, Papandreou C, Logothetis C, McConkey DJ (2003) Differential effects of the proteasome inhibitor bortezomib on apoptosis and angiogenesis in human prostate tumor xenografts. Mol Cancer Ther 2: 835–843

Wood JM, Bold G, Buchdunger E, Cozens R, Ferrari S, Frei J, Hofmann F, Mestan J, Mett H, O'Reilly T, Persohn E, Rosel J, Schnell C, Stover D, Theuer A, Towbin H, Wenger F, Woods-Cook K, Menrad A, Siemeister G, Schirner M, Thierauch KH, Schneider MR, Drevs J, Martiny-Baron G, Totzke F (2000) PTK787/ZK 222584, a novel and potent inhibitor of vascular endothelial growth factor receptor tyrosine kinases, impairs vascular endothelial growth factor-induced responses and tumor growth after oral administration. Cancer Res 60: 2178–2189

Zorick TS, Mustacchi Z, Bando SY, Zatz M, Moreira-Filho CA, Olsen B, Passos-Bueno MR (2001) High serum endostatin levels in Down syndrome: implications for improved treatment and prevention of solid tumours. Eur J Hum Genet 9:811–814

10 Metronomic Chemotherapy: Principles and Lessons Learned from Applications in the Treatment of Metastatic Prostate Cancer

Urban Emmenegger, Giulio Francia, Yuval Shaked, and Robert S. Kerbel

Abstract By frequent and protracted administration of conventional cytotoxic drugs without prolonged interruptions, the primary treatment target shifts from the tumor cell population to the tumor vasculature. This "metronomic" way of chemotherapy administration results in antivascular effects, the mechanistic basis of which remains to be fully elucidated. We outline the basic aspects of the metronomic concept, describe the results of clinical applications of such chemotherapy by focusing on studies in metastatic prostate cancer, and discuss certain shortcomings. Based on preclinical findings, we finally point to the possible ways to address these shortcomings in order to bring this novel and promising use of conventional anticancer agents to full fruition.

U. Emmenegger (✉)
Department of Medicine, Division of Medical Oncology, and Department of Medical Biophysics, Division of Molecular and Cellular Biology, Sunnybrook Health Sciences Centre, University of Toronto, 2075, Bayview Avenue, Toronto, ON, Canada, M4N3M5
e-mail: urban.emmenegger@sri.utoronto.ca

10.1 Introduction

The concept of using antiangiogenic therapies as an anticancer strategy was formulated in 1971 by Folkman (1971) and clinically validated three decades later with the first successful application of an antiangiogenic agent, that is, the vascular endothelial growth factor (VEGF) targeting monoclonal antibody bevacizumab (Hurwitz et al. 2004). During this period, a sometimes tortuous path of discoveries led to an ever-increasing understanding of the complex process of tumor angiogenesis (Kerbel 2000). At present, the use of antiangiogenic agents is considered (part of) the standard of care for the treatment of colorectal, nonsmall cell lung, breast, kidney, and hepatocellular cancer, and involves the use of drugs such as bevacizumab and the antiangiogenic small molecule receptor tyrosine kinase inhibitors sunitinib and sorafenib (Kerbel 2006; Zhu 2008).

One interesting finding of the development of antiangiogenic therapies was that some targeted agents that were originally not developed as antiangiogenic drugs have been found to have "accidental" antiangiogenic properties (Kerbel et al. 2000). Furthermore, most conventional cytotoxic drugs can exert significant

R. Liersch et al. (eds.), *Angiogenesis Inhibition,* Recent Results in Cancer Research,
DOI: 10.1007/978-3-540-78281-0_10, © Springer Verlag Berlin Heidelberg 2010

antiangiogenic effects (Miller et al. 2001). However, when chemotherapeutics are used in a conventional manner (i.e., bolus drug administration followed by a 3–4-week drug-free period to allow the host to recover from the adverse side effects), the vascular damage inflicted by the cytotoxic drug(s) is thought to be rapidly repaired during the recovery period, thus negating any significant overall antiangiogenic effects. Conversely, Browder et al. showed that by shortening the drug-free break period between individual chemotherapy administrations, the net antiangiogenic effects of conventional cytotoxic drugs can be largely augmented (Browder et al. 2000). In addition, we showed that this form of antiangiogenic chemotherapy, commonly referred to as metronomic chemotherapy (Hanahan et al. 2000), is more potent when combined with targeted antiangiogenic agents, especially drugs that interfere with the endothelial cell survival activity of VEGF (Klement et al. 2000). As summarized by Kerbel and Kamen (2004), metronomic chemotherapy protocols are generally characterized by:

- Frequent (dose-dense) and regular (metronomic) – often daily – chemotherapy administration without any prolonged interruptions.
- Absence of a dose-escalation up to the maximal tolerated dose (MTD).
- Absence of the need for hematopoietic growth factor support.
- Preference for oral, outpatient regimens by using drugs such as cyclophosphamide (CPA).
- Low incidence or absence of treatment-related side effects.
- Potential for delayed emergence of resistance.

Because of mostly inconsequential side effects, metronomic regimens can be coadministered with targeted therapies for prolonged periods of time. Furthermore, the use of inexpensive, off-patent drugs such as CPA results in reduced costs compared to many MTD chemotherapy regimens (Bocci et al. 2005).

The feasibility and clinical benefits of this novel use of conventional cytotoxic drugs have been shown in various Phase II trials involving diverse tumor types such as breast, prostate, and ovarian cancer as well as non-Hodgkin's lymphomas among others (Colleoni et al. 2002; Glode et al. 2003; Burstein et al. 2005; Bottini et al. 2006; Buckstein et al. 2006; Colleoni et al. 2006; Young et al. 2006; Lord et al. 2007; Garcia et al. 2008). These findings remain to be confirmed in Phase III trials. Furthermore, important questions remain to be addressed such as the optimal dose and most effective dosing interval, improved monitoring of the antiangiogenic effects, the choice of cytotoxic drugs used for a given tumor type, and the most efficacious way to integrate metronomic chemotherapy into standard therapy protocols.

We provide an overview of the molecular mechanisms behind the antivascular effects of metronomic chemotherapy, and discuss clinical results as well as some shortcomings of the metronomic concept by focusing on published applications for the treatment of metastatic castration-resistant prostate cancer (CRPC). Finally, we discuss the potential future role of metronomic as compared to conventional MTD chemotherapy.

10.2 Mechanisms of Action of Metronomic Chemotherapy

Experimental evidence that chemotherapy administered in a condensed schedule slows down the repair of the drug-induced damage to the tumor vasculature was first reported in 2000. Browder et al. showed that CPA administered every 6 days produced more sustained antiangiogenic effects compared to conventional every 3-week MTD CPA administration (Browder et al. 2000). Intriguingly, CPA was even effective in tumors that had been made resistant in vivo to a conventional CPA regimen, further suggesting that mechanisms other than direct antitumor effects are the basis of the antitumor effects seen with metronomic protocols. In addition, when mice bearing large, established human neuroblastoma xenografts were treated by Klement et al. with twice weekly metronomic administrations of vinblastine combined with DC101, a monoclonal antibody blocking the murine vascular endothelial cell growth factor receptor 2 (VEGFR2), this combination therapy resulted in a significant therapeutic benefit (Klement et al. 2000). Tumors completely regressed over time and did not relapse during a 7-month period of uninterrupted therapy. Both studies suggest that metronomic regimens act largely by inhibiting tumor angiogenesis.

10.2.1 Preferential Antiproliferative Effects of Metronomic Chemotherapy Toward Endothelial Cells

In vitro studies indicated that a 6-day continuous exposure of human micro- and macrovascular endothelial cells to low concentrations of chemotherapy drugs such as paclitaxel or the CPA precursor 4-hydroperoxy-CPA resulted in preferential endothelial cell growth inhibition compared to other cell types, for example, human fibroblast and breast cancer cells (Bocci et al. 2002). These results provided further evidence that metronomic regimens using various chemotherapy drugs may have a highly selective effect against rapidly dividing vascular endothelial cells.

Subsequently, we reported that protracted in vitro exposure of endothelial cells to low concentrations of several cytotoxic agents causes a marked induction in the expression of thrombospondin-1 (TSP-1) at the mRNA and protein level (Bocci et al. 2003). TSP-1 is a potent endogenous inhibitor of angiogenesis, which acts primarily by binding to endothelial cells expressing the CD36 receptor, resulting in the induction of endothelial cell death (Volpert et al. 2002; Yap et al. 2005). TSP-1 also exerts indirect antiangiogenic effects by binding and sequestering VEGF (Gupta et al. 1999). With regard to metronomic chemotherapy in vivo, induction of circulating TSP-1 plasma levels was observed in mice bearing human xenografts that were treated with metronomic CPA (Bocci et al. 2003). Further evidence for the role of TSP-1 was obtained by administering metronomic CPA to TSP-1 knockout mice bearing Lewis lung carcinoma. Compared to wild-type mice, the metronomic regimen lost its antitumor activity in the knockout mice. However, when CPA was administered at the MTD, retention of the antitumor effects in both wild-type and TSP-1 deficient mice was observed. Similar results were obtained by another group when CPA was administered on a weekly basis to TSP-1 knock-out mice bearing B16 mouse melanoma, and others (Hamano et al. 2004; Damber et al. 2006; Ma and Waxman 2007; Ma and Waxman 2008). Interestingly, the antitumor effects of metronomic regimens were retained in mice that were unable to produce either endostatin or tumstatin, both of which are other endogenous inhibitors of angiogenesis (Hamano et al. 2004). Taken together, these results suggested that TSP-1 is a mediator of the antiangiogenic effects of at least some metronomic regimens and confers endothelial cell specificity.

10.2.2 Circulating Bone Marrow-Derived Endothelial Precursor Cells as Targets of Metronomic Chemotherapy

In addition to *angiogenesis* mediated by local sprouting of rapidly dividing endothelial cells from pre-existing capillaries, the tumor vasculature also depends on *vasculogenesis* mediated by circulating endothelial precursor cells (CEPs) originating from the bone marrow. Following mobilization, CEPs enter the blood circulation and subsequently home to sites of active angiogenesis, where they differentiate and incorporate into the lumen of growing blood vessels and proliferate (Bertolini et al. 2006). A number of preclinical studies suggest that certain tumors are highly dependent on this vasculogenic support, namely lymphomas, Ewing's sarcomas, and inflammatory carcinomas of the breast (Bertolini et al. 2003; de Bont et al. 2001; Bolontrade et al. 2002; Shirakawa et al. 2002). For example, using NOD SCID mice bearing Namalwa or Granta 519 human lymphomas, Bertolini et al. demonstrated that shortly after the administration of an intensive MTD course of CPA, levels of CEPs were substantially reduced for the first few days, followed by a marked rebound during the drug-free break period. This rebound and its timing are reminiscent of the process of hematopoietic recovery after myelosuppressive therapy (Bertolini et al. 2003). In contrast, when CPA was administered in a metronomic regimen, that is, either injected i.p. every 6 days (Browder et al. 2000) or continuously via drinking water (Man et al. 2002), levels of CEPs gradually declined and remained suppressed during the entire treatment period. The degree of mobilization of CEPs and their viability during treatment with MTD versus metronomic CPA is depicted in Fig. 10.1.

Interestingly, we reported a similar or even more important CEP rebound after treatment with vascular disrupting agents (VDAs) (Shaked et al. 2006). As opposed to antiangiogenic agents, this class of drugs causes an acute occlusion of tumor blood vessels, which subsequently results in tumor cell death. However, some remaining viable tumor tissue is usually observed at the rim, from which tumor growth rapidly resumes. We have shown that CEPs can be mobilized from the bone marrow in a matter of hours of treatment with a VDA, and subsequently home to the viable tumor rim. CEPs then incorporate into the tumor blood vessels and promote angiogenesis, which results in rapid tumor repopulation. Taken together, the surge of CEPs following MTD chemotherapy or treatment with a VDA could contribute to the vascular repair process referred to by Browder et al. (2000). Conversely, the metronomic administration of cytotoxic drugs may inhibit the CEP rebound phenomenon and promote the antiangiogenic effects of such chemotherapy. Suppression of the CEP surge is one of the mechanisms that might account for the beneficial effects seen when metronomic or other antiangiogenic therapies are combined with MTD chemotherapy (Kerbel 2006).

10.2.2.1 Benefit of Combined Bolus and Metronomic Chemotherapy Administration

One aspect of the aforementioned study by Bertolini et al. (2003) was whether the combination of metronomic with intermittent bolus dose chemotherapy administration could be effective as a long-term antitumor treatment strategy. We hypothesized that the metronomic regimen might inhibit the CEP rebound following bolus chemotherapy administration. Using three different tumor models, that is, human prostate cancer xenografts (PC-3), Friend virus-induced murine erythroleukemia, and murine breast cancer (EMT-6), we demonstrated that the combination of bolus dose CPA (in our case one-third of the conventional MTD administered every 3 or 6 weeks) plus metronomic CPA was more effective than MTD or metronomic monotherapy (Shaked et al. 2005b). Importantly, the levels of CEPs remained suppressed despite bolus CPA administration. In another study, Pietras and Hanahan reported similar findings. Briefly, a "chemo-switch" regimen (defined by upfront MTD CPA, followed by metronomic CPA combined with targeted antiangiogenic agents) produced significant antitumor responses and survival benefits in a mouse pancreatic cancer model (Pietras and Hanahan 2005).

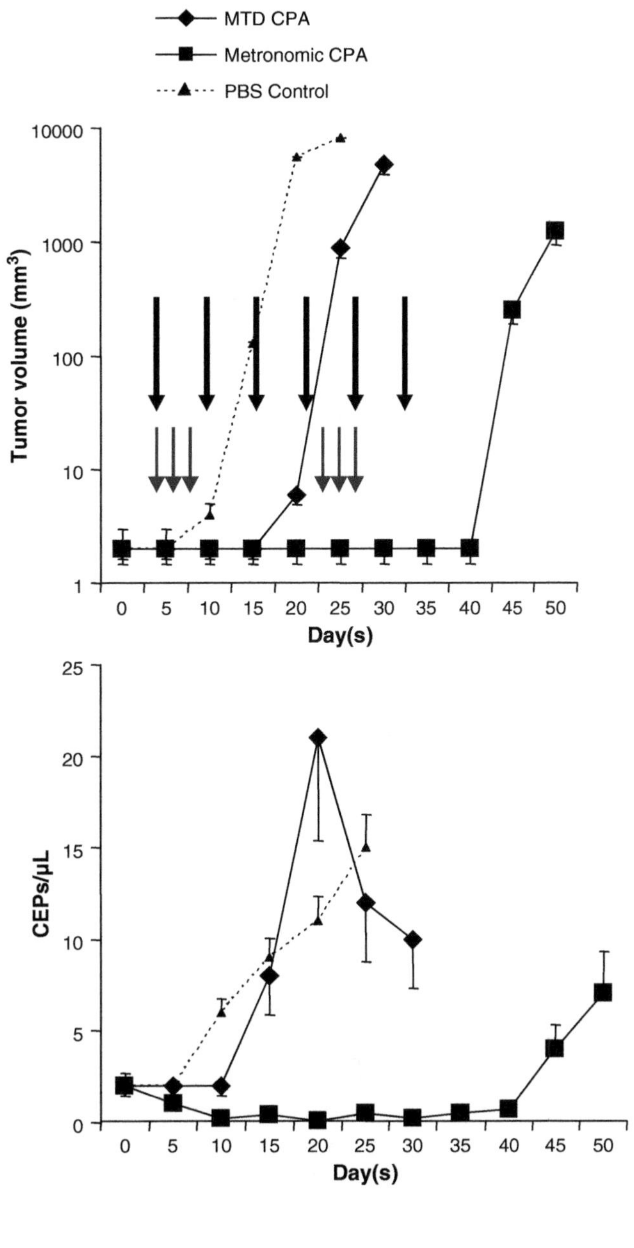

Fig. 10.1 The effect of metronomic and MTD chemotherapy regimens on CEP levels. Human Namalwa lymphoma bearing NOD/SCID mice were treated with CPA administered either at the MTD for this mouse strain, i.e., 75 mg/kg i.p. injection every other day for three doses per cycle (*purple arrows*), or as a metronomic regimen, i.e., 170 mg/kg i.p. injection every 6 days (*black arrows*). Tumor volumes (*upper graph*) and levels of CEPs detected in peripheral blood (*lower graph*) were monitored regularly (adopted with minor modifications from Bertolini et al. 2003, with permission from the publisher)

10.2.2.2 CEPs and Optimal Biological Dose of Antiangiogenic Agents

Evidence for antivasculogenic effects of metronomic chemotherapy was also reported in our study that sought to determine whether CEPs can serve as a pharmacodynamic biomarker to determine the optimal biological (=antiangiogenic) dose of antiangiogenic drugs or treatment strategies. The fact that CEPs gradually declined after treatment with metronomic CPA

(Bertolini et al. 2003) led us to investigate whether the levels of such circulating cells may reflect the level of antivascular activity in mice. A previous study had demonstrated that various mouse strains exhibit different levels of angiogenic responsiveness as measured by the corneal micropocket assay (Rohan et al. 2000). The angiogenic stimulus, that is, basic fibroblast growth factor (bFGF), was implanted into the corneas of different mouse strains and vessel growth/sprouting was evaluated. Strains such as C57Bl/6 exhibited a low number of sprouting vessels (indicating a low level of angiogenic responsiveness), whereas others strains, for example, BALB/c or 129, showed a very strong angiogenic response. In our studies, we evaluated the baseline CEP levels in different mouse strains and found a striking correlation between the number of such cells in peripheral blood and the angiogenic responsiveness previously determined for the same strains with the corneal micropocket assay (Shaked et al. 2005a). These results suggest that CEPs might be used as a biomarker to determine the level of angiogenic activity in mice. Subsequently, CEP levels were measured 1 week after treatment with antiangiogenic drugs such as DC101 or ABT-510, a TSP-1 mimetic peptide (Shaked et al. 2005a). In both cases, we found that the drug doses producing maximum antitumor activity also caused the greatest decline in viable CEPs. Similar results were obtained with metronomic regimens using various chemotherapy drugs, for example, CPA, vinblastine, vinorelbine, cisplatinum, ABI-007 (Abraxane®, a cremophor-free nanoparticle paclitaxel preparation), and UFT (Uftoral®, tegafur-uracil), administered to mice bearing various human tumor xenografts (Shaked et al. 2005c; Munoz et al. 2006; Ng et al. 2006). In fact, after a single week of treatment we found a striking correlation between the metronomic drug dose resulting in maximal antitumor activity without overt toxicity and the greatest decline in CEP levels in peripheral blood (Shaked et al. 2005c).

10.2.3 Mechanisms of Action Summarized

Figure 10.2 demonstrates some of the possible mechanisms of action of metronomic chemotherapy regimens. Thus far, such regimens have mostly been investigated with respect to their antivascular effects involving the inhibition of both the locally dividing activated endothelial cells and the systemic vasculogenic process mediated by CEPs. However, much needs to be learned about the effects of metronomic therapy on other bone marrow cell types that might promote angiogenesis or tumor growth via different mechanisms, possible direct effects of metronomic regimens on tumor cells, potential immunomodulatory activities of drugs like CPA, in particular when used in a protracted manner (Ghiringhelli et al. 2007), and possible adverse side effects (Fig. 10.3).

10.3 Metronomic Chemotherapy for the Treatment of Metastatic Castration-Resistant Prostate Cancer

Protracted cytotoxic drug administration was studied as early as in the 1970s (Vogelzang 1984). However, such chemotherapy regimens often included regular treatment-free breaks and the dosing was oriented toward maximizing the cytotototoxic effects. Since the first preclinical descriptions in 2000 (Browder et al. 2000; Klement et al. 2000), the results of more than 50 clinical trials embracing the metronomic concept have been published. Breast and prostate cancer are among the best studied tumor types in this respect (Colleoni et al. 2002; Glode et al. 2003; Burstein et al. 2005; Bottini et al. 2006; Colleoni et al. 2006; Lord et al. 2007).

CRPC is particularly well suited for a metronomic chemotherapy type of treatment strategy. The role of angiogenesis in prostate cancer in

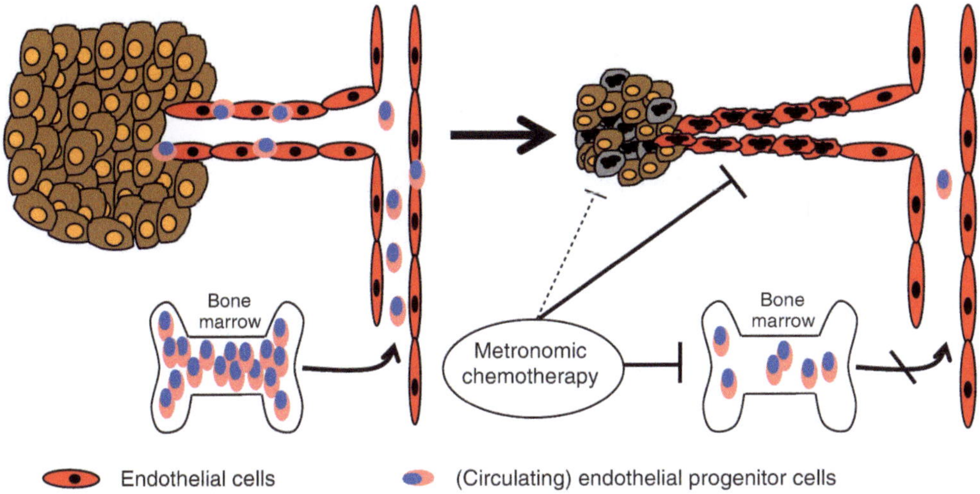

Fig. 10.2 Antivascular effects of metronomic chemotherapy. Metronomic chemotherapy affects dividing, activated tumor endothelial cells and inhibits the mobilization and/or the viability of bone marrow derived CEPs, which can contribute to tumor neoangiogenesis. Furthermore, drugs like CPA used in a protracted, low-dose manner might also exert immunomodulatory effects. Direct anti-tumor effects seem not to play a major role in most instances when chemotherapy is given in a metronomic manner (modified from Shaked et al. 2005c, with permission from the publisher)

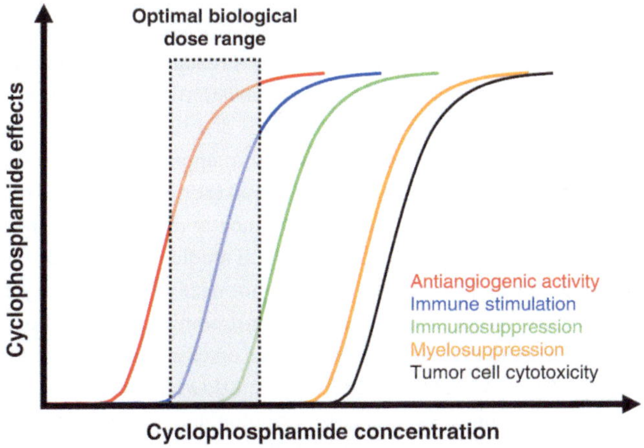

Fig. 10.3 Hypothetical dose-response curves of various metronomic CPA effects. When given at the optimal biological dose, metronomic CPA results in antiangiogenic and possibly also immunostimulatory effects. Higher CPA doses increase the risk of immuno/myelosuppression, likely without added benefit as far as antiangiogenic effects are concerned

general, and in the castration-resistant stage in particular, is well documented (Nicholson and Theodorescu 2004). Furthermore, CRPC is mainly a disease of the elderly where treatment-related adverse effects may limit the use of overly toxic approaches (Pienta and Smith 2005). Historically, the focus on quality of life aspects rather than improving overall survival has been a necessity in the treatment of CRPC in the absence of therapies impacting on the latter (Tannock et al. 1996). The current standard MTD chemotherapy approach, that is, 3-weekly administration of docetaxel-based chemotherapy (Petrylak et al. 2004; Tannock et al. 2004), results in prolonged overall survival, improved pain control, and better quality of life. However, the impact on survival is only a modest 2–3 month increase compared to the former standard therapy of mitoxantrone/prednisone (Tannock et al. 1996). Thus, there is a clear need for novel strategies in patients that are not considered suitable for docetaxel chemotherapy or those that develop severe docetaxel-related side effects. In addition, there is an unmet need for new approaches in the maintenance setting following maximal response to docetaxel (Lin et al. 2007). Metronomic and other antiangiogenic therapies might meet these needs and are also an interesting option in early CRPC, where the possible benefits of conventional cytotoxic therapy do not outweigh the risk of adverse side-effects and their potential impact on the quality of life.

10.3.1 From Bench to Bedside

Given the lack of feasible metastatic prostate cancer models, the benefit of using metronomic chemotherapy in advanced metastatic disease has thus far been studied preclinically in spontaneous metastatic breast cancer and melanoma models (Munoz et al. 2006; Cruz-Munoz et al. 2008). An unexpected lesson from such studies is that the primary tumor response is not necessarily indicative of the effects of metronomic treatment strategies against metastatic disease. Briefly, breast cancer xenografts were allowed to grow in mice as primary, orthotopically implanted tumors, or to develop (following surgical removal of primary tumors) into visceral metastatic disease. Both primary tumors and metastases were then treated with metronomic CPA and UFT, administered as monotherapies or in combination. The results showed that the combination of CPA and UFT did not improve primary tumor response compared to CPA alone. However, the same combination was highly efficacious against metastatic disease involving multiple organs. Similar results were obtained with vinblastine and CPA in a metastatic melanoma model (Cruz-Munoz, Man and Kerbel, unpublished observations). Thus, had the analysis been carried out only on a primary tumor model, it would likely have suggested the erroneous interpretation that UFT (or vinblastine) was ineffective in improving the anticancer benefits of metronomic CPA monotherapy. These results highlight the importance of consideration that is needed to identify new metronomic combinations, and the importance of assessing them in appropriate disease models including metastatic cancer. Restricting studies to primary tumors may result in novel metronomic regimens being erroneously discarded as ineffective. For the same reason, it is therefore important that better metastatic prostate cancer models be developed to carry out similar studies in prostate cancer.

In attempting to develop improved metronomic therapies and compare them to conventional chemotherapy administration, another factor might be relatively overlooked, that is, the lack of significant observable host toxicity resulting from metronomic regimens, particularly when compared to conventional MTD chemotherapy. The limited preclinical studies of metronomic regimens against metastatic disease have thus far confirmed this finding. The toxicity aspect has hitherto been little appreciated because host toxicity is seldom a limiting factor in the design and execution of preclinical studies involving primary tumor xenografts. If the impact of treatment-related toxicity is not considered, the benefit of metronomic treatment on survival in preclinical metastatic disease might be underappreciated when compared to standard MTD regimens. Although this assumption remains yet to be formally tested in metastatic models, there already is confirmatory evidence from long-term therapy studies involving metronomic vs. MTD dosing in primary tumor models by du Manoir et al. and Shaked et al. (2005b; du

Manoir et al. 2006). Thus du Manoir et al. treated a human breast cancer model with trastuzumab (Herceptin®) plus CPA, where the alkylating agent was administered either metronomically or in a MTD fashion. Shaked et al. described a detailed comparison of MTD CPA with a metronomic CPA regimen that included interspersed bolus administrations of CPA at one third of the MTD in order to minimize toxicity. Both studies showed tumor responses that are schematically shown in Figs.10.4a, b. When tumor volume measurements were analyzed, there was indication that MTD CPA therapy was more effective against primary tumor growth than the metronomic-based regimen, particularly over a short treatment period (e.g., less than 50 days). This is important since currently most preclinical studies are completed within a relatively short time frame in which it is not unusual for the treatment to involve only one or two cycles of MTD therapy. However, over a longer treatment period, the mice on the MTD therapy had to be sacrificed. This was not because of complications arising from tumor growth, but because of overt toxicity, exemplified by weight loss (Fig. 10.4c). When the toxicity and tumor response were jointly considered in a Kaplan–Meier analysis, as done by du Manoir et al. (du Manoir et al. 2006), MTD CPA therapy did not show as significant an advantage over the metronomic-based regimen. Indeed, the fact that the mice on the MTD-based regimen died after three cycles of MTD actually made the metronomic regimen look better in the Kaplan–Meier plot comparison (Fig. 10.4d). On the other hand, in the study by Shaked et al. it was noted that mice on the MTD CPA regimen bearing human prostate cancer xenografts died after nine treatment cycles

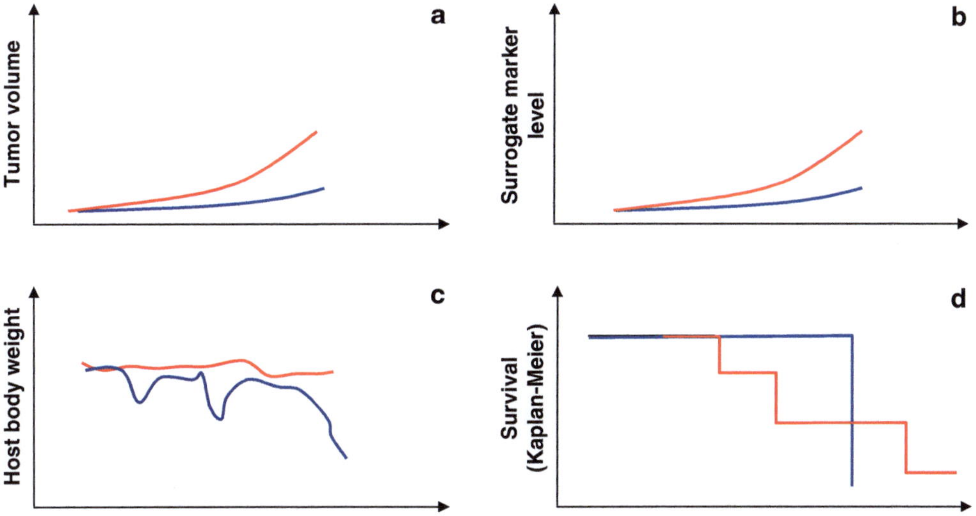

Fig. 10.4 Potential pitfalls in the design and interpretation of preclinical studies in mice using metronomic regimens. A number of studies have shown that in some cases, particularly over short periods of time, MTD (*blue lines*) can be more effective than metronomic (*red lines*) chemotherapy. This is something that would be assessed by (caliper based) tumor measurements (**a**), or surrogate marker analysis (**b**). However, such studies risk failing assessment of the relative impact of host toxicity which may only appear after a number of cycles of MTD administration, e.g., exemplified by progressive weight loss (**c**). This can be appreciated in a Kaplan–Meier plot (**d**), in which both toxicity and tumor growth are taken into account

due to toxicity (Shaked et al. 2005b). This is in sharp contrast to the metronomic CPA monotherapy regimen, which did not give rise to toxicity in the same mouse strain, even after several months of drug administration (Emmenegger et al. 2004; Emmenegger et al. 2006). Future preclinical metastasis studies reporting tumor size parameters and Kaplan–Meier plots will better define the contrast between MTD and metronomic dosing.

In clinical trials, parallel considerations may arise if a metronomic regimen proves equally effective to an MTD regimen in terms of survival, yet without the degree of toxicity that is often associated with MTD dosing (Rivera et al. 2008). To date, a number of clinical trials have reported the low incidence of high-grade toxic side effects with metronomic regimens (Colleoni et al. 2002; Bottini et al. 2006; Colleoni et al. 2006; Lord et al. 2007). Thus, one interesting possibility which would conceivably emerge is that metronomic chemotherapy protocols may be established as a valid alternative to MTD regimens, not because they are superior in prolonging survival, but because of an improved overall therapeutic benefit.

10.3.2 Key Findings of Metronomic Trials in Castration-Resistant Prostate Cancer and Emerging Questions

Table 10.1 summarizes the key findings of published metronomic CRPC trials (Nishimura et al. 2001; Glode et al. 2003; Nicolini et al. 2004; Di Lorenzo et al. 2007; Lord et al. 2007). With the exception of the study by Lord et al. (2007), many of the study subjects enrolled onto these trials had been previously exposed to conventional cytotoxic therapy. One of the drugs administered in all these studies is CPA, an agent that has been commonly used in the past for the treatment of CRPC using various nonmetronomic intravenous and oral regimens (Mike et al. 2006; Winquist et al. 2006). The applied CPA dose varied from 50 mg/day – the dose most commonly used in metronomic trials involving CPA (Kerbel and Kamen 2004; Gille et al. 2005) – to alternating 100/150 mg/day (Nicolini et al. 2004). Although PSA responses of >50% were typically rare, clinical benefit in the form of either minor PSA responses <50% or PSA stabilization were commonly seen and maintained for several months.

Toxicity has not been a major issue in metronomic trials for CRPC. In fact, grade 3–4 side effects are rare, the only exception being G3 lymphopenias seen in one-third of the patients in the study by Lord et al. (2007). The rather high daily CPA dose of 50 mg/m^2 used by these authors (representing ~100 mg/day for most patients) might be an explanation for this unexpected high rate of lymphopenia. However, it is reassuring that the lymphopenias described did not result in opportunistic infections. Although lymphopenias have been described as a consequence of metronomic CPA therapy in mice at the optimal biological dose (Emmenegger et al. 2004), the commonly used CPA dose in metronomic clinical trials of 50 mg/day seems to be devoid of this side-effect despite clear evidence of clinical activity (Colleoni et al. 2002; Glode et al. 2003; Burstein et al. 2005; Bottini et al. 2006; Buckstein et al. 2006; Colleoni et al. 2006; Garcia et al. 2008).

In the study by Lord et al., 22 patients received fewer than 8 weeks of CPA therapy. Most of them had to be removed from the study because of rapid disease progression (Lord et al. 2007). This is a reminder that this type of therapy needs to be used with caution in patients with rapidly progressive disease. An alternative might be to consider an initial intravenous bolus dose of CPA (or another cytotoxic agent) before commencing metronomic scheduling (Fontana et al. 2007).

In summary, metronomic studies in CRPC show reasonable clinical activity combined with a very appealing toxicity profile, findings that need to be confirmed in Phase III trials. Similarly,

Table 10.1 Metronomic Chemotherapy Trials in CRPC

Reference	Lord et al. 2007	Glode et al. 2003	Nishimura et al. 2001	Di Lorenzo et al. 2007	Nicolini et al. 2004
CRPC stage	Early	*Early*-advanced	*Early*-advanced	Advanced	Early-*advanced*
N=(evaluable)	80(58)	34(32)	21(21)	16(16)	8(8)
Treatment	CPA 50 mg/m^2 o.d.	CPA 50 mg o.d. Dexamethasone 1 mg o.d.	CPA 50 mg b.i.d UFT 200 mg b.i.d. EMP 280 mg b.i.d	CPA 50 mg o.d. THD 100 or 200 mg o.d.	CPA alternating 100 or 150 mg o.d. Mesna 400 mg p.o. 3/4 weeks
PSA response (%)	3	69	57	15	25
PSA stabilization (%)	N/A	6	24	8	37.5
Clinical benefit (%)	45	75	81	23	62.5
Grade 3–4 toxicities	Lymphopenia G3 32.8% Neutropenia G3 1.7% Anemia G3 1.7%	N/A	Leucopenia G3 14% Hemorrhagic cystitis G3 3.5% G3.5%	Neutropenia 20% Anemia 10%	N/A
Median response duration (range)	7.5 months (3–18)	8 months (95% CI: 4–10)	7 months (2–15)	Median survival 15 weeks (9–19)	9 months (8–31)
Comments	22 patients did not finish at least two treatment cycles (8 weeks) and were not included in the analysis	Retrospective analysis; treatment interruption in four patients (mainly for hematological toxicity); CPA withdrawn in 1 patient (gastro-intestinal symptoms)		All patients post two lines of cytotoxic therapy; only combined G3/G4 toxicity data presented	Best PSA response 3, 5, 7, 8, and 31 months after treatment initiation

CRPC castration-resistant prostate cancer; *N* number of patients; *CPA* cyclophosphamide; *UFT* tegafur-uracil; *EMP* estramustine phosphate; *THD* thalidomide; *N/A* not available; *clinical benefit*=complete response+partial response+stable disease positive observations have been reported with other tumor types (Bottini et al. 2006; Buckstein et al. 2006; Colleoni et al. 2006; Garcia et al. 2008). However, these studies also raise many questions such as: What is the best choice of drug(s) used in such regimens? What is the optimal biological dose of a given drug? What are the most efficacious drugs or drug combinations to be used in metronomic protocols? How can metronomic regimens be integrated into current standards of practice?

10.3.2.1 Choice of Cytotoxic Drugs Used in Metronomic Regimens

CPA is an obvious choice for metronomic use in CRPC in that (a) the beneficial effects of metronomic CPA are well documented (pre)clinically (Man et al. 2002; Emmenegger et al. 2006), (b) the potential (long-term) side effects of CPA are well known from immunosuppressive protocols using CPA, albeit at higher daily doses than typically applied in metronomic regimens (Hoffman et al. 1992; Haubitz et al. 1998), and (c) CPA is available in an oral form. Furthermore, CPA has been used in the past for the treatment of CRPC, either orally or administered intravenously, albeit applying more conventional dosing schedules (Mike et al. 2006; Winquist et al. 2006). Interestingly, cytotoxic drugs successfully used in a conventional manner for a certain tumor type often also show clinical activity in metronomic protocols for the same tumor type. It remains to be seen whether this reflects certain tumor-related characteristics or whether it is rather a bias dictated by the experience of the prescribing oncologists. In fact, it is currently not known whether certain agents are more active in certain tumor types when used metronomically. Similarly, further study is needed to define whether the sequential use of cytotoxic drugs in metronomic regimens might be able to delay or overcome resistance (Kieran et al. 2005).

There is limited evidence that cytotoxics are not interchangeable when used as antiangiogenics. In fact, while inhibition of proliferation of endothelial cells seems to be likely a universal consequence of the metronomic use of chemotherapeutic agents (Bocci et al. 2002; Wang et al. 2003), other biological effects might be more drug-specific, such as the (a) TSP-1 induction by CPA and various microtubule inhibitors (Bocci et al. 2003; Hamano et al. 2004), (b) anti-Hif-1α activities of topoisomerase I inhibitors and microtubule inhibitors (Rapisarda et al. 2004; Escuin et al. 2005), and (c) the induction of CD95 on endothelial cells by agents such as doxorubicin and CPA (Quesada et al. 2005; Yap et al. 2005). Furthermore, pharmacokinetic characteristics might make certain chemotherapeutics drugs more or less suitable for metronomic use (Hahnfeldt et al. 2003).

Besides the question of which drug to use, it is also important to define patient and/or tumor characteristics that predict prolonged benefit from metronomic therapies. As an example, Orlando et al. have described advanced breast cancer patients receiving metronomic CPA/methotrexate with a median time to progression of almost 2 years (Orlando et al. 2006). In this study, patients achieving remissions or stable disease for 12 months or more comprised 15.7% of the entire study population.

10.3.2.2 Optimal Biological Dose

Preclinically, metronomic dosing often implies the frequent administration of ~1/3rd to 1/10th of the MTD of a given cytotoxic drug (Kerbel and Kamen 2004; Gille et al. 2005; Lam et al. 2006). More recently, a less empirical way to characterize the optimal biological dose was determined preclinically, that is, the dose with maximal CEP suppression in the absence of significant toxicity such as myelosuppression and body weight loss, as described earlier

(Shaked et al. 2005c). Unfortunately, the use of CEP levels for individual dosing is hampered in humans because of the lower number of such cells compared to mice (Bertolini et al. 2007).

Takahashi proposed the concept of the *individualized maximum repeatable dose* (Takahashi et al. 2005). Briefly, the weekly dose of gemcitabine was titrated to a dose resulting in stable Grade 1 toxicity despite prolonged gemcitabine use. As appealing as such an approach might be, it would likely be restricted to situations of metronomic monotherapy. As an alternative, the assessment of pharmacokinetic and/or pharmacodynamic parameters might become a way to tailor individual dosing in the future (Kamen et al. 2006; Emmenegger et al. 2007). However, despite major efforts there continues to be a lack of validated pharmacodynamic surrogate markers for antiangiogenic activity (Jubb et al. 2006).

Even when more sophisticated metronomic dosing might become feasible in the future, practical aspects need to be considered as well. As an example, in the metronomic clinical trial by Colleoni et al. in metastatic breast cancer, a daily CPA dose of 50 and 2.5 mg of methotrexate b.i.d. on Day 1 and 2 of every week were administered (Colleoni et al. 2002). The choice of these doses was driven by practical considerations such as available tablet size, and was assumed to facilitate a high level of patient compliance.

10.3.2.3
Combination Therapies

High levels of proangiogenic cytokines can confer endothelial cell resistance to the effects of cytotoxic drugs (Tran et al. 2002). Therefore, by combination with targeted antiangiogenic agents such as inhibitors of the VEGF pathway, the effects of metronomic chemotherapy can be augmented and vice versa (Klement et al. 2000; Burstein et al. 2005; Pietras and Hanahan 2005). In contrast to combinations involving MTD chemotherapy, which are generally limited to 6–10 continuous cycles, protocols involving targeted antiangiogenics combined with metronomic chemotherapy might be used for prolonged periods of time, given the excellent safety profile of such regimens (Bottini et al. 2006; Buckstein et al. 2006; Colleoni et al. 2006; Garcia et al. 2008). However, much needs to be learned about what type of drugs should be combined. For example, the combination of metronomic chemotherapy (CPA/methotrexate and CPA/vinblastine) with thalidomide or minocycline, respectively, two agents known to inhibit angiogenesis, seem not to be superior to metronomic chemotherapy alone (Colleoni et al. 2006; Young et al. 2006). On the other hand, the combination of bevacizumab with metronomic CPA has yielded very promising results in breast and ovarian cancer (Burstein et al. 2005; Garcia et al. 2008). Indeed, in the randomized Phase II trial of advanced breast cancer by Burstein et al. the bevacizumab plus metronomic CPA/methotrexate arm was superior compared to CPA/methotrexate therapy alone in terms of response rate and median time to progression (Burstein et al. 2005).

Besides doublet metronomic chemotherapy involving CPA and methotrexate, combinations of CPA and fluorinated pyrimidines are also showing promising clinical activity. The combination of metronomic CPA and UFT was clearly superior to monotherapy with either CPA or UFT in a preclinical model of advanced metastatic breast cancer (Munoz et al. 2006). A similar metronomic doublet of CPA and capecitabine combined with bevacizumab has been successfully applied for the treatment of advanced breast cancer, and seems to confirm the preclincial findings of Munoz et al. (2006). As far as the treatment of CRPC is concerned, Nishimura et al. successfully combined CPA with UFT and estramustine in a nonrandomized Phase II trial (Table 10.1) (Nishimura et al. 2001).

10.3.3 Integration of Metronomic Chemotherapy into Current Standards of Practice for Prostate Cancer

Metronomic chemotherapy has been generally studied in situations of advanced disease stages, with metastatic CRPC being a typical example (Kerbel and Kamen 2004; Gille et al. 2005). Such applications will likely continue to dominate in the near future. However, the results of a few studies suggest other indications worthy to be pursued.

For instance, metronomic chemotherapy might be considered as an adjunct to docetaxel chemotherapy, similar to other clinical trials which are comparing docetaxel monotherapy with docetaxel plus various antiangiogenics as first-line therapy in CRPC (Ryan et al. 2006). In fact, concomitant conventional and metronomic chemotherapy administration has shown to be beneficial preclinically (Shaked et al. 2005b) and clinically (Ellis et al. 2002; Casanova et al. 2004). As far as clinical results are concerned, the pilot study by Casanova et al. demonstrated the feasibility and activity of MTD vinorelbine and daily oral CPA in children with refractory or recurrent sarcomas. Furthermore, Ellis et al. described the use of continuous CPA combined with dose-dense doxorubicin in the adjuvant therapy of node-positive breast cancer patients, a promising regimen that is being further pursued in a Phase III trial.

An alternative to concomitant administration is the sequential use of MTD and metronomic chemotherapy, as preclinically described by Pietras and Hanahan (2005). Indeed, maintenance strategies following initial tumor debulking are actively studied in CRPC (Lin et al. 2007). Metronomic chemotherapy is an interesting treatment option in this respect, besides the use of various targeted agents.

Finally, beneficial effects of metronomic temozolomide combined with radiation therapy have been described for pediatric brain tumors (Sterba et al. 2002). Similarly, metronomic therapy might find a place in the CRPC setting when given concomitantly with radiation therapy.

Earlier stages of prostate cancer could also be considered for metronomic chemotherapy applications. While a metronomic combination of CPA and methotrexate is being studied in the adjuvant setting involving patients with ER- and PR-negative breast cancer (IBCSG 22-00, www.ibcsg.org), no such studies are yet underway for locally advanced prostate cancer following definite local therapy. Interestingly, adjuvant androgen deprivation therapy (ADT), the standard therapy in this setting, seems to act through antiangiogenic mechanisms (Nicholson and Theodorescu 2004). Thus, a strategy of combined ADT plus metronomic chemotherapy might be an interesting alternative to other approaches currently being studied which involve MTD chemotherapy (Glode 2006). For similar reasons, metronomic chemotherapy might also become an option for the treatment of hormone-sensitive prostate cancer, either concomitant with ADT or sequentially (in ADT-free intervals) when intermittent ADT is applied.

10.4 Conclusions and Perspectives

Over the last few years, beneficial effects of antiangiogenic tumor therapies have been described in several tumor types (Ferrara and Kerbel 2005). It also became increasingly clear that by changing the way of administration, the primary cellular target of cytotoxic drugs can shift from the tumor cell population to the tumor neovasculature, representing a potent antiangiogenic treatment approach. Metronomic chemotherapy is unlikely to replace conventional MTD chemotherapy administration when rapid tumor cell killing is needed. However, given the particular mode of action and the beneficial safety profile, it is likely to become a valuable alternative in combination therapies involving targeted (antiangiogenic) agents and in the palliative setting. Because many aspects of the metronomic approach remain empirical, major efforts are still needed to bring this novel and emerging concept to full fruition. Furthermore, the long-term administration of oral drugs involves new challenges such as treatment adherence and possibly an increased risk of interference with comedications (Emmenegger et al. 2007). Despite these drawbacks, metronomic chemotherapy has already come a long way from its description less than 10 years ago. It is hoped that the exciting Phase II trial results will be confirmed in future Phase III trials.

Acknowledgments The work summarized in this review was supported by grants from the National Cancer Institute of Canada, the Canadian Institutes for Health Research, and the National Institutes of Health, USA, to Robert S. Kerbel, and by sponsored research agreements with ImClone Systems, New York, and Taiho Pharmaceuticals, Japan. Urban Emmenegger is supported by the Ontario Institute for Cancer Research through funding provided by the Province of Ontario. We thank Cassandra Cheng for her excellent secretarial assistance.

References

Bertolini F, Mancuso P, Shaked Y, Kerbel RS (2007) Molecular and cellular biomarkers for angiogenesis in clinical oncology. Drug Discov Today 12:806–812

Bertolini F, Paul S, Mancuso P, Monestiroli S, Gobbi A, Shaked Y, Kerbel RS (2003) Maximum tolerable dose and low-dose metronomic chemotherapy have opposite effects on the mobilization and viability of circulating endothelial progenitor cells. Cancer Res 63:4342–4346

Bertolini F, Shaked Y, Mancuso P, Kerbel RS (2006) The multifaceted circulating endothelial cell in cancer: towards marker and target identification. Nat Rev Cancer 6:835–845

Bocci G, Francia G, Man S, Lawler J, Kerbel RS (2003) Thrombospondin 1, a mediator of the antiangiogenic effects of low-dose metronomic chemotherapy. Proc Natl Acad Sci U S A 100: 12917–12922

Bocci G, Nicolaou KC, Kerbel RS (2002) Protracted low-dose effects on human endothelial cell proliferation and survival in vitro reveal a selective antiangiogenic window for various chemotherapeutic drugs. Cancer Res 62:6938–6943

Bocci G, Tuccori M, Emmenegger U, Liguori V, Falcone A, Kerbel RS, Del Tacca M (2005) Cyclophosphamide-methotrexate 'metronomic' chemotherapy for the palliative treatment of metastatic breast cancer. A comparative pharmacoeconomic evaluation. Ann Oncol 16:1243–1252

Bolontrade MF, Zhou RR, Kleinerman ES (2002) Vasculogenesis plays a role in the growth of Ewing's sarcoma in vivo. Clin Cancer Res 8: 3622–3627

Bottini A, Generali D, Brizzi MP, Fox SB, Bersiga A, Bonardi S, Allevi G, Aguggini S, Bodini G, Milani M, Dionisio R, Bernardi C, Montruccoli A, Bruzzi P, Harris AL, Dogliotti L, Berruti A (2006) Randomized phase II trial of letrozole and letrozole plus low-dose metronomic oral cyclophosphamide as primary systemic treatment in elderly breast cancer patients. J Clin Oncol 24: 3623–3628

Browder T, Butterfield CE, Kraling BM, Shi B, Marshall B, O'Reilly MS, Folkman J (2000) Antiangiogenic scheduling of chemotherapy improves efficacy against experimental drug-resistant cancer. Cancer Res 60:1878–1886

Buckstein R, Kerbel RS, Shaked Y, Nayar R, Foden C, Turner R, Lee CR, Taylor D, Zhang L, Man S, Baruchel S, Stempak D, Bertolini F, Crump M (2006) High-dose celecoxib and metronomic "low-dose" cyclophosphamide is an effective and safe therapy in patients with relapsed and refractory aggressive histology non-Hodgkin's lymphoma. Clin Cancer Res 12:5190–5198

Burstein HJ, Spigel D, Kindsvogel K, Parker LM, Bunnel CA, Partridge AH, Come SE, Ryan PD, Gelman R, Winer EP (2005) Metronomic chemotherapy with and without bevacizumab for advanced breast cancer: a randomized phase II study. In: San Antonio Breast Cancer Symposium. Breast Cancer Res Treat 94(Suppl 1):S6, Abstract 4

Casanova M, Ferrari A, Bisogno G, Merks JH, De Salvo GL, Meazza C, Tettoni K, Provenzi M, Mazzarino I, Carli M (2004) Vinorelbine and low-dose cyclophosphamide in the treatment of pediatric sarcomas: pilot study for the upcoming European Rhabdomyosarcoma Protocol. Cancer 101:1664–1671

Colleoni M, Orlando L, Sanna G, Rocca A, Maisonneuve P, Peruzzotti G, Ghisini R, Sandri MT, Zorzino L, Nole F, Viale G, Goldhirsch A (2006) Metronomic low-dose oral cyclophosphamide and methotrexate plus or minus thalidomide in metastatic breast cancer: antitumor activity and biological effects. Ann Oncol 17: 232–238

Colleoni M, Rocca A, Sandri MT, Zorzino L, Masci G, Nole F, Peruzzotti G, Robertson C, Orlando L, Cinieri S, de BF, Viale G, Goldhirsch A (2002) Low-dose oral methotrexate and cyclophosphamide in metastatic breast cancer: antitumor activity and correlation with vascular endothelial growth factor levels. Ann Oncol 13:73–80

Cruz-Munoz W, Man S, Kerbel RS. Effective Treatment of Advanced Human Melanoma Metastasis in Immunodeficient Mice Using Combination Metronomic Chemotherapy Regimens. Clin Cancer Res. 2009 Jul 21. [Epub ahead of print]

Cruz-Munoz W, Man S, Xu P, Kerbel RS (2008) Development of a preclinical model of spontaneous human melanoma CNS metastasis. Cancer Res 68(12):4500–4505

Damber JE, Vallbo C, Albertsson P, Lennernas B, Norrby K (2006) The anti-tumour effect of low-dose continuous chemotherapy may partly be mediated by thrombospondin. Cancer Chemother Pharmacol 58:354–360

de Bont ES, Guikema JE, Scherpen F, Meeuwsen T, Kamps WA, Vellenga E, Bos NA (2001) Mobilized human CD34+ hematopoietic stem cells enhance tumor growth in a nonobese diabetic/severe combined immunodeficient mouse model of human non-Hodgkin's lymphoma. Cancer Res 61:7654–7659

Dellapasqua S, Bertolini F, Bagnardi V, Campagnoli E, Scarano E, Torrisi R, Shaked Y, Mancuso P, Goldhirsch A, Rocca A, Pietri E, Colleoni M. Metronomic cyclophosphamide and capecitabine combined with bevacizumab in advanced breast cancer. J Clin Oncol. 2008;26:4899-905

Di Lorenzo G, Autorino R, De Laurentiis M, Forestieri V, Romano C, Prudente A, Giugliano F, Imbimbo C, Mirone V, De Placido S (2007) Thalidomide in combination with oral daily cyclophosphamide in patients with pretreated hormone refractory prostate cancer: a phase I clinical trial. Cancer Biol Ther 6:313–317

du Manoir JM, Francia G, Man S, Mossoba M, Medin JA, Viloria-Petit A, Hicklin DJ, Emmenegger U, Kerbel RS (2006) Strategies for delaying or treating in vivo acquired resistance to trastuzumab in human breast cancer xenografts. Clin Cancer Res 12:904–916

Ellis GK, Livingston RB, Gralow JR, Green SJ, Thompson T (2002) Dose-dense anthracycline-based chemotherapy for node-positive breast cancer. J Clin Oncol 20:3637–3643

Emmenegger U, Man S, Shaked Y, Francia G, Wong JW, Hicklin DJ, Kerbel RS (2004) A comparative analysis of low-dose metronomic cyclophosphamide reveals absent or low-grade toxicity on tissues highly sensitive to the toxic effects of maximum tolerated dose regimens. Cancer Res 64:3994–4000

Emmenegger U, Morton GC, Francia G, Shaked Y, Franco M, Weinerman A, Man S, Kerbel RS (2006) Low-dose metronomic daily cyclophosphamide and weekly tirapazamine: a well-tolerated combination regimen with enhanced efficacy that exploits tumor hypoxia. Cancer Res 66:1664–1674

Emmenegger U, Shaked Y, Man S, Bocci G, Spasojevic I, Francia G, Kouri A, Coke R, Cruz-Munoz W, Ludeman SM, Colvin OM, Kerbel RS (2007) Pharmacodynamic and pharmacokinetic study of chronic low-dose metronomic cyclophosphamide therapy in mice. Mol Cancer Ther 6:2280–2289

Escuin D, Kline ER, Giannakakou P (2005) Both microtubule-stabilizing and microtubule-destabilizing drugs inhibit hypoxia-inducible factor-1alpha accumulation and activity by disrupting microtubule function. Cancer Res 65:9021–9028

Ferrara N, Kerbel RS (2005) Angiogenesis as a therapeutic target. Nature 438:967–974

Folkman J (1971) Tumor angiogenesis: therapeutic implications. N Engl J Med 285:1182–1186

Fontana A, Bocci G, Galli L, Fontana E, Galli C, Landi L, Fioravanti A, Orlandi P, Del Tacca M, Falcone A (2007) Low-dose metronomic cyclophosphamide (CTX) plus celecoxib (C) and dexamethasone (DEX) in advanced hormone-refractory prostate cancer (HRPC): A phase II clinical trial with evaluation of clinical and pharmacodynamic effects of the combination. In: ASCO GU Proceedings 2007, abstract 215

Garcia AA, Hirte H, Fleming G, Yang D, Tsao-Wei DD, Roman L, Groshen S, Swenson S, Markland F, Gandara D, Scudder S, Morgan R, Chen H, Lenz HJ, Oza AM (2008) Phase II clinical trial of bevacizumab and low-dose metronomic oral cyclophosphamide in recurrent ovarian cancer: a trial of the California, Chicago, and Princess Margaret Hospital phase II consortia. J Clin Oncol 26:76–82

Ghiringhelli F, Menard C, Puig PE, Ladoire S, Roux S, Martin F, Solary E, Le Cesne A, Zitvogel L, Chauffert B (2007) Metronomic cyclophosphamide regimen selectively depletes CD4(+)CD25 (+) regulatory T cells and restores T and NK effector functions in end stage cancer patients. Cancer Immunol Immunother 56: 641–648

Gille J, Spieth K, Kaufmann R (2005) Metronomic low-dose chemotherapy as antiangiogenic therapeutic strategy for cancer. J Dtsch Dermatol Ges 3:26–32

Glode LM (2006) The case for adjuvant therapy for prostate cancer. J Urol 176:S30–S33

Glode LM, Barqawi A, Crighton F, Crawford ED, Kerbel R (2003) Metronomic therapy with cyclophosphamide and dexamethasone for prostate carcinoma. Cancer 98:1643–1648

Gupta K, Gupta P, Wild R, Ramakrishnan S, Hebbel RP (1999) Binding and displacement of vascular endothelial growth factor (VEGF) by thrombospondin: effect on human microvascular endothelial cell proliferation and angiogenesis. Angiogenesis 3:147–158

Hahnfeldt P, Folkman J, Hlatky L (2003) Minimizing long-term tumor burden: the logic for metronomic chemotherapeutic dosing and its antiangiogenic basis. J Theor Biol 220:545–554

Hamano Y, Sugimoto H, Soubasakos MA, Kieran M, Olsen BR, Lawler J, Sudhakar A, Kalluri R (2004) Thrombospondin-1 associated with tumor microenvironment contributes to low-dose cyclophosphamide-mediated endothelial cell apoptosis and tumor growth suppression. Cancer Res 64:1570–1574

Hanahan D, Bergers G, Bergsland E (2000) Less is more, regularly: metronomic dosing of cytotoxic drugs can target tumor angiogenesis in mice. J Clin Invest 105:1045–1047

Haubitz M, Schellong S, Gobel U, Schurek HJ, Schaumann D, Koch KM, Brunkhorst R (1998) Intravenous pulse administration of cyclophosphamide versus daily oral treatment in patients with antineutrophil cytoplasmic antibody-associated vasculitis and renal involvement: a prospective, randomized study. Arthritis Rheum 41: 1835–1844

Hoffman GS, Kerr GS, Leavitt RY, Hallahan CW, Lebovics RS, Travis WD, Rottem M, Fauci AS (1992) Wegener granulomatosis: an analysis of 158 patients. Ann Intern Med 116:488–498

Hurwitz H, Fehrenbacher L, Novotny W, Cartwright T, Hainsworth J, Heim W, Berlin J, Baron A, Griffing S, Holmgren E, Ferrara N, Fyfe G, Rogers B, Ross R, Kabbinavar F (2004) Bevacizumab plus irinotecan, fluorouracil, and leucovorin for metastatic colorectal cancer. N Engl J Med 350: 2335–2342

Jubb AM, Oates AJ, Holden S, Koeppen H (2006) Predicting benefit from anti-angiogenic agents in malignancy. Nat Rev Cancer 6:626–635

Kamen BA, Glod J, Cole PD (2006) Metronomic therapy from a pharmacologist's view. J Pediatr Hematol Oncol 28:325–327

Kerbel RS (2000) Tumor angiogenesis: past, present and the near future. Carcinogenesis 21: 505–515

Kerbel RS (2006) Antiangiogenic therapy: a universal chemosensitization strategy for cancer? Science 312:1171–1175

Kerbel RS, Kamen BA (2004) The anti-angiogenic basis of metronomic chemotherapy. Nat Rev Cancer 4:423–436

Kerbel RS, Viloria-Petit A, Klement G, Rak J (2000) 'Accidental' anti-angiogenic drugs. anti-oncogene directed signal transduction inhibitors and conventional chemotherapeutic agents as examples. Eur J Cancer 36:1248–1257

Kieran MW, Turner CD, Rubin JB, Chi SN, Zimmerman MA, Chordas C, Klement G, Laforme A, Gordon A, Thomas A, Neuberg D, Browder T, Folkman J (2005) A feasibility trial of antiangiogenic (metronomic) chemotherapy in pediatric patients with recurrent or progressive cancer. J Pediatr Hematol Oncol 27:573–581

Klement G, Baruchel S, Rak J, Man S, Clark K, Hicklin DJ, Bohlen P, Kerbel RS (2000) Continuous low-dose therapy with vinblastine and VEGF receptor-2 antibody induces sustained tumor regression without overt toxicity. J Clin Invest 105:R15–R24

Lam T, Hetherington JW, Greenman J, Maraveyas A (2006) From total empiricism to a rational design of metronomic chemotherapy phase I dosing trials. Anticancer Drugs 17:113–121

Lin AM, Ryan CJ, Small EJ (2007) Intermittent chemotherapy for metastatic hormone refractory

10

prostate cancer. Crit Rev Oncol Hematol 61: 243–254

Lord R, Nair S, Schache A, Spicer J, Somaihah N, Khoo V, Pandha H (2007) Low dose metronomic oral cyclophosphamide for hormone resistant prostate cancer: a phase II study. J Urol 177: 2136–2140; discussion 2140

Ma J, Waxman DJ (2007) Collaboration between hepatic and intratumoral prodrug activation in a P450 prodrug-activation gene therapy model for cancer treatment. Mol Cancer Ther 6:2879–2890

Ma J, Waxman DJ (2008) Modulation of the antitumor activity of metronomic cyclophosphamide by the angiogenesis inhibitor axitinib. Mol Cancer Ther 7:79–89

Man S, Bocci G, Francia G, Green SK, Jothy S, Hanahan D, Bohlen P, Hicklin DJ, Bergers G, Kerbel RS (2002) Antitumor effects in mice of low-dose (metronomic) cyclophosphamide administered continuously through the drinking water. Cancer Res 62:2731–2735

Mike S, Harrison C, Coles B, Staffurth J, Wilt TJ, Mason MD (2006) Chemotherapy for hormone-refractory prostate cancer. Cochrane Database Syst Rev: CD005247

Miller KD, Sweeney CJ, Sledge GW Jr (2001) Redefining the target: chemotherapeutics as antiangiogenics. J Clin Oncol 19:1195–1206

Munoz R, Man S, Shaked Y, Lee CR, Wong J, Francia G, Kerbel RS (2006) Highly efficacious nontoxic preclinical treatment for advanced metastatic breast cancer using combination oral UFT-cyclophosphamide metronomic chemotherapy. Cancer Res 66:3386–3391

Ng SS, Sparreboom A, Shaked Y, Lee C, Man S, Desai N, Soon-Shiong P, Figg WD, Kerbel RS (2006) Influence of formulation vehicle on metronomic taxane chemotherapy: albumin-bound versus cremophor EL-based paclitaxel. Clin Cancer Res 12:4331–4338

Nicholson B, Theodorescu D (2004) Angiogenesis and prostate cancer tumor growth. J Cell Biochem 91:125–150

Nicolini A, Mancini P, Ferrari P, Anselmi L, Tartarelli G, Bonazzi V, Carpi A, Giardino R (2004) Oral low-dose cyclophosphamide in metastatic hormone refractory prostate cancer (MHRPC). Biomed Pharmacother 58:447–450

Nishimura K, Nonomura N, Ono Y, Nozawa M, Fukui T, Harada Y, Imazu T, Takaha N, Sugao H, Miki T, Okuyama A (2001) Oral combination of cyclophosphamide, uracil plus tegafur and estramustine for hormone-refractory prostate cancer. Oncology 60:49–54

Orlando L, Cardillo A, Rocca A, Balduzzi A, Ghisini R, Peruzzotti G, Goldhirsch A, D'Alessandro C, Cinieri S, Preda L, Colleoni M (2006) Prolonged clinical benefit with metronomic chemotherapy in patients with metastatic breast cancer. Anticancer Drugs 17:961–967

Petrylak DP, Tangen CM, Hussain MH, Lara PN Jr, Jones JA, Taplin ME, Burch PA, Berry D, Moinpour C, Kohli M, Benson MC, Small EJ, Raghavan D, Crawford ED (2004) Docetaxel and estramustine compared with mitoxantrone and prednisone for advanced refractory prostate cancer. N Engl J Med 351:1513–1520

Pienta KJ, Smith DC (2005) Advances in prostate cancer chemotherapy: a new era begins. CA Cancer J Clin 55: 300–318; quiz 323–305

Pietras K, Hanahan D (2005) A multitargeted, metronomic, and maximum-tolerated dose "chemo-switch" regimen is antiangiogenic, producing objective responses and survival benefit in a mouse model of cancer. J Clin Oncol 23: 939–952

Quesada AJ, Nelius T, Yap R, Zaichuk TA, Alfranca A, Filleur S, Volpert OV, Redondo JM (2005) In vivo upregulation of CD95 and CD95L causes synergistic inhibition of angiogenesis by TSP1 peptide and metronomic doxorubicin treatment. Cell Death Differ 12:649–658

Rapisarda A, Zalek J, Hollingshead M, Braunschweig T, Uranchimeg B, Bonomi CA, Borgel SD, Carter JP, Hewitt SM, Shoemaker RH, Melillo G (2004) Schedule-dependent inhibition of hypoxia-inducible factor-1alpha protein accumulation, angiogenesis, and tumor growth by topotecan in U251-HRE glioblastoma xenografts. Cancer Res 64:6845–6848

Rivera E, Mejia JA, Arun BK, Adinin RB, Walters RS, Brewster A, Broglio KR, Yin G, Esmaeli B, Hortobagyi GN, Valero V (2008) Phase 3 study comparing the use of docetaxel on an every-3-week versus weekly schedule in the treatment of metastatic breast cancer. Cancer 112:1455–1461

Rocca A, Dellapasqua A, Pietri E, Dettori M, D'Alessandro C, Ghisini R, Colombo A, Goldhirsch A, Colleoni M (2007) Metronomic chemotherapy with capecitabine and oral cyclophosphamide in combination with bevacizumab in metastatic breast cancer (mbc): evidence of activity of an antiangiogenic treatment. In: ASCO Annual Meeting Proceedings Part I. J Clin Oncol 25(18S): abstract 11501

Rohan RM, Fernandez A, Udagawa T, Yuan J, D'Amato RJ (2000) Genetic heterogeneity of angiogenesis in mice. Faseb J 14:871–876

Ryan CJ, Lin AM, Small EJ (2006) Angiogenesis inhibition plus chemotherapy for metastatic hormone refractory prostate cancer: history and rationale. Urol Oncol 24:250–253

Shaked Y, Bertolini F, Man S, Rogers MS, Cervi D, Foutz T, Rawn K, Voskas D, Dumont DJ, Ben-David Y, Lawler J, Henkin J, Huber J, Hicklin DJ, D'Amato RJ, Kerbel RS (2005a) Genetic heterogeneity of the vasculogenic phenotype parallels angiogenesis; Implications for cellular surrogate marker analysis of antiangiogenesis. Cancer Cell 7:101–111

Shaked Y, Ciarrocchi A, Franco M, Lee CR, Man S, Cheung AM, Hicklin DJ, Chaplin D, Foster FS, Benezra R, Kerbel RS (2006) Therapy-induced acute recruitment of circulating endothelial progenitor cells to tumors. Science 313:1785–1787

Shaked Y, Emmenegger U, Francia G, Chen L, Lee CR, Man S, Paraghamian A, Ben-David Y, Kerbel RS (2005b) Low-dose metronomic combined with intermittent bolus-dose cyclophosphamide is an effective long-term chemotherapy treatment strategy. Cancer Res 65:7045–7051

Shaked Y, Emmenegger U, Man S, Cervi D, Bertolini F, Ben-David Y, Kerbel RS (2005c) Optimal biologic dose of metronomic chemotherapy regimens is associated with maximum antiangiogenic activity. Blood 106:3058–3061

Shirakawa K, Furuhata S, Watanabe I, Hayase H, Shimizu A, Ikarashi Y, Yoshida T, Terada M, Hashimoto D, Wakasugi H (2002) Induction of vasculogenesis in breast cancer models. Br J Cancer 87:1454–1461

Sterba J, Pavelka Z, Slampa P (2002) Concomitant radiotherapy and metronomic temozolomide in pediatric high-risk brain tumors. Neoplasma 49: 117–120

Takahashi Y, Mai M, Sawabu N, Nishioka K (2005) A pilot study of individualized maximum repeatable dose (iMRD), a new dose finding system, of weekly gemcitabine for patients with metastatic pancreas cancer. Pancreas 30:206–210

Tannock IF, de Wit R, Berry WR, Horti J, Pluzanska A, Chi KN, Oudard S, Theodore C, James ND, Turesson I, Rosenthal MA, Eisenberger MA (2004) Docetaxel plus prednisone or mitoxantrone plus prednisone for advanced prostate cancer. N Engl J Med 351:1502–1512

Tannock IF, Osoba D, Stockler MR, Ernst DS, Neville AJ, Moore MJ, Armitage GR, Wilson JJ, Venner PM, Coppin CM, Murphy KC (1996) Chemotherapy with mitoxantrone plus prednisone or prednisone alone for symptomatic hormone-resistant prostate cancer: a Canadian randomized trial with palliative end points. J Clin Oncol 14:1756–1764

Tran J, Master Z, Yu JL, Rak J, Dumont DJ, Kerbel RS (2002) A role for survivin in chemoresistance of endothelial cells mediated by VEGF. Proc Natl Acad Sci U S A 99:4349–4354

Vogelzang NJ (1984) Continuous infusion chemotherapy: a critical review. J Clin Oncol 2:1289–1304

Volpert OV, Zaichuk T, Zhou W, Reiher F, Ferguson TA, Stuart PM, Amin M, Bouck NP (2002) Inducer-stimulated Fas targets activated endothelium for destruction by anti-angiogenic thrombospondin-1 and pigment epithelium-derived factor. Nat Med 8:349–357

Wang J, Lou P, Lesniewski R, Henkin J (2003) Paclitaxel at ultra low concentrations inhibits angiogenesis without affecting cellular microtubule assembly. Anticancer Drugs 14:13–19

Winquist E, Waldron T, Berry S, Ernst DS, Hotte S, Lukka H (2006) Non-hormonal systemic therapy in men with hormone-refractory prostate cancer and metastases: a systematic review from the Cancer Care Ontario Program in Evidence-based Care's Genitourinary Cancer Disease Site Group. BMC Cancer 6:112

Yap R, Veliceasa D, Emmenegger U, Kerbel RS, McKay LM, Henkin J, Volpert OV (2005) Metronomic low-dose chemotherapy boosts CD95-dependent antiangiogenic effect of the thrombospondin peptide ABT-510: a complementation antiangiogenic strategy. Clin Cancer Res 11: 6678–6685

Young SD, Whissell M, Noble JC, Cano PO, Lopez PG, Germond CJ (2006) Phase II clinical trial results involving treatment with low-dose daily oral cyclophosphamide, weekly vinblastine, and rofecoxib in patients with advanced solid tumors. Clin Cancer Res 12:3092–3098

Zhu AX (2008) Development of sorafenib and other molecularly targeted agents in hepatocellular carcinoma. Cancer 112:250–259

Targeting Inflammatory Cells to Improve Anti-VEGF Therapies in Oncology

11

Hans-Peter Gerber, Ezogelin Olazoglu, and Iqbal S. Grewal

Abstract Vascular endothelial growth factor A (VEGF-A) is a well-characterized regulator of physiological and pathological angiogenesis. Multiple therapeutic compounds interfering with VEGF-A-regulated signal transduction pathways are currently being developed for the treatment of neoplasias and other malignancies associated with pathological angiogenesis. A major challenge in developing anti-VEGF therapies are tumor intrinsic refractoriness and the emergence of treatment-induced resistance. A variety of molecular and cellular mechanisms contribute to tumor angiogenesis, including the recruitment of bone marrow (BM)-derived endothelial cell progenitors (EPCs) and inflammatory cells to the tumor mass. Among the latter, two types of tumor infiltrating, inflammatory cells were recently identified to mediate refractoriness to anti-VEGF treatment: CD11b + Gr1+ myeloid derived suppressor cells (MDSC) and tumor-associated macrophages (TAMs). In this chapter, we review some of the inflammatory components regulating tumor angiogenesis and their roles in mediating refractoriness toward anti-VEGF treatment. In addition, we discuss potential therapeutic strategies targeting angiogenic pathways regulated by inflammatory cells. A better understanding of the biological and molecular events involved in mediating refractoriness to anti-VEGF treatment may help to further improve therapeutic strategies targeting tumor angiogenesis.

11.1 Role of Bone Marrow-Derived Tumor Infiltrating Cells in Tumor Angiogenesis

Traditionally, tumor cells were recognized as the major source of angiogenic factors, and therapeutic compounds targeting tumor-derived growth factors or signaling pathways regulated by these factors induced tumor growth inhibition in preclinical and clinical studies. More recently, it has become apparent that cancer development largely depends on the ability of tumor cells to engage and exploit normal physiological processes of the host, including the recruitment and activation of untransformed stromal cells. Many of the stromal cells that were shown to play important roles during tissue regeneration were also found to regulate tumor angiogenesis and to contribute to the development of refractoriness toward anti-VEGF therapy. Primary inducers of recruitment

H. P. Gerber (✉)
Sr Dir Discovery Tumor Prog,
Pharma, Research & Development, Pearl River, NY,
e-mail: gerberh@wyeth.com

R. Liersch et al. (eds.), *Angiogenesis Inhibition,* Recent Results in Cancer Research,
DOI: 10.1007/978-3-540-78281-0_11, © Springer Verlag Berlin Heidelberg 2010

of inflammatory cells to sites of tissue injury are ischemia, hypoglycemia, and tissue necrosis. Many of these conditions are also part of the pathophysiological changes observed in tumors treated with anti-VEGF (Gerber and Ferrara 2005). Therefore, it is tempting to speculate that anti-VEGF refractoriness may be caused by misguided inflammatory cells responding to stress signals induced by anti-VEGF treatment, initiating physiological changes associated with tissue regeneration (Dvorak 1986).

The production of angiogenic activities by tumor infiltrating stromal cells was attributed to fibroblasts (Dong et al. 2004; Orimo et al. 2005), endothelial progenitor cells (EPCs) (Asahara et al. 1997; Nolan et al. 2007; Shi et al. 1998), mesenchymal stem cells (MSCs) (Kanehira et al. 2007), and leukocytes (reviewed by (de Visser and Coussens 2006)). Hematopoietic cells exerting angiogenic functions include tumor-associated macrophages (TAMs) (De Palma et al. 2005; Yang et al. 2004), T- and B-lymphocytes (Freeman et al. 1995), vascular leukocytes (Conejo-Garcia et al. 2005), dendritic cells (Conejo-Garcia et al. 2004), neutrophils (Coussens et al. 2000), mast-cells (Coussens et al. 1999), and myeloid cells (Shojaei et al. 2007a; Yang et al. 2004) (Fig. 11.1). Such tumor-infiltrating leukocytes are variably loaded with chemokines, cytokines, cytotoxic mediators including reactive oxygen species (ROS), serine-cysteines and metalloproteases, membrane performing agents, interleukins, and interferons (Tlsty and Coussens 2006). Many of these factors were shown to be either pro- or anti-angiogenic, depending on the experimental model employed. Recent preclinical studies conducted with compounds interfering with VEGF signaling identified a novel role for tumor-infiltrating leukocytes in mediating refractoriness to anti-VEGF treatment (Fischer et al. 2007; Shojaei et al. 2007a; Shojaei et al. 2007b). The identification of a key role of inflammatory cells in mediating refractoriness toward anti-VEGF treatment validates these cells as potential targets for tumor therapy. Despite the important contributions of inflammatory cells to tumor angiogenesis identified in various preclinical studies, their overall role for tumor development in cancer patients remains controversial (reviewed in (Coussens and Werb 2002)). Here, we review some of the key features associated with tumor-infiltrating leukocytes and the preclinical and clinical evidence in support of their potential role during tumor angiogenesis and escape from anti-VEGF treatment.

11.2 Endothelial Progenitor Cells (EPCs) and Circulatory Endothelial Progenitor Cells (CEPs)

Studies conducted with a large variety of experimental tumors in mice demonstrated that BM-derived EPCs are important for blood vessel formation through a process known as vasculogenesis (reviewed in Rafii et al. 2002). In this process, EPCs are mobilized to the peripheral circulation, from where they home as circulatory endothelial cells (CEPs) to distal sites of neovascularization, followed by their in situ differentiation to mature endothelial cells. Vasculogenesis does not only contribute to tumor angiogenesis, but also to tissue revascularization and regeneration in preclinical models of wound healing, hind-limb ischemia, postmyocardial infarction, atherosclerosis, and retinal and lymphoid organ neovascularization (reviewed in Rafii and Lyden 2003).

EPCs and CEPs were originally defined as cells expressing the hematopoietic stem cell markers CD34, CD133 and the endothelial marker VEGF receptor-2 (VEGFR-2). Studies with such triple positive EPCs demonstrated that their recruitment to the tumor vasculature is required for vascularization of certain experimental tumors (Table 11.1, (Asahara et al. 1997; Shi et al. 1998)). Initial preclinical studies demonstrating the requirement of EPCs for tumor angiogenesis were conducted in Id-mutant mice, which failed to generate CEPs and did not support tumor

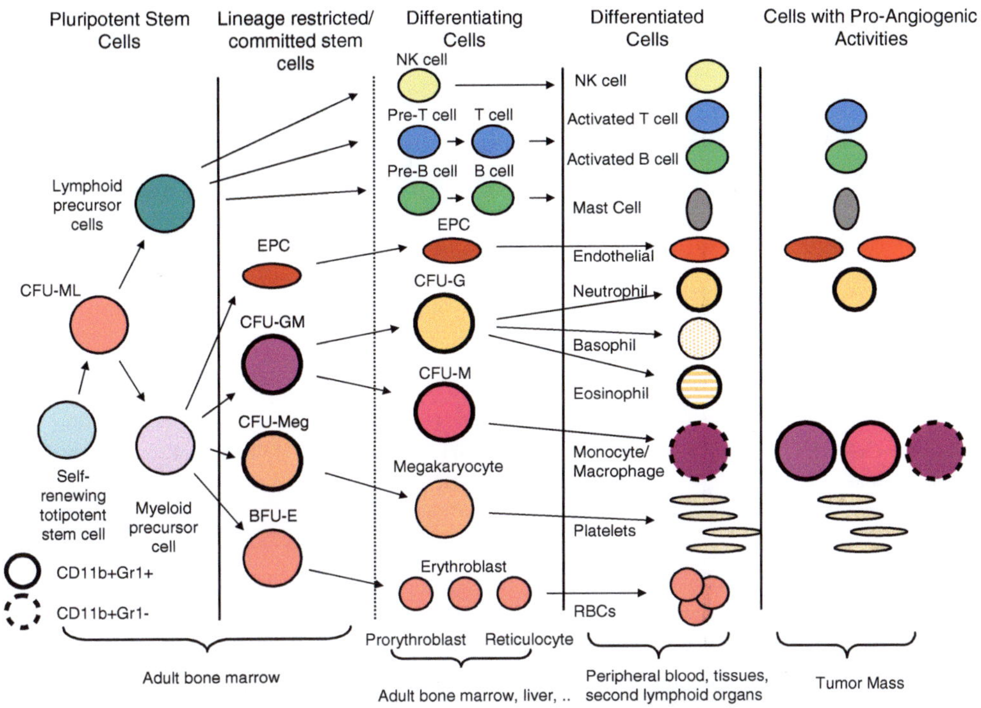

Fig. 11.1 Differentiation of hematopoietic lineages. Self-renewing totipotent stem cells in the bone marrow give rise to cells of the immune system. Colony-forming unit-myeloid-lymphoid (CFU-ML) precursor cells divide to produce two types of stem cells: Lymphoid precursor cells giving rise to NK cell, T cells and B cells, and myeloid precursor cells give rise to CFU-GM, CFU-Meg and BFU-E which eventually differentiates to granulocytes/monocytes, megakaryocytes producing platelets and erythrocytes, respectively. After encounter with an antigen, T cells become activated and differentiate to effector cells while B cells differentiate into antibody-secreting plasma cells. CFU-GM are the precursor cells giving rise to CFU-M and CFU-G, which are phenotypically CD11b+Gr-1+. CFU-M differentiates to monocytes that travel to the blood and eventually become macrophages in the tissue, these cells are phenotypically CD11b+Gr-1-. While monocytes are in the bone marrow, they are CD11b+ , whereas Gr-1 is expressed only transiently. CFU-G is the precursor that eventually differentiates to neutrophils, basophils and eosinophils. They are termed granulocytes due to cytoplasmic granules and irregular shape of nuclei and they maintain CD11b+ and Gr-1+ on their cell surface. Mast cells arise from an unknown precursor and complete their maturation in the tissues and are known to be CD11b+, the expression of Gr-1 on these cells has not been assessed

angiogenesis and growth (Lyden et al. 2001). The consensus marker expression for EPCs in men and mice is defined as CD133+CD34+VEGFR2+ cells, which facilitates the direct comparisons between their angiogenic activities when tested in different experimental models (Urbich and Dimmeler 2004). In general, failure of EPCs to migrate from the BM to the tumor vasculature resulted in reduced tumor angiogenesis and growth (reviewed in (Luttun et al. 2002b)). The frequencies of EPCs within the vasculature of experimental tumors varies significantly, ranging from 0–100%, depending on the type of tumor, host, and stage of tumor growth (Lyden et al. 2001; Natori et al. 2002; Peters et al. 2005; Shaked et al. 2005). Despite the important roles

Table 11.1 Potential therapeutic targets to interfere with anti-VEGF refractoriness of solid tumors

Cell type targeted	Migration from bone marrow to circulation	Homing to tumors	Tumor mass
TAMs		CD51, CCL2, CCL3, CCL4,CCL5, CCL8, VEGF-A	PlGF, VEGF-A, bFGF, TNF-α, IL-8, MMP-2, MMP-7, MMP-9, MMP12, Cox2, uPA
EPCs	VEGF-A, PlGF, SDF-1α, GM-CSF, Ang1, elastase, cathepsin G, MMPs, Kit-ligand, e-NOS	MMP-9, integrin, αvβ3 and αvβ5, E-and P-selectin, glycoprotein ligand-1	
Neutrophils			VEGF-A, IL-8, MMP-2, MMP-9, elastase
CD11b + Gr1 + MDSCs	Gr1	Gr1	Bv8, Gr1
Mast cell and lymphocytes		CD20	CD20, VEGF, bFGF, IL-8 and TNF-α

of EPCs for growth of experimental tumors in mice, the frequencies of EPCs in advanced stage tumors in patients are low, ranging from 1 to 12% and averaged 4.9% (Peters et al. 2005). Some of the discrepancies between the frequencies of EPCs in the tumor vasculature between clinical and preclinical studies may be caused by the rapid kinetics of EPC recruitment to tumor vasculature, with maximum levels during the first couple of days post tumor implantation in animals. In contrast, the patient tumors analyzed in various studies represent mostly advanced-stage tumors.

The molecular mechanisms regulating the mobilization of EPCs from the BM to peripheral circulation are only incompletely understood. Initial experiments revealed that distinct classes of genes and environmental factors contribute to this process (reviewed in (Papayannopoulou 2004; Urbich and Dimmeler 2004)). Among them, local tissue ischemia is considered a predominant signal-inducing event, leading to mobilization of EPCs to sites of tissue injury or tumors (Akita et al. 2003) (reviewed in (Kawamoto et al. 2002)). Local hypoxia was shown to induce EPC-mobilizing cytokines within tumors, including VEGF-A, PlGF, SDF-1α (Yamaguchi et al. 2003), granulocyte macrophage colony-stimulating factor (GM-CSF) (Rehman et al. 2003), and angiopoietin-1 (Hattori et al. 2001). In addition, activation of proteinases such as elastase, cathepsin G, matrix metalloproteinases (MMPs), cleavage of Kit ligand (Heissig et al. 2002), and expression of endothelial-nitric oxide synthetase (e-NOS) (Aicher et al. 2003; Ii et al. 2005; Wassmann et al. 2006) was also associated with the mobilization of EPCs from the BM to the peripheral circulation.

Homing of CEPs is initiated in specific "hot-spot" regions within the tumor microvasculature, followed by their extravasation into the tumor interstitium and the formation of multicellular clusters, ultimately giving rise to functional vascular networks (Vajkoczy et al. 2003). Several genes that were found upregulated on the tumor vasculature are associated with the regulation of circulatory EPCs (cEPCs) homing and extravasation, including MMP-9, integrins $\alpha_v\beta_3$ and $\alpha_v\beta_5$, E-and P-selectin and glycoprotein ligand-1 (Urbich and Dimmeler 2004). Many of these genes were independently identified as downstream targets of VEGF signaling in endothelial cells (Hesser et al. 2004).

The relevance of EPCs to anti-VEGF refractoriness was investigated by using VEGF blocking compounds and experimental models employing genetically marked BM progenitor cells. Nolan et al. demonstrated critical roles for these cells during the early stages of tumor development. At later stages, however, vessels consisting of BM-derived EPCs became diluted with non-BM-derived vessels from the periphery (Nolan et al. 2007). Importantly, selective ablation of EPCs shortly after tumor implantation resulted in a marked tumor growth delay, suggesting that targeting EPC during early stages, but not at later stages of tumor progression, may be most beneficial. Lack of BM-derived EPCs in the tumor vasculature during later stages of tumor growth was confirmed independently by Shojaei et al., who investigated the recruitment of EPCs to tumor vasculature in mice treated with an VEGF-A selective antibody (G6-23), or a compound blocking VEGF-A, PlGF, and VEGF-B combined by using Flt-IgG. When assessed between Days 14 and 18 post tumor cell implantation, the frequencies of EPCs were low, and no differences in the numbers of EPCs in the vasculature of anti-VEGF sensitive and refractory tumors were discernable, irrespective of the treatment modality (Shojaei et al. 2007a). Combined, these finding suggest that recruitment of BM derived EPCs may not contribute significantly to refractoriness of late stage tumors to anti-VEGF treatment. These observations may help to enhance our understanding of some of the controversial reports regarding the frequencies and functional relevance of EPCs for tumor angiogenesis reported for different experimental models.

11.3 Tumor-Associated Macrophages

Macrophages are derived from CD34+ BM progenitors, which shed their progeny into the blood stream as promonocytes. They then develop into monocytes and extravasate to tissues where they differentiate into specific types of resident tissue macrophages, with marked phenotypic differences between different tissues. Resident macrophages share a set of common functions, including the defense against microbial infections, the regulation of normal cell turnover and tissue remodeling, and repair at sites of injury. Recruitment of macrophages to sites of tissue injury or tumor growth is a well- documented phenomenon, and environmental conditions including hypoxia, lack of nutrients, inflammation, and cell death were described as key stimulators of macrophage recruitment (Leek et al. 1999; Leek et al. 1996; Negus et al. 1997; Ohno et al. 2004). TAMs secrete a variety of cytokines and proteolytic enzymes that are capable of promoting tumor progression by stimulating tumor-cell proliferation, angiogenesis and by inducing alterations in the extracellular matrix favorable for tumor growth (reviewed in Knowles et al. 2004). Despite the angiogenic functions of macrophages identified in various preclinical models, the role of tumor-associated macrophages in cancer patients remains controversial (Bingle et al. 2002; Ohno et al. 2003). A positive correlation between the relative numbers of TAMs in breast, prostate, and kidney tumors and clinical prognosis was inferred from clinical studies. While a few reports correlated high TAM numbers with good prognosis, such as in the case of stomach, colorectal, and melanoma tumors, the majority of the clinical studies linked high TAM numbers with reduced patient survival (Lewis and Pollard 2006). In most human tumors studied, infiltration of high numbers of macrophages correlated with increased angiogenesis (Leek et al. 1996; Lin and Pollard 2007), and poor prognosis (Bingle et al. 2002). Combined, these findings led to the proposal to consider cytokine blockades as a potential strategy to modulate angiogenesis during inflammation and in cancer (Crivellato and Ribatti 2005). However, other preclinical studies associated inhibitory activities on tumor growth with increased levels of macrophages within tumors (reviewed in Kohchi et al. 2004). Thus, depending on the specific type of inflammatory cells recruited to tumors, immune cell infiltration may either antagonize tumor formation and growth (Dunn et al. 2004; Lin and Pollard 2004) or promote tumor growth by stimulating angiogenesis and tumor-cell proliferation (Coussens and Werb 2002; de Visser et al. 2005).

In the context of solid tumors, circulating monocytes are shown to be recruited to the tumor vicinity by a number of tumor-derived chemoattractants, including colony-stimulating factor-1 (CSF-1), CC chemokines such as CCL2, CCL3, CCL4, CCL5, CCL8, and VEGF (Murdoch et al. 2004; Sica et al. 2006) . TAMs were described as a significant source of proangiogenic activities in solid tumors and they play important roles in mediating tumor angiogenesis. TAMs release potent proangiogenic cytokines and growth factors, including VEGF-A, bFGF, TNF-α, and IL-8 (Lewis et al. 1995; Mantovani et al. 2002; Sunderkotter et al. 1991). They also upregulate other genes associated with the regulation of angiogenesis, including MMP- 2, MMP-7, MMP-9, MMP-12, and cyclooxygenase-2 (Cox-2, reviewed in (Lewis and Pollard 2006)). To sum up, the many proangiogenic activities produced by TAMs render them likely candidates for mediating escape from anti-VEGF treatment.

One of the key problems in defining the role of TAMs during tumor development is the lack of a common definition for their phenotypic markers or functional properties. TAMs have been characterized inconsistently by low expression levels of differentiation-associated macrophage antigens, carboxypeptidase M and CD51, high constitutive expression of interleukin (IL)-1, IL-6 and low expression of TNF-α, and the presence of the myeloid marker F4/80 in mice or CD68 in humans (Bingle et al. 2002). Macrophages derived from experimental or human tumors display greatly reduced immuno-stimmulatory activities on cytotoxic T-cells and NK cells. It was suggested that this may be the result of their exposure to IL-4 and IL-10 within the tumors, inducing TAMs to develop into polarized Type II or M2 macrophages (Mantovani et al. 2004).

Early macrophage ablation studies provided experimental evidence that TAMs are essential for the growth of certain experimental tumors in mice (Polverini and Leibovich 1987). Based on these findings, a model was proposed, wherein macrophages are capable of modulating angiogenesis (Sunderkotter et al. 1991). From studies conducted in a genetic model of mammary tumor, a correlation between the recruitment of TAMs to premalignant lesions before the onset of angiogenesis and transition to malignancy was identified. Depletion of macrophages in this model was associated with a significant reduction in vessel formation and an increase in hypoxic and necrotic areas in the tumors (Lewis and Pollard 2006).

More recently, a novel role for TAMs in the development of refractoriness toward treatment with anti-VEGF compounds was reported. When comparing the antitumor effects of therapeutic compounds blocking either PlGF selectively, or PlGF and VEGF-A combined with other antineoplastic agents, improved antitumor activity for the anti-PlGF selective compound was noted. The improved antitumor activity observed for the combination treatment correlated with a similar fold reduction in the numbers of tumor associated, F4/80 positive macrophages in anti-PlGF treated mice when compared to anti-VEGF treatment alone. Importantly, compounds blocking VEGFR-2 signaling induced different pharmacodynamic alterations, and gene expression analysis of tumors treated with anti-VEGF compounds revealed a shift toward a proangiogenic rescue/ antiangiogenesis escape signature. In contrast, anti-PlGF treatment did not induce such escape signature, providing an advantage of anti-PLGF compounds by potentially circumventing the development of refractoriness to antiangiogenic treatment (Fischer et al. 2007). In conclusion, the effects of blocking VEGF in combination with compounds targeting TAMs will be of relevance for future clinical development of anti-VEGF compounds.

11.4 CD11b+ Gr1+ Myeloid-Derived Suppressor Cells

CD11b+ Gr1+ myeloid cells, also termed myeloid suppressor cells (MSCs) or myeloid-derived suppressor cells (MDSC, (Gabrilovich et al. 2001)), were originally described based on their immuno-suppressive characteristics, enabling tumors to escape from immune surveillance (reviewed in Vieweg et al. 2007). Recently, preclinical studies identified potent proangiogenic activities by CD11b+Gr1+ cells in the context of experimental tumor models, enabling refractoriness toward anti-VEGF treatment (Shojaei et al. 2007a; Shojaei et al. 2007b). MDSC were investigated intensively within the context of their anti-inflammatory activities. MDSCs can exert immunosuppressive functions within the tumor environment by inhibiting the activation of CD4+ and CD8+ T-cells. Several other immunosuppressive mechanisms are employed by MDSCs, including the inhibition of antigen-specific T-cell functions via CD80 or B7-H1 expression, nitric oxide production, or the L-arginine metabolism. Thus, in addition to providing proangiogenic stimuli, the presence of MDSCs within solid tumors may significantly inhibit desirable antitumor adaptive immune responses. By definition, MDSCs express Gr1 and CD11b, which are typical markers of the myeloid precursor derived lineages, MDSCs display reduced expression on mature myeloid cells such as monocytes or macrophages, which differentiates these cells from TAMs described earlier (Fig. 11.1). When analyzed in BM cell isolates, most of the cells within the CD11b+Gr1+ population belong to the class of neutrophils and only a minority are representing monocytic lineages (Shojaei et al. 2007a; Shojaei et al. 2007b). Thus, MDSCs are rather heterogeneous and variable in their phenotype and functional properties. The precise nature of MDSCs depends on the tumor-type and the nature of the tumor-derived factors. Therefore, different tumor-types may contain MDSCs expressing different phenotypic markers and exerting different functional potencies. Given the difficulties in determining the nature of MDSCs, a proposal was made to standardize the phenotypic markers to CD11b+Gr1+ cells. Such consensus phenotype allows for the direct comparison between different experimental models and facilitates the use of a common term of "myeloid derived suppressor cells" (MDSCs) to describe these cells (Gabrilovich et al. 2007).

Importantly, ablation of CD11b+Gr1+ cells by means of an antibody binding to Gr1 resulted in improved antitumor effects when tested in combination with anti-VEGF compounds, compared to the antitumor effects obtained for single-agent treatments. These studies validated MDSCs as therapeutic targets for combination treatments with anti-VEGF in solid tumors (Shojaei et al. 2007a). In the clinic, accumulation of immature myeloid suppressor cells in peripheral blood of cancer patients was observed (Almasri et al. 2004; Serafini et al. 2004). Therefore, quantification of circulatory MDSCs in the peripheral blood of cancer patients and analysis of potential correlations with response to anti-VEGF therapy may represent a valuable diagnostic approach to identify patients with optimal responses. Lastly, the methods and cell surface makers used to identify TAMs in experimental or patient tumors frequently overlap with the phenotypic markers used to define MDSCs. Therefore, some of the activities reported for TAMs may be attributable to MDSCs, and vice versa. Further investigations regarding the identity of MDSCs and TAMs may help to better understand some of the similarities in the biological functions reported for these cell types.

11.5 Lymphocytes and Mast Cells (MCs)

Experiments conducted in genetic models of cancer in mice demonstrated that T- and/or B-cell deficiency is associated with significant alterations in tumor growth rates compared to tumors grown in immune-competent mice. Activation of the adaptive immune system identified CD8+ T cells to be necessary for the improvement of the antitumor immune responses in mice (Zitvogel et al. 2006). However, cancer burden, incidence, and angiogenesis of tumors developing in the skin and cervix were variable and dependent on the location and genetic background of the tumors (reviewed in de Visser et al. 2006). In a genetic model of mouse squamous cell carcinoma of the skin, B- and T-cell deficiency was associated with a marked decrease in the infiltration of innate immune cells and a decrease in tumor formation and progression. Transfer of B-cells or serum from immuno-competent, tumor-bearing mice was sufficient to restore tumorigenicity, demonstrating that soluble mediators derived from B-cells are critical for the stimulation of tumor growth (de Visser et al. 2005). In contrast, adoptive transfer of tumor-associated B-cells yielded opposite effects, stimulating tumor invasion and metastasis through antibody–antigen complex-mediated granulocye and macrophage induction (Barbera-Guillem et al. 1999). Thus, different elements of the adaptive immune-system can introduce confounding effects on tumor growth, depending on the tumor type and the model used. Importantly, the potential of B- and T-cells to mediate refractoriness toward anti-VEGF treatment has been addressed experimentally in SCID beige mice, which are deficient in B- and T-cell lineages and have low granulocytes. Tumor-growth experiments in these mice implanted with either anti-VEGF refractory or sensitive tumor cell lines revealed that anti-VEGF refractoriness is T- or B-cell independent (Shojaei et al. 2007a).

The presence of tumor-infiltrating mast cells (MCs) was described in a variety of human cancers, including breast carcinomas (Kankkunen et al. 1997), colorectal cancer (Lachter et al. 1995), basal cell carcinomas (Yamamoto et al. 1997), nonsmall cell lung cancer (Shijubo et al. 2003), and pulmonary adenocarcinomas (Imada et al. 2000). Experiments in preclinical tumor models revealed important roles for MCs in the induction of tumor angiogenesis (Hiromatsu and Toda 2003; Toda et al. 2000). Activated MCs represent a source for many known angiogenic factors, including VEGF-A, bFGF, IL-8, and TNF-α. In addition, histamine and heparin stored in the secretory granules of MCs were shown to stimulate endothelial cell proliferation. The angiogenic potential of the granules of MCs was significantly reduced in presence of neutralizing compounds targeting VEGF-A or bFGF. Genetic depletion of MCs in mice resulted in reduced tumor angiogenesis of subcutaneously grown, syngeneic mouse tumors (Starkey et al. 1988), and reduced progression of malignant squamous cell carcinomas. Depletion of MCs was associated with diminished premalignant angiogenesis and reduced carcinoma incidence in a skin carcinoma model (Coussens et al. 1999; Coussens et al. 2000). Combined, these studies identified a critical role for the adaptive immune system, specifically B-cells, in the development of angiogenic responses in tumors. However, the role of MCs in mediating refractoriness to anti-VEGF treatment has not been addressed experimentally.

11.6 Neutrophils

Neutrophils play an active role in enhancing tumor angiogenesis, either directly via the release of vesicle-stored growth factors, cytokines such as VEGF-A or IL-8 (Schaider et al. 2003) and proteolytic activities, including matrix metalloproteinases (MMP-2) (Masson et al. 2005), MMP-9 (Coussens et al. 2000) and elastases (Iwatsuki et al. 2000). In general, neutrophil recruitment precedes the induction of angiogenesis in several preclinical tumor models, including genetic models (Coussens et al.

2000) or heterotransplant models of human cancers in nude mice (Gutschalk et al. 2006; Obermueller et al. 2004). The release of VEGF-A by neutrophils appears to be a key mechanism underlying the angiogenesis-promoting capacity of neutrophils, as depletion of neutrophils abrogated the angiogenic response to stimulation with CXCL1/MIP-2 in vivo (Scapini et al. 2004). Importantly, the angiogenic activities of MMP-9 positive neutrophils were potently suppressed by anti-VEGF compounds, indicating that these cells may not be part of the mechanism inducing refractoriness toward anti-VEGF treatment (Vosseler et al. 2005). The essential role of neutrophils during tumor angiogenesis was further supported by studies conducted with the Rip-Tag2 model of pancreatic islet carcinogenesis. In this model, transient depletion of neutrophils reduced the frequency of the angiogenic switch in dysplastic islets (Nozawa et al. 2006). Most of the proangiogenic activity produced by neutrophils was mediated by MMP-9, which releases matrix bound VEGF-A from the ECM and promotes VEGF-A binding and activation of VEGFR-2 on the tumor vasculature. In addition to the regulation of proangiogenic activities, an important role of neutrophils in the modulation of the phenotypes of TAMs was described (Gutschalk et al. 2006; Obermueller et al. 2004). Combined, these findings clearly demonstrated VEGF-dependent regulation of angiogenesis by neutrophils.

11.7 Therapeutic Targets to Overcome Anti-VEGF Refractoriness

11.7.1 Bv8

Bv8 is an endothelial cell mitogen that also induces haematopoietic cell mobilization and increases the production of granulocytic and monocytic colonies in BM colony formation assays in vitro (LeCouter et al. 2003; LeCouter et al. 2004). Several human tumor-cell lines implanted into nude mice are infiltrated with CD11b+Gr1+ myeloid cells expressing high levels of Bv8. Pharmacological studies blocking Bv8 along with VEGF-A revealed improved antitumor effects. An increase in CD11b+Gr1+ cells could be observed within anti-VEGF treated tumors, which correlated with the onset of central tumor necrosis. These findings suggested that the pathophysiological changes induced by anti-VEGF treatment, including local hypoxia and/or necrosis of the tumor, increases Bv8 production and induces resistance to anti-VEGF treatment. In contrast, anti-VEGF treatment in syngeneic tumor models in mice did not increase the numbers of CD11b+ Gr1+ cells in the tumors. These finding suggest that tumor intrinsic refractoriness and treatment-induced resistance to anti-VEGF may be the result of the differences in the experimental models used. Alternatively, the differences between intrinsic versus and treatment-induced refractoriness may indicate that upregulation of Bv8 is treatment induced, whereas the recruitment of inflammatory cells to the tumor is tumor intrinsic. In conclusion, these studies demonstrated that blocking proangiogenic factors produced by tumor infiltrating, BM-derived CD11b+Gr1+ myeloid cells improved antiangiogenic therapy.

11.8 VEGF-B, -C, -D, and PIGF

VEGF-A, a member of the platelet-derived growth factor family, is among the most potent angiogenic factors described so far. Other family members are VEGF-B, VEGF-C, VEGF-D, VEGF-E, and placental growth factor (PIGF). VEGF-A promotes angiogenesis by binding to two receptor tyrosine-kinases, VEGFR-1 and

VEGFR-2, found predominantly on the surface of vascular endothelial cells. Studies show, however, that VEGFR-2, not VEGFR-1, is the principle receptor for VEGF signaling (reviewed in (Ferrara 2004)). VEGF-A and PlGF exhibit additional regulatory functions on nonendothelial cells, including the stimulation of hematopoietic stem cell survival (Gerber et al. 2002) and EPC recruitment to the circulation (Hattori et al. 2001; Hattori et al. 2002). Increased expression of VEGFR-1, VEGF-A, VEGF-B, and PlGF was reported in different models of tumor growth (Autiero et al. 2003b; Lyden et al. 2001). Studies using VEGFR-1 blocking antibodies also identified a critical role for VEGFR-1 in EPC recruitment to peripheral circulation (Autiero et al. 2003a; Autiero et al. 2003b; Lyden et al. 2001). Blocking PlGF was shown to be anti-inflammatory, consistent with the fact that PlGF is a chemoattractant for VEGFR-1+ macrophages (Luttun et al. 2002a; Pipp et al. 2003). The efficacy of VEGFR-1 blockade during tumor growth in mice, however, is variable (Luttun et al. 2002c), and was most pronounced in tumors expressing high endogenous or ectopic levels of ligands activating VEGFR-1 (Stefanik et al. 2001).

To investigate the roles of different VEGF family members in the recruitment of myeloid cells to experimental tumors, the effects of anti-VEGF compounds blocking either VEGF-A along (G6-23-IgG), or combined with VEGF-B and PlGF (mFlt(1–3)-IgG) were determined in syngeneic tumors or human tumor xenografts grown in mice (Shojaei et al. 2007a; Shojaei et al. 2007b). Both compounds induced comparable tumor growth delays in mice implanted with anti-VEGF-sensitive or refractory tumors, suggesting that endogenous levels of PlGF and VEGF-B are redundant during VEGF-A blockade. However, these observations did not exclude the possibility that PlGF or VEGF-B may potentially contribute to EPC recruitment in conditions when VEGF-A is not neutralized.

The effects of a neutralizing antibody selectively blocking PlGF were tested in experimental tumor models in mice, when administered either alone or in combination with anti-VEGF or cytotoxic agents (Fischer et al. 2007). Improved therapeutic effects were noted when the anti-PlGF antibody was combined with anti-VEGF compounds or chemotherapy, relative to single agent treatment groups. Interestingly, such increase in efficacy inversely correlated with the frequency of TAMs in treated tumors. Moreover, treatment with the anti-VEGF compound induced a set of angiogenic factors, which was not observed in anti-PlGF treated tumors (Fischer et al. 2007). Combined, these findings suggest that PlGF not only represents an important regulator of EPC recruitment to pathologic vasculature, but is also a key regulator of TAM recruitment to anti-VEGF resistant tumors. Therefore, compounds blocking PlGF may have therapeutic utility for the treatment of carcinomas.

11.9 Targeting MDSCs and TAMs

Recent experiments demonstrated a critical role of MDSCs and TAMs in mediating refractoriness to anti-VEGF treatment. These experiments were conducted with compounds inducing either systemic ablation of inflammatory cells or blocking of specific angiogenic activities produced by these cells. However, gene knock-out or pharmacological experiments demonstrated that prolonged ablation of more differentiated monocytes or macrophage lineages in mice resulted in severe toxicity and mortality due to secondary infections. Therefore, identification of therapeutic targets that interfere selectively with a subset of tumor-associated monocytic cells or with proangiogenic activities produced by these cells may be required to circumvent these limitations (Table 11.1).

11.10 Targeting EPCs

Blocking of the genes involved in the homing of EPCs to tumor vasculature carries the potential to improve antiangiogenic and antitumor effects. However, due to rapid kinetics of EPC recruitment to tumor vasculature, EPCs may represent promising targets in prevention type anticancer treatment strategies, which are initiated during the earliest stages of tumor development. Due to the low incidents of EPCs in advanced tumors, targeting EPCs in already established tumors may induce only limited antiangiogenic effects.

11.11 Conclusions

The identification of tumor-infiltrating inflammatory cells as key mediators of refractoriness to anti-VEGF treatment validates MDSCs and TAMs as potential targets for therapeutic intervention in combination with anti-VEGF modalities and eventually other antineoplastic agents. Conceptually, interference with tumor-associated inflammatory cells can occur at three stages during leukocyte differentiation and development: (1) interference with migration of progenitors from the BM to the peripheral circulation. (2) Interference with endothelial cell transmigration of leukocytes from the peripheral circulation to tumors. (3) Interference with proangiogenic functions of leukocytes within tumors.

Several therapeutic strategies targeting different subsets of inflammatory cells for the treatment of autoimmune and inflammatory diseases are currently undergoing clinical development and some have gained approval. Targeting inflammatory cells has revealed some challenges. For example, prolonged treatment with compounds inducing systemic leukopenia or neutropenia frequently leads to discontinuation of treatment due to secondary infections. On the other hand, chronic use of anti-inflammatory agents, specifically COX-2 inhibitors, induced promising antitumor effects in preclinical and clinical studies (Clevers 2004; Turini and DuBois 2002). Pharmacological studies targeting COX-2 provided evidence that targeting inflammatory processes in cancer can be beneficial. Inflammatory cells display a remarkable plasticity with regard to their surface marker expression and functional potencies, and the specific type of cells and the expression of phenotypic marker of inflammatory cells is largely dependent on the tumor type and the environment. Thus, careful selection of the most relevant inflammatory cell type and/or molecular targets for each cancer indication will be critical to optimize the therapeutic benefit.

References

Aicher A, Heeschen C, Mildner-Rihm C, Urbich C, Ihling C, Technau-Ihling K, Zeiher AM, Dimmeler S (2003) Essential role of endothelial nitric oxide synthase for mobilization of stem and progenitor cells. Nat Med 9:1370–1376

Akita T, Murohara T, Ikeda H, Sasaki K, Shimada T, Egami K, Imaizumi T (2003) Hypoxic preconditioning augments efficacy of human endothelial progenitor cells for therapeutic neovascularization. Lab Invest 83:65–73

Almasri NM, Habashneh MA, Khalidi HS (2004) Non-Hodgkin lymphoma in Jordan. Types and patterns of 111 cases classified according to the WHO classification of hematological malignancies. Saudi Med J 25:609–614

Asahara T, Murohara T, Sullivan A, Silver M, van der Zee R, Li T, Witzenbichler B, Schatteman G, Isner JM (1997) Isolation of putative progenitor endothelial cells for angiogenesis. Science 275: 964–967

Autiero M, Luttun A, Tjwa M, Carmeliet P (2003a) Placental growth factor and its receptor, vascular endothelial growth factor receptor-1: novel targets for stimulation of ischemic tissue revascularization and inhibition of angiogenic and inflammatory disorders. J Thromb Haemost 1: 1356–1370

Autiero M, Waltenberger J, Communi D, Kranz A, Moons L, Lambrechts D, Kroll J, Plaisance S, De Mol M, Bono F et al (2003b) Role of PlGF in the intra- and intermolecular cross talk between the VEGF receptors Flt1 and Flk1. Nat Med 9: 936–943

Barbera-Guillem E, May KF Jr, Nyhus JK, Nelson MB (1999) Promotion of tumor invasion by cooperation of granulocytes and macrophages activated by anti-tumor antibodies. Neoplasia 1:453–460

Bingle L, Brown NJ, Lewis CE (2002) The role of tumour-associated macrophages in tumour progression: implications for new anticancer therapies. J Pathol 196:254–265

Clevers H (2004) At the crossroads of inflammation and cancer. Cell 118:671–674

Conejo-Garcia JR, Benencia F, Courreges MC, Kang E, Mohamed-Hadley A, Buckanovich RJ, Holtz DO, Jenkins A, Na H, Zhang L et al (2004) Tumor-infiltrating dendritic cell precursors recruited by a beta-defensin contribute to vasculogenesis under the influence of Vegf-A. Nat Med 10:950–958

Conejo-Garcia JR, Buckanovich RJ, Benencia F, Courreges MC, Rubin SC, Carroll RG, Coukos G (2005) Vascular leukocytes contribute to tumor vascularization. Blood 105:679–681

Coussens LM, Raymond WW, Bergers G, Laig-Webster M, Behrendtsen O, Werb Z, Caughey GH, Hanahan D (1999) Inflammatory mast cells up-regulate angiogenesis during squamous epithelial carcinogenesis. Genes Dev 13:1382–1397

Coussens LM, Tinkle CL, Hanahan D, Werb Z (2000) MMP-9 supplied by bone marrow-derived cells contributes to skin carcinogenesis. Cell 103: 481–490

Coussens LM, Werb Z (2002) Inflammation and cancer. Nature 420:860–867

Crivellato E, Ribatti D (2005) Involvement of mast cells in angiogenesis and chronic inflammation. Curr Drug Targets Inflamm Allergy 4:9–11

De Palma M, Venneri MA, Galli R, Sergi Sergi L, Politi LS, Sampaolesi M, Naldini L (2005) Tie2 identifies a hematopoietic lineage of proangiogenic monocytes required for tumor vessel formation and a mesenchymal population of pericyte progenitors. Cancer Cell 8:211–226

de Visser KE, Coussens LM (2006) The inflammatory tumor microenvironment and its impact on cancer development. Contrib Microbiol 13:118–137

de Visser KE, Eichten A, Coussens LM (2006) Paradoxical roles of the immune system during cancer development. Nat Rev Cancer 6:24–37

de Visser KE, Korets LV, Coussens LM (2005) De novo carcinogenesis promoted by chronic inflammation is B lymphocyte dependent. Cancer Cell 7:411–423

Dong J, Grunstein J, Tejada M, Peale F, Frantz G, Liang WC, Bai W, Yu L, Kowalski J, Liang X et al (2004) VEGF-null cells require PDGFR alpha signaling-mediated stromal fibroblast recruitment for tumorigenesis. Embo J 23:2800–2810

Dunn GP, Old LJ, Schreiber RD (2004) The immunobiology of cancer immunosurveillance and immunoediting. Immunity 21:137–148

Dvorak HF (1986) Tumors: wounds that do not heal. Similarities between tumor stroma generation and wound healing. N Engl J Med 315: 1650–1659

Ferrara N (2004) Vascular endothelial growth factor as a target for anticancer therapy. Oncologist 9(Suppl 1):2–10

Fischer C, Jonckx B, Mazzone M, Zacchigna S, Loges S, Pattarini L, Chorianopoulos E, Liesenborghs L, Koch M, De Mol M et al (2007) Anti-PlGF inhibits growth of VEGF(R)-inhibitor-resistant tumors without affecting healthy vessels. Cell 131: 463–475

Freeman MR, Schneck FX, Gagnon ML, Corless C, Soker S, Niknejad K, Peoples GE, Klagsbrun M (1995) Peripheral blood T lymphocytes and lymphocytes infiltrating human cancers express vascular endothelial growth factor: a potential role for T cells in angiogenesis. Cancer Res 55:4140–4145

Gabrilovich DI, Bronte V, Chen SH, Colombo MP, Ochoa A, Ostrand-Rosenberg S, Schreiber H (2007) The terminology issue for myeloid-derived suppressor cells. Cancer Res 67:425; author reply:426

Gabrilovich DI, Velders MP, Sotomayor EM, Kast WM (2001) Mechanism of immune dysfunction in cancer mediated by immature Gr-1+ myeloid cells. J Immunol 166:5398–5406

Gerber HP, Ferrara N (2005) Pharmacology and pharmacodynamics of bevacizumab as monotherapy or in combination with cytotoxic therapy in preclinical studies. Cancer Res 65:671–680

Gerber HP, Malik AK, Solar GP, Sherman D, Liang XH, Meng G, Hong K, Marsters JC, Ferrara N (2002) VEGF regulates haematopoietic stem cell survival by an internal autocrine loop mechanism. Nature 417:954–958

Gutschalk CM, Herold-Mende CC, Fusenig NE, Mueller MM (2006) Granulocyte colony-stimulating factor and granulocyte-macrophage colony-stimulating factor promote malignant growth of cells from head and neck squamous cell carcinomas in vivo. Cancer Res 66:8026–8036

Hattori K, Dias S, Heissig B, Hackett NR, Lyden D, Tateno M, Hicklin DJ, Zhu Z, Witte L, Crystal RG et al (2001) Vascular endothelial growth factor and angiopoietin-1 stimulate postnatal hematopoiesis by recruitment of vasculogenic and hematopoietic stem cells. J Exp Med 193:1005–1014

Hattori K, Heissig B, Wu Y, Dias S, Tejada R, Ferris B, Hicklin DJ, Zhu Z, Bohlen P, Witte L et al (2002) Placental growth factor reconstitutes hematopoiesis by recruiting VEGFR1(+) stem cells from bone-marrow microenvironment. Nat Med 8:841–849

Heissig B, Hattori K, Dias S, Friedrich M, Ferris B, Hackett NR, Crystal RG, Besmer P, Lyden D, Moore MA et al (2002) Recruitment of stem and progenitor cells from the bone marrow niche requires MMP-9 mediated release of kit-ligand. Cell 109:625–637

Hesser BA, Liang XH, Camenisch G, Yang S, Lewin DA, Scheller R, Ferrara N, Gerber HP (2004) Down syndrome critical region protein 1 (DSCR1), a novel VEGF target gene that regulates expression of inflammatory markers on activated endothelial cells. Blood 104:149–158

Hiromatsu Y, Toda S (2003) Mast cells and angiogenesis. Microsc Res Tech 60:64–69

Ii M, Nishimura H, Iwakura A, Wecker A, Eaton E, Asahara T, Losordo DW (2005) Endothelial progenitor cells are rapidly recruited to myocardium and mediate protective effect of ischemic preconditioning via "imported" nitric oxide synthase activity. Circulation 111:1114–1120

Imada A, Shijubo N, Kojima H, Abe S (2000) Mast cells correlate with angiogenesis and poor outcome in stage I lung adenocarcinoma. Eur Respir J 15:1087–1093

Iwatsuki K, Kumara E, Yoshimine T, Nakagawa H, Sato M, Hayakawa T (2000) Elastase expression by infiltrating neutrophils in gliomas. Neurol Res 22:465–468

Kanehira M, Xin H, Hoshino K, Maemondo M, Mizuguchi H, Hayakawa T, Matsumoto K, Nakamura T, Nukiwa T, Saijo Y (2007) Targeted delivery of NK4 to multiple lung tumors by bone marrow-derived mesenchymal stem cells. Cancer Gene Ther 14: 894–903

Kankkunen JP, Harvima IT, Naukkarinen A (1997) Quantitative analysis of tryptase and chymase containing mast cells in benign and malignant breast lesions. Int J Cancer 72:385–388

Kawamoto A, Asahara T, Losordo DW (2002) Transplantation of endothelial progenitor cells for therapeutic neovascularization. Cardiovasc Radiat Med 3:221–225

Knowles H, Leek R, Harris AL (2004) Macrophage infiltration and angiogenesis in human malignancy. Novartis Found Symp 256:189–200; discussion 200–204, 259–269

Kohchi C, Inagawa H, Hino M, Oda M, Nakata K, Yoshida A, Hori H, Terada H, Makino K, Takiguchi K, Soma G (2004) Utilization of macrophages in anticancer therapy: the macrophage network theory. Anticancer Res 24:3311–3320

Lachter J, Stein M, Lichtig C, Eidelman S, Munichor M (1995) Mast cells in colorectal neoplasias and premalignant disorders. Dis Colon Rectum 38: 290–293

LeCouter J, Lin R, Tejada M, Frantz G, Peale F, Hillan KJ, Ferrara N (2003) The endocrine-gland-derived VEGF homologue Bv8 promotes angiogenesis in the testis: Localization of Bv8 receptors to endothelial cells. Proc Natl Acad Sci U S A 100:2685–2690

LeCouter J, Zlot C, Tejada M, Peale F, Ferrara N (2004) Bv8 and endocrine gland-derived vascular endothelial growth factor stimulate hematopoiesis and hematopoietic cell mobilization. Proc Natl Acad Sci U S A 101:16813–16818

Leek RD, Landers RJ, Harris AL, Lewis CE (1999) Necrosis correlates with high vascular density and focal macrophage infiltration in invasive carcinoma of the breast. Br J Cancer 79:991–995

Leek RD, Lewis CE, Whitehouse R, Greenall M, Clarke J, Harris AL (1996) Association of macrophage infiltration with angiogenesis and prognosis in invasive breast carcinoma. Cancer Res 56:4625–4629

Lewis CE, Leek R, Harris A, McGee JO (1995) Cytokine regulation of angiogenesis in breast cancer: the role of tumor-associated macrophages. J Leukoc Biol 57:747–751

Lewis CE, Pollard JW (2006) Distinct role of macrophages in different tumor microenvironments. Cancer Res 66:605–612

Lin EY, Pollard JW (2004) Role of infiltrated leucocytes in tumour growth and spread. Br J Cancer 90:2053–2058

Lin EY, Pollard JW (2007) Tumor-associated macrophages press the angiogenic switch in breast cancer. Cancer Res 67:5064–5066

Luttun A, Brusselmans K, Fukao H, Tjwa M, Ueshima S, Herbert JM, Matsuo O, Collen D, Carmeliet P, Moons L (2002a) Loss of placental growth factor protects mice against vascular permeability in pathological conditions. Biochem Biophys Res Commun 295:428–434

Luttun A, Carmeliet G, Carmeliet P (2002b) Vascular progenitors: from biology to treatment. Trends Cardiovasc Med 12:88–96

Luttun A, Tjwa M, Moons L, Wu Y, Angelillo-Scherrer A, Liao F, Nagy JA, Hooper A, Priller J, De Klerck B et al (2002c) Revascularization of ischemic tissues by PlGF treatment, and inhibition of tumor angiogenesis, arthritis and atherosclerosis by anti-Flt1. Nat Med 8:831–840

Lyden D, Hattori K, Dias S, Costa C, Blaikie P, Butros L, Chadburn A, Heissig B, Marks W, Witte L et al (2001) Impaired recruitment of bone-marrow-derived endothelial and hematopoietic precursor cells blocks tumor angiogenesis and growth. Nat Med 7:1194–1201

Mantovani A, Allavena P, Sica A (2004) Tumour-associated macrophages as a prototypic type II polarised phagocyte population: role in tumour progression. Eur J Cancer 40:1660–1667

Mantovani A, Sozzani S, Locati M, Allavena P, Sica A (2002) Macrophage polarization: tumor-associated macrophages as a paradigm for polarized M2 mononuclear phagocytes. Trends Immunol 23: 549–555

Masson V, de la Ballina LR, Munaut C, Wielockx B, Jost M, Maillard C, Blacher S, Bajou K, Itoh T, Itohara S et al (2005) Contribution of host MMP-2 and MMP-9 to promote tumor vascularization and invasion of malignant keratinocytes. FASEB J 19:234–236

Murdoch C, Giannoudis A, Lewis CE (2004) Mechanisms regulating the recruitment of macrophages into hypoxic areas of tumors and other ischemic tissues. Blood 104:2224–2234

Natori T, Sata M, Washida M, Hirata Y, Nagai R, Makuuchi M (2002) G-CSF stimulates angiogenesis and promotes tumor growth: potential contribution of bone marrow-derived endothelial progenitor cells. Biochem Biophys Res Commun 297:1058–1061

Negus RP, Stamp GW, Hadley J, Balkwill FR (1997) Quantitative assessment of the leukocyte infiltrate in ovarian cancer and its relationship to the expression of C-C chemokines. Am J Pathol 150:1723–1734

Nolan DJ, Ciarrocchi A, Mellick AS, Jaggi JS, Bambino K, Gupta S, Heikamp E, McDevitt MR, Scheinberg DA, Benezra R, Mittal V (2007) Bone marrow-derived endothelial progenitor cells are a major determinant of nascent tumor neovascularization. Genes Dev 21:1546–1558

Nozawa H, Chiu C, Hanahan D (2006) Infiltrating neutrophils mediate the initial angiogenic switch in a mouse model of multistage carcinogenesis. Proc Natl Acad Sci U S A 103:12493–12498

Obermueller E, Vosseler S, Fusenig NE, Mueller MM (2004) Cooperative autocrine and paracrine functions of granulocyte colony-stimulating factor and granulocyte-macrophage colony-stimulating factor in the progression of skin carcinoma cells. Cancer Res 64:7801–7812

Ohno S, Ohno Y, Suzuki N, Kamei T, Koike K, Inagawa H, Kohchi C, Soma G, Inoue M (2004) Correlation of histological localization of tumor-associated macrophages with clinicopathological features in endometrial cancer. Anticancer Res 24:3335–3342

Ohno S, Suzuki N, Ohno Y, Inagawa H, Soma G, Inoue M (2003) Tumor-associated macrophages: foe or accomplice of tumors? Anticancer Res 23: 4395–4409

Orimo A, Gupta PB, Sgroi DC, Arenzana-Seisdedos F, Delaunay T, Naeem R, Carey VJ, Richardson AL, Weinberg RA (2005) Stromal fibroblasts present in invasive human breast carcinomas promote tumor growth and angiogenesis through elevated SDF-1/CXCL12 secretion. Cell 121:335–348

Papayannopoulou T (2004) Current mechanistic scenarios in hematopoietic stem/progenitor cell mobilization. Blood 103:1580–1585

Peters BA, Diaz LA, Polyak K, Meszler L, Romans K, Guinan EC, Antin JH, Myerson D, Hamilton SR, Vogelstein B et al (2005) Contribution of bone marrow-derived endothelial cells to human tumor vasculature. Nat Med 11: 261–262

Pipp F, Heil M, Issbrucker K, Ziegelhoeffer T, Martin S, van den Heuvel J, Weich H, Fernandez B, Golomb G, Carmeliet P et al (2003) VEGFR-1-selective VEGF homologue PlGF is arteriogenic: evidence for a monocyte-mediated mechanism. Circ Res 92:378–385

Polverini PJ, Leibovich SJ (1987) Effect of macrophage depletion on growth and neovascularization of hamster buccal pouch carcinomas. J Oral Pathol 16:436–441

Rafii S, Lyden D (2003) Therapeutic stem and progenitor cell transplantation for organ vascularization and regeneration. Nat Med 9:702–712

Rafii S, Lyden D, Benezra R, Hattori K, Heissig B (2002) Vascular and haematopoietic stem cells: novel targets for anti-angiogenesis therapy? Nat Rev Cancer 2:826–835

Rehman J, Li J, Orschell CM, March KL (2003) Peripheral blood "endothelial progenitor cells" are derived from monocyte/macrophages and secrete angiogenic growth factors. Circulation 107: 1164–1169

Scapini P, Morini M, Tecchio C, Minghelli S, Di Carlo E, Tanghetti E, Albini A, Lowell C, Berton G, Noonan DM, Cassatella MA (2004) CXCL1/macrophage inflammatory protein-2-induced angiogenesis in vivo is mediated by neutrophil-derived vascular endothelial growth factor-A. J Immunol 172:5034–5040

Schaider H, Oka M, Bogenrieder T, Nesbit M, Satyamoorthy K, Berking C, Matsushima K, Herlyn M (2003) Differential response of primary and metastatic melanomas to neutrophils attracted by IL-8. Int J Cancer 103:335–343

Serafini P, De Santo C, Marigo I, Cingarlini S, Dolcetti L, Gallina G, Zanovello P, Bronte V (2004) Derangement of immune responses by myeloid suppressor cells. Cancer Immunol Immunother 53: 64–72

Shaked Y, Bertolini F, Man S, Rogers MS, Cervi D, Foutz T, Rawn K, Voskas D, Dumont DJ, Ben-David Y et al (2005) Genetic heterogeneity of the vasculogenic phenotype parallels angiogenesis; Implications for cellular surrogate marker analysis of antiangiogenesis. Cancer Cell 7: 101–111

Shi Q, Rafii S, Wu MH, Wijelath ES, Yu C, Ishida A, Fujita Y, Kothari S, Mohle R, Sauvage LR et al (1998) Evidence for circulating bone marrow-derived endothelial cells. Blood 92:362–367

Shijubo N, Kojima H, Nagata M, Ohchi T, Suzuki A, Abe S, Sato N (2003) Tumor angiogenesis of non-small cell lung cancer. Microsc Res Tech 60: 186–198

Shojaei F, Wu X, Malik AK, Zhong C, Baldwin ME, Schanz S, Fuh G, Gerber HP, Ferrara N (2007a) Tumor refractoriness to anti-VEGF treatment is mediated by CD11b+Gr1+ myeloid cells. Nat Biotechnol 25:911–920

Shojaei F, Wu X, Zhong C, Yu L, Liang XH, Yao J, Blanchard D, Bais C, Peale FV, van Bruggen N et al (2007b) Bv8 regulates myeloid-cell-dependent tumour angiogenesis. Nature 450:825–831

Sica A, Schioppa T, Mantovani A, Allavena P (2006) Tumour-associated macrophages are a distinct M2 polarised population promoting tumour progression: potential targets of anti-cancer therapy. Eur J Cancer 42:717–727

Starkey JR, Crowle PK, Taubenberger S (1988) Mast-cell-deficient W/Wv mice exhibit a decreased rate of tumor angiogenesis. Int J Cancer 42:48–52

Stefanik DF, Fellows WK, Rizkalla LR, Rizkalla WM, Stefanik PP, Deleo AB, Welch WC (2001) Monoclonal antibodies to vascular endothelial growth factor (VEGF) and the VEGF receptor, FLT-1, inhibit the growth of C6 glioma in a mouse xenograft. J Neurooncol 55:91–100

Sunderkotter C, Goebeler M, Schulze-Osthoff K, Bhardwaj R, Sorg C (1991) Macrophage-derived angiogenesis factors. Pharmacol Ther 51: 195–216

Tlsty TD, Coussens LM (2006) Tumor stroma and regulation of cancer development. Annu Rev Pathol 1:119–150

Toda S, Tokuda Y, Koike N, Yonemitsu N, Watanabe K, Koike K, Fujitani N, Hiromatsu Y, Sugihara H (2000) Growth factor-expressing mast cells accumulate at the thyroid tissue-regenerative site of subacute thyroiditis. Thyroid 10:381–386

Turini ME, DuBois RN (2002) Cyclooxygenase-2: a therapeutic target. Annu Rev Med 53:35–57

Urbich C, Dimmeler S (2004) Endothelial progenitor cells: characterization and role in vascular biology. Circ Res 95:343–353

Vajkoczy P, Blum S, Lamparter M, Mailhammer R, Erber R, Engelhardt B, Vestweber D, Hatzopoulos AK (2003) Multistep nature of microvascular recruitment of ex vivo-expanded embryonic endothelial progenitor cells during tumor angiogenesis. J Exp Med 197:1755–1765

Vieweg J, Su Z, Dahm P, Kusmartsev S (2007) Reversal of tumor-mediated immunosuppression. Clin Cancer Res 13:727s–732s

Vosseler S, Mirancea N, Bohlen P, Mueller MM, Fusenig NE (2005) Angiogenesis inhibition by vascular endothelial growth factor receptor-2 blockade reduces stromal matrix metalloproteinase expression, normalizes stromal tissue, and reverts epithelial tumor phenotype in surface heterotransplants. Cancer Res 65:1294–1305

Wassmann S, Werner N, Czech T, Nickenig G (2006) Improvement of endothelial function by systemic transfusion of vascular progenitor cells. Circ Res 99:e74–e83

Yamaguchi J, Kusano KF, Masuo O, Kawamoto A, Silver M, Murasawa S, Bosch-Marce M, Masuda H, Losordo DW, Isner JM, Asahara T (2003) Stromal cell-derived factor-1 effects on ex vivo expanded endothelial progenitor cell recruitment for ischemic neovascularization. Circulation 107:1322–1328

Yamamoto T, Katayama I, Nishioka K (1997) Expression of stem cell factor in basal cell carcinoma. Br J Dermatol 137:709–713

Yang L, DeBusk LM, Fukuda K, Fingleton B, Green-Jarvis B, Shyr Y, Matrisian LM, Carbone DP, Lin PC (2004) Expansion of myeloid immune suppressor Gr+CD11b+ cells in tumor-bearing host directly promotes tumor angiogenesis. Cancer Cell 6:409–421

Zitvogel L, Tesniere A, Kroemer G (2006) Cancer despite immunosurveillance: immunoselection and immunosubversion. Nat Rev Immunol 6: 715–727

Antibody-Based Vascular Tumor Targeting

12

Christoph Schliemann and Dario Neri

Abstract The inhibition of angiogenesis represents a major step toward a more selective and better-tolerated therapy of cancer. An alternative way to take advantage of a tumor's absolute dependence on a functional neovasculature is illustrated by the strategy of "antibody-based vascular tumor targeting." This technology aims at the selective delivery of bioactive molecules to the tumor site by their conjugation to a carrier antibody reactive with a tumor-associated vascular antigen. A number of high-affinity monoclonal antibodies are nowadays available which have demonstrated a remarkable ability to selectively localize to the tumor vasculature. Indeed, some of them have already progressed from preclinical animal experiments to clinical studies in patients with cancer, acting as vehicles for the site-specific pharmacodelivery of proinflammatory cytokines or radionuclides.

In this chapter, we present a selection of well-characterized markers of angiogenesis which have proven to be suitable targets for antibody-based vascular targeting approaches. Furthermore, different transcriptomic and proteomic methodologies for the discovery of novel vascular tumor markers are described. In the last two sections, we focus on the discussion of antibody-based vascular tumor targeting strategies for imaging and therapy applications in oncology.

D. Neri (✉)
Institute of Pharmaceutical Sciences,
Department of Chemistry and Applied Biosciences,
Swiss Federal Institute of Technology Zürich,
Wolfgang-Pauli-Strasse 10, CH-8093, Zürich,
Switzerland
e-mail: dario.neri@pharma.ethz.ch

12.1 Concept and Definitions

Conventional pharmaceuticals currently in use for the treatment of cancer often suffer from a lack of specificity, leading to the unintentional exposure of normal tissues and – in some cases – life-threatening side effects. The development of more selective and better-tolerated cancer therapeutics is possibly one of the most important goals in modern oncology. As we have seen in the previous chapters, the inhibition of critical angiogenic pathways may represent an attractive therapeutic approach without the disadvantages of classical cytotoxic cancer therapies. Alternatively, one may prefer to target the tumoral neovasculature by the development of monoclonal antibodies, which are able to discriminate between a mature blood vessel and a tumor blood vessel, thus potentially acting as "delivery vehicles." This approach is generally termed "antibody-based vascular

R. Liersch et al. (eds.), *Angiogenesis Inhibition,* Recent Results in Cancer Research,
DOI: 10.1007/978-3-540-78281-0_12,

tumor targeting" and involves the selective delivery of bioactive agents to the tumor site by their conjugation to an antibody specific to a tumor-associated vascular antigen. The targeting to the tumor vasculature results in increased local concentrations of the delivered compound in the tumor tissue, while minimizing side effects to healthy organs. Indeed, the favorable toxicity profile of site-specific vascular-targeted therapeutics may open new avenues in the treatment of cancer, allowing the systemic administration of highly potent and promising agents, such as interleukin-12, whose clinical application has been to date compromised by unacceptable toxicities when administered in a nontargeted fashion (Cohen 1995; Halin et al. 2002b).

In principle, ligand-based tumor targeting applications fundamentally rely on good-quality markers of pathology, which allow a clear-cut discrimination between tumor and healthy tissues. It is not surprising at first sight that most efforts in the field have been made using targets expressed on the surface of cancer cells. However, targeting of antigens on tumor cells is a complex task and associated with a number of physical and kinetic barriers such as interstitial hypertension, long diffusion distances, or antigen heterogeneity, all significantly hindering deep-tissue penetration (Heldin et al. 2004; Jain 1999). Considering these obstacles, target molecules expressed in tumor-associated blood vessels seem particularly attractive in view of their inherent accessibility for blood-borne agents, their selective, abundant and stable expression, and their wide range of therapeutic options that they allow, from the recruitment of immune effector cells to intraluminal blood coagulation. Furthermore, as angiogenesis is a common feature of virtually all malignant tumors, including hematological malignancies, a single vascular targeting compound should, in principle, be applicable to a number of different tumor entities.

In this chapter, we refer to "vascular tumor targeting" as the targeted delivery of a bioactive agent (the effector molecule, typically a cytokine, procoagulant factor, drug, radionuclide or toxin) or an imaging molecule to the tumor site using an antibody specific for a tumor-associated vascular marker (the target molecule, either expressed on the surface of endothelial cells or in the subendothelial extracellular matrix). It is of significance that there is a fundamental conceptual difference between the targeted inhibition of an angiogenesis-related signaling pathway and the concept of vascular targeting as defined here. While the first strategy aims at the inhibition of target molecules involved in the process of new vessel development, the latter takes advantage of the target molecule as an easily accessible binding site for specific ligands capable of delivering bioactive molecules to the tumor site. The difference between both concepts becomes more obvious in light of the fact that the pathophysiological function of some well-characterized target molecules, proven to be excellently suitable for vascular targeting applications, is still largely unclear and possibly redundant (e.g., the extra domains of fibronectin). Depending on the properties of the selected effector function, the main therapeutic effect of a vascular targeting compound can be primarily directed either against the tumor cells themselves (whenever a vascular targeting approach is used to improve the therapeutic index of an otherwise less specific pharmaceutical) or against the endothelial cells of the vasculature (to destroy the tumor`s blood supply). An example for the first scenario would be the delivery of immunostimulatory cytokines to the tumor environment. The latter scenario is illustrated by the targeted delivery of a toxin to the tumor vascular endothelium as reported in a proof-of-principle study by Burrows and Thorpe (1993) or by the delivery of an α-particle emitting radionuclide with a near-acting range to a target on the luminal aspect of endothelial cells (Singh Jaggi et al. 2007). Of note, many effector molecules such as β-emitters exert overlapping actions against both cell types, thereby combining vascular disruption with direct cytotoxicity against tumor cells.

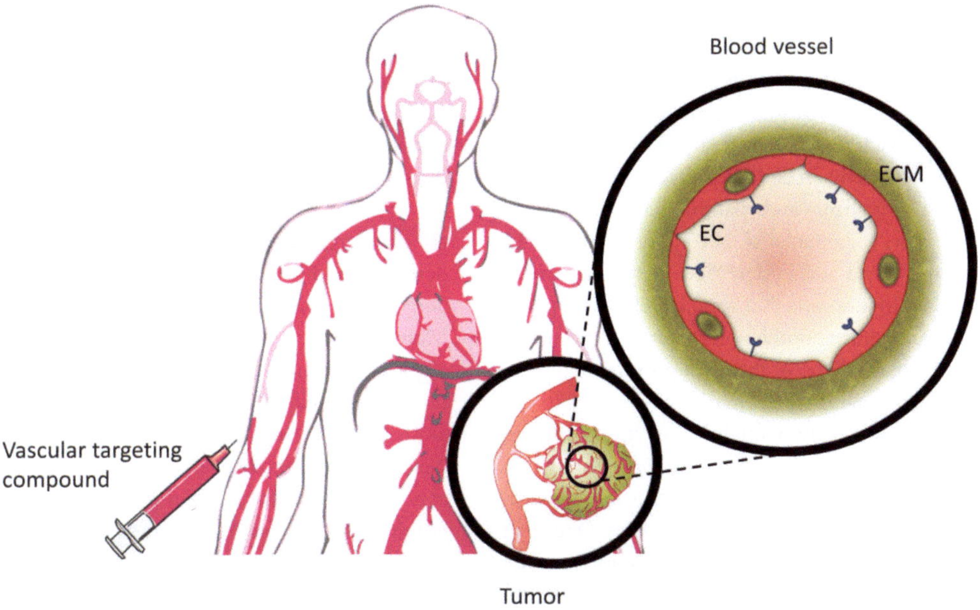

Fig. 12.1 *Concept of antibody-based vascular tumor targeting.* The vascular targeting agent, consisting of an antibody as a carrier molecule and an effector molecule, is administered systemically and homes to the tumor-specific vascular antigen, leading to the accumulation of the delivered pharmaceutical at the tumor site. As shown in the close-up, vascular antigens can be expressed on the luminal aspect of vascular endothelial cells (EC) or in the subendothelial extracellular matrix (ECM)

The general concept of antibody-based vascular tumor targeting is illustrated in Fig. 12.1.

12.2 Discovery of Novel Vascular Targets

Until recently, most efforts for the identification of novel tumor-associated vascular antigens were based on the study of in vitro cultures of endothelial cells, exposed to culture conditions which would mimic cell proliferation or quiescence. Another popular strategy has been to use endothelial cultures for the generation of antibodies either by immunization or phage display approaches. Major advances have arisen in the last years with the accessibility of full genome transcriptomic technologies, in particular, serial analyzes of gene expression (SAGE) in combination with bioinformatics, and, more recently, with perfusion-based proteomic technologies.

- The SAGE approach is based on the serial sequencing of short tags that are unique to each and every gene. These gene-specific tags are produced by a series of molecular biological manipulations and concatenated for automated sequencing. St. Croix and colleagues constructed SAGE libraries using isolated endothelial cells derived from normal and tumoral tissues and identified a number of genes that were specifically upregulated in the tumor endothelium, leading to the identification of several novel tumor endothelial markers (TEMs) (St Croix et al. 2000; Velculescu et al. 1995). Since target accessibility from the bloodstream is of fundamental

12

importance for vascular targeting approaches, further work has focused on those genes that encode proteins with predicted transmembrane domains. In a recent analysis, a SAGE approach revealed differences in gene expression patterns in endothelial cells derived from physiological and pathological angiogenic events (Seaman et al. 2007). Interestingly, 13 transcripts were identified in tumor-derived endothelial cells that were undetectable in the angiogenic endothelium of normal, regenerating tissue. One of the most promising tumor-specific endothelial markers was CD276.
- The increasing availability of transcriptome databanks has facilitated the *in silico* search for novel endothelial cell-specific tumor markers by comparative bioinformatics. One such approach applied a subtractive algorithm to the sequence tag expression data available in public databases and identified magic roundabout (Robo4) and an endothelial-specific protein disulfide isomerase (EndoPDI) as potential TEMs (Huminiecki and Bicknell 2000).

In general, transcriptomic analyzes are able to provide precise information on the quality and quantity of messenger RNAs that are expressed in the cell types and tissues of interest. However, a subsequent validation of the findings is of particular importance, since endothelium-associated targets identified in transcriptomic analyzes are not necessarily equally expressed at the protein level and surface-accessible for targeting agents. Thus, the most direct way to identify novel vascular antigens would involve the in vivo labeling of vascular structures, followed by the isolation and comparative proteomic analysis of proteins.

- Schnitzer and coworkers have demonstrated the use of colloidal silica for the in vivo coating of the vasculature, allowing the isolation of silica-coated luminal endothelial plasma membranes by subcellular fractionation, which are then analyzed by two-dimensional gel electrophoresis or multidimensional mass spectrometry techniques to produce high-resolution protein maps (Durr et al. 2004; Jacobson et al. 1992; Oh et al. 2004). Differential spot analysis, mass spectrometry of tryptic peptides, database searching and immunoblotting then allow the characterization of differentially expressed proteins. As an example, annexin A1 was found to be preferentially expressed on the surface of tumor-endothelial cells and was demonstrated to be suitable marker for antibody-based targeting applications (see below).
- More recently, a technology for the in vivo chemical labeling of vascular proteins based on the terminal perfusion of tumor-bearing animals with reactive derivatives of biotin has been described (Roesli et al. 2006; Rybak et al. 2005). This approach allows the biotinylation of proteins on the surface of endothelial cells or in the vessel-associated subendothelial matrix, which are readily accessible from the bloodstream. The purification of biotinylated proteins on a streptavidin column and comparative proteomic analyses based on LC-MS/MS methodologies subsequently permit the identification of hundreds of accessible vascular proteins and are able to reveal both quantitative and qualitative differences in the recovery of biotinylated antigens between the tumor and normal organs. Recently, this approach has been extended to the ex vivo perfusion of surgically resected human organs with tumors. The biotinylation of resected human kidneys bearing renal cell carcinomas led to the identification of a total of 637 proteins, 184 of which were exclusively expressed in the tumor vasculature, such as isoforms of periostin, versican, annexin A4 or MG50 (Castronovo et al. 2006).

12.3 Validated Markers of the Tumor Vasculature

In principle, vascular antigens can be either expressed on the surface of endothelial cells or in the subendothelial extracellular matrix (ECM)

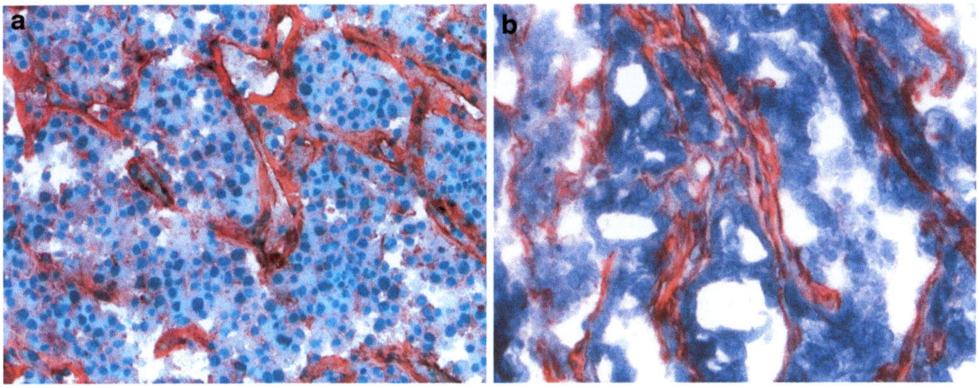

Fig. 12.2 *Immunohistochemical stainings of tumor sections with an anti-EDB antibody.* Sections of a human glioblastoma xenograft (U87) (**a**) and a human colorectal carcinoma (**b**) were stained with L19. Expression of extra domain B (EDB) fibronectin clearly associates with tumor vascular structures

of tumor blood vessels. The intuitive impression that antigens expressed on the luminal aspect of endothelial cells may be superior for targeting applications may not be valid in general. Indeed, luminal markers are easily reached from the circulation, but may carry the disadvantage of a relatively low abundance, precluding the accumulation of large quantities of the vascular targeting compound. In contrast, antigens expressed in the remodeled perivascular matrix offer the convenience of a typically more abundant and stable expression. Although they might seem less accessible, extravasation enables the ligand to bind to its antigen. In this section, we will discuss a selection of well-characterized targets of the tumor vasculature.

12.3.1 Extra Domains of Fibronectin

The extra domain B (EDB) is a type III homology domain of fibronectin which is not present in the fibronectin molecule under physiological, quiescent conditions but becomes inserted during tissue remodeling and angiogenesis by alternative splicing (Zardi et al. 1987). EDB fibronectin is virtually absent in normal adult tissues (exception made for the endometrium in the proliferative phase and some vessels in the ovary), but is highly abundant in the subendothelial matrix of the neovasculature of many aggressive tumors (Fig. 12.2) (Birchler et al. 2003; Carnemolla et al. 1989; Castellani et al. 1994; Khan et al. 2005). The EDB sequence is completely identical in mouse, rat, rabbit, monkey and man. This feature facilitates animal experiments in immunocompetent syngeneic settings, but has, so far, prevented the generation of antibodies using hybridoma technology. However, synthetic human antibody phage libraries have allowed the isolation of specific EDB-antibodies (Carnemolla et al. 1996; Neri et al. 1997). These include the high-affinity antibody L19, which has been shown to efficiently localize to tumor-associated angiogenic blood vessels in various animal models (Borsi et al. 2002; Tarli et al. 1999) and in patients with cancer (Birchler et al. 2007; Santimaria et al. 2003). Among more than 30 L19-based fusion proteins that have been developed and investigated in animal models, L19 fused to interleukin-2 (L19-IL2), L19 fused to tumor necrosis factor (L19-TNF) and L19 in small immunoprotein format (SIP) labeled with ^{131}I are three therapeutic derivatives of the L19 antibody that have moved to clinical trials in patients with different types of cancer (Menrad and Menssen 2005).

Recently, the extra domain A (EDA) of fibronectin has been identified as a marker of primary tumors and metastatic lesions using a combination of in vivo vascular biotinylation and mass spectrometry (Rybak et al. 2007a). The human monoclonal antibody F8, directed against EDA, exhibited an impressive preferential localization at the tumor site, comparable to the targeting performance of L19 in the tumor models and antibody formats analyzed so far (Villa et al. 2008). Further comparative studies will assess which fibronectin antibody is the best suited targeting agent for a given tumor type, based on antigen expression data and quantitative biodistribution analyses.

12.3.2 Large Isoforms of Tenascin C

Tenascin C is a high molecular mass glycoprotein of the extracellular matrix. Alternative splicing generates several isoforms by insertion of additional domains (Siri et al. 1991). Although not completely absent from normal tissues, these large isoforms of tenascin C exhibit a more restricted pattern of expression as compared to the isoforms without extra domains (Borsi et al. 1992). Radiolabeled derivatives of monoclonal antibodies specific to the domains A1 and D have been used for imaging and radioimmunotherapy in patients with cancer for over a decade (Paganelli et al. 1999; Reardon et al. 2006; Riva et al. 1999). Among all domains, the C domain of tenascin C features the most restricted expression: while being essentially undetectable in normal human tissues, it is highly abundant in high grade astrocytomas and lung cancer. The tumor-targeting performance of the human high-affinity antibody G11, specific to the domain C of tenascin C, has been demonstrated in an orthotopic rat glioma model (Silacci et al. 2006). Similarly, the recently described human monoclonal antibody F16, specific to the domain A1 of tenascin C, exhibited an excellent tumor-targeting performance in quantitative biodistribution experiments (Brack et al. 2006). A F16-based immunocytokine ("F16-IL2") has entered clinical trials for the treatment of metastatic breast, ovarian and lung cancer in combination with chemotherapy.

12.3.3 Phosphatidylserine

Phosphatidylserine (PS), an anionic phospholipid, is an essential component of the cell membrane, which is preferentially found in the inner leaflet of the lipid bilayer under normal conditions. Under conditions such as cellular stress, apoptosis, and proliferation, PS becomes exposed on the outer surface of the plasma membrane of angiogenic endothelial cells, rendering it accessible for targeting agents (Ran et al. 2002). Targeting experiments using monoclonal antibodies specific to PS have confirmed the accessibility of the antigen on the external surface of vascular endothelial cells in tumors (Ran et al. 2002, 2005). The PS-antibody 3G4 has been shown to exhibit potent single-agent activity as a naked antibody (by antibody-dependent cellular cytotoxicity against endothelial cells) (Ran et al. 2005) and to enhance the efficacy of chemotherapy in rodent models of cancer (Huang et al. 2005). Recently, the plasma protein β-2-glycoprotein 1, a member of the complement control protein family, has been identified as a critical cofactor mediating the interaction between 3G4 and surface-exposed PS (Luster et al. 2006). A chimeric version of 3G4, Bavituximab, is currently being investigated in Phase II clinical studies (Peregrine Pharmaceuticals, Inc.).

12.3.4 Annexin A1

Annexins are cytosolic proteins that can associate with plasma membranes in a calcium-dependent manner. Some annexins translocate the lipid bilayer to the outer cell surface. Using the methodology described above, Schnitzer and coworkers discovered annexin A1 as a target for vascular targeting applications (Oh et al. 2004). A monoclonal antibody to this antigen has been successfully used for the radioimmunoscintigraphic detection of solid tumors in a rat model. Furthermore, relatively low doses of the antibody labeled with ^{125}I (50 μCi as a single injection) showed therapeutic efficacy in the same animal model.

12.3.5 Prostate-Specific Membrane Antigen (PSMA)

PSMA, a membrane glycoprotein with proteolytic activity, has been originally found to be overexpressed in prostate cancer. However, several studies have documented that PSMA is also expressed in the neovasculature of several solid tumors (Chang et al. 1999; Liu et al. 1997; Silver et al. 1997), whereas its expression in healthy tissues appears to be restricted to prostatic, duodenal and breast epithelium and renal tubules. Of particular importance for vascular targeting strategies, it is virtually absent in normal blood vessels. The monoclonal-PSMA antibody J591 labeled with different radionuclides has demonstrated promising targeting efficacy in patients not only with prostate cancer but also with solid tumors in general (Bander et al. 2005; Milowsky et al. 2007; Morris et al. 2007).

12.3.6 Endoglin

Endoglin (CD105) is a homodimeric transmembrane glycoprotein which is overexpressed in neovascular endothelial cells of various solid tumors (Burrows et al. 1995; Wang et al. 1993). Although immunohistochemical studies revealed that endoglin is also significantly detectable in normal organs (Balza et al. 2001; Minhajat et al. 2006), monoclonal anti-endoglin antibodies have been used in biodistribution studies and for imaging and therapy purposes in rodent and dog models of cancer (Bredow et al. 2000; Fonsatti et al. 2000; Korpanty et al. 2007; Matsuno et al. 1999).

12.3.7 Integrins

Integrins represent a class of cell-surface proteins which are critically involved in endothelial cell adhesion to the ECM or cellular receptor proteins. Due to their significant involvement in angiogenesis events, integrins have gained significant attention as targets for the pharmacological inhibition of angiogenesis (for details see Chap. 6).

In addition, integrins have been proposed as targets for the ligand-based delivery of therapeutic agents to the tumoral neovasculature. A murine antibody specific to the integrin $\alpha_v\beta_3$ (LM609), selectively labeled neovessels in a breast cancer model and was shown to localize at the tumor site in a magnetic resonance imaging setup in rabbits (Sipkins et al. 1998). A humanized and affinity-matured version of LM609, the high-affinity antibody Abegrin (Medi-522, MedImmune, Inc.), has completed Phase II clinical trials as an antiangiogenic agent (McNeel et al. 2005; Mulgrew et al. 2006). However, when used as a ligand for antibody-based targeting applications, only moderate targeting results have been observed using ^{64}Cu-labeled Abegrin in quantitative biodistribution experiments in an orthotopic mouse model of human breast cancer (Cai et al. 2006). As an alternative ligand for α_v integrins, the peptide RGD has been isolated by in vivo phage display (Pasqualini et al. 1997) and a variety of RGD derivatives have been evaluated both for imaging and therapy applications (Temming et al. 2005).

12

12.3.8 Vascular Endothelial Growth Factors (VEGFs) and Receptors

As key mediators in the regulation of pathological angiogenesis, VEGFs have been successfully exploited for antiangiogenesis approaches. In addition, the VEGF/VEGFR signaling system is also being recognized as a potential target for vascular targeting approaches. The in vivo localization of monoclonal antibodies to VEGF-A, VEGF receptor 2, and the VEGF/VEGFR-2 complex has been studied. However, the absolute amounts of antibodies accumulating at the tumor site were often only modest, which possibly reflects kinetic limitations in the targeting of antigens of low abundance, even though they are easily accessible from the bloodstream (Cooke et al. 2001; Jayson et al. 2002; Stollman et al. 2008). Interestingly, in a very recent study using radiolabeled preparations of the anti-VEGF monoclonal antibody bevacizumab, an inverse correlation between the administered dose of radiolabeled antibody and the tumor targeting performance was observed (Stollman et al. 2008). The highest tumor uptake (as expressed in percent injected dose per gram of tissue) and the highest tumor-to-blood ratios were observed at protein doses as low as 1–3 μg (20–25% ID/g), while at doses exceeding 100 μg the absolute tumor uptake was lower than 3% ID/g.

12.3.9 Nucleolin

Porkka and coworkers discovered a synthetic 31-amino acid peptide (F3) which may be suitable for the targeted delivery of therapeutic effector molecules into tumors, because it is internalized into tumor-associated endothelial cells and tumor cells upon binding to the cell surface (Porkka et al. 2002). Later, the receptor protein which is recognized by F3 was identified as nucleolin. Originally described as a nuclear protein involved in the regulation of cell proliferation and nucleogenesis, nucleolin is also expressed on the surface of proliferating endothelial cells but restricted to the nucleus in resting endothelium (Christian et al. 2003). However, although nucleolin seems to feature a restricted expression pattern and the ability to internalize binding molecules, quantitative biodistribution studies using antibodies specific to nucleolin have not been reported yet.

12.4 Vascular Tumor Targeting: Imaging Applications

As we have seen in the previous sections, a number of high-affinity monoclonal antibodies are nowadays available, which selectively localize to angiogenic blood vessels upon systemic administration and allow a clear-cut discrimination between proliferating and quiescent vasculature. In principle, these antibodies may represent valuable tools for the macroscopic imaging of active angiogenesis in vivo, not only for the diagnosis and staging of cancer but also for monitoring response to therapy, especially with angiogenesis inhibitors. From a theoretical point of view, two essential requirements for the successful visualization of a ligand homing to neovascular structures are necessary:

- a suitable chemical modification strategy which makes the ligand visible for the corresponding physical detection system;
- a target molecule which is abundant enough to compensate the small contribution of the vasculature to the overall tumor mass.

In practice, the ability of radiolabeled antibodies to image tumors in vivo using SPECT or PET or methodologies is very well established (Verel et al. 2005). Furthermore, antibodies conjugated with near-infrared fluorophores have been shown to be suitable for in vivo and ex vivo photodetection procedures in both animal models and patients with cancer (Bremer et al. 2003; Neri et al. 1997; Pelegrin et al. 1991). However, while yielding high resolutions in the detection of superficial lesions and transparent structures of the body (e.g., for angiogenesis-related ocular disorders), fluorescence-based imaging techniques are limited in the detection of deeper lesions, even when diffuse optical tomography procedures are used. In both cases, the antibody label (a radionuclide or a fluorophore) is relatively small and does not significantly influence the pharmacokinetic properties of the antibody. As long as antigens expressed on the luminal aspect of endothelial serve as targets, also larger structures such as microbubbles or paramagnetic nanoparticles for contrast-enhanced ultrasound or MRI imaging can be used for in vivo molecular imaging (Korpanty et al. 2007; Sipkins et al. 1998). However, it is not obvious at the time whether antibodies equipped with microbubbles, magnetic nanoparticles or luminescent quantum dots can efficiently bind to targets "behind" the endothelial cell layer, particularly in light of experiences of our group suggesting that antibody derivatives >250 kDa or with extreme p*I* values lose their tumor targeting ability in vivo, while retaining the antigen binding properties of the parental antibody in vitro (Halin et al. 2002a, 2003; Melkko et al. 2002; Niesner et al. 2002). In contrast to our observations, anti-PSMA antibodies labeled with encapsulated quantum dots have been suggested as suitable compounds for the direct in vivo imaging of PSMA-positive prostate cancer cells (Gao et al. 2004). In this study, the accumulation of antibody-quantum dot conjugates at the tumor site was primarily attributed to the active targeting of cancer cells. However, as no convincing microscopic analyzes have been reported that the conjugate was able to extravasate and reach the tumor cells in vivo, the expression of PSMA on vascular endothelial cells (see above) may have contributed to the promising targeting performance as seen in the macroscopic imaging experiments. Thus, the issue remains controversial and it may well be possible that vascular-targeted imaging applications based on larger antibody labels may only be feasible with antibodies specific to antigens which are expressed on the inner surface of vascular structures.

12.5 Vascular Tumor Targeting: Therapeutic Applications

The selective localization of a targeting agent onto neovascular structures at the site of disease is an essential feature for the development of superior biopharmaceuticals, but it does not elicit a therapeutic response *per se*. Most often, ligands need to be coupled to suitable bioactive molecules, in order to mediate a therapeutic action. Before discussing the various therapeutic strategies which have been conceived and implemented experimentally over the years, it is useful to consider a few pharmacokinetic aspects related to vascular targeting.

After intravenous injection, a vascular targeting antibody (or antibody derivative) rapidly distributes in the body, while mainly remaining confined to vascular structures. The rates of elimination from blood greatly differ among the various molecular formats which can be considered. Two extreme cases may be represented by full immunoglobulins in IgG formats (which may remain in circulation for several weeks) and by the small scFv antibody fragments (for which the alpha phase accounts for over 95% of the biphasic clearance profile, with a typical half-life of 15–20 min) (Borsi et al. 2002). Similarly, clearance routes highly depend on the molecular features of the vascular targeting agent. While antibody derivatives with size below 60 kDa are rapidly filtered through the kidneys, larger antibody derivatives are typically eliminated via the hepatobiliary route. Also intact IgGs, which display long serum half-lives as a result of FcRn-mediated recirculation properties, are eventually cleared via the liver. Similar long circulatory half-lives can be obtained by PEG-modification of biopharmaceuticals, by their covalent fusion with serum albumin, or by a suitable modification with albumin-binding molecules (Dennis et al. 2007; Dumelin et al. 2008). For good quality tumor-associated vascular targets, high-affinity antibody derivatives display increasingly favorable tumor-to-blood and tumor-to-organ ratios at later time points after injection (Neri and Bicknell 2005). These ratios may be greater at early time points for small biopharmaceuticals, but the absolute amount delivered to tumoral lesions is typically larger for biopharmaceuticals which display longer circulatory half-lives (Adams et al. 2006; Borsi et al. 2002; Wu and Senter 2005). These considerations should not be forgotten when planning a therapeutic strategy. Certain antibody derivatives start mediating toxic events immediately after injection (e.g., radiolabeled antibodies) when the biopharmaceutical has distributed to all tissues, and only gradually gain in selectivity, as the agent clears from all organs except tumors. By contrast, other strategies appear to be ideally suited for matching the slow build-up of a preferential antibody accumulation at the tumor site. For example, antibody-drug conjugates with suitable cleavable linkers may continue releasing the drug at the tumor site for a long time period, while most of the biopharmaceutical has cleared from blood and normal tissues. In most cases, special care will have to be devoted to the minimization of the toxic effects to the organs responsible for clearance (e.g., liver or kidney).

Figure 12.3 summarizes some of the antibody modification strategies which have been

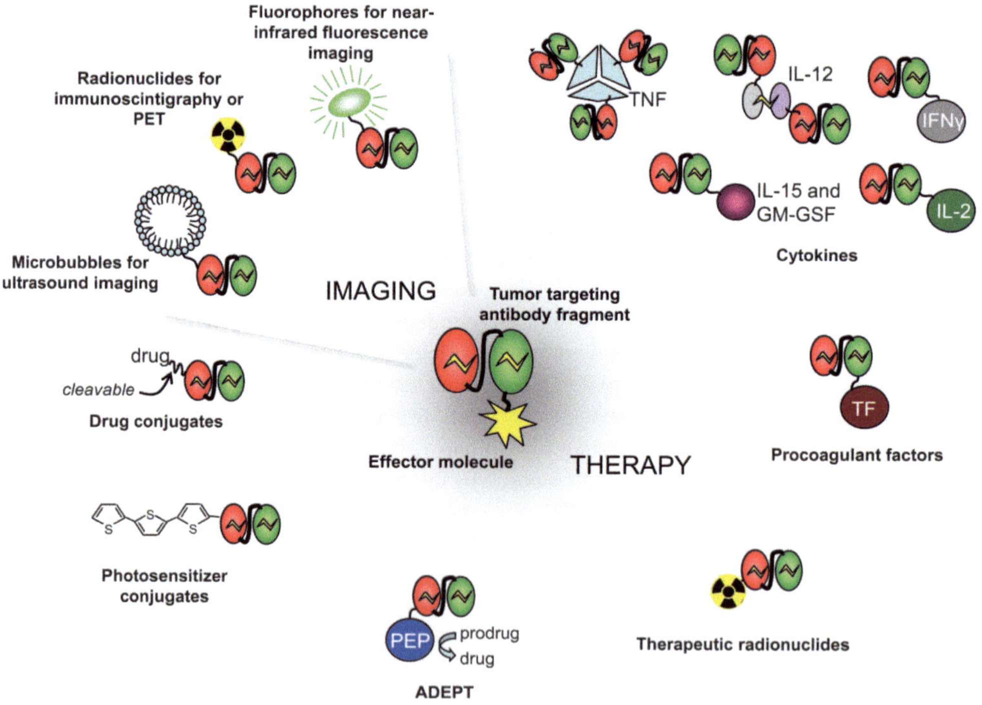

Fig. 12.3 *Schematic representation of antibody modification strategies.* A variety of L19-derivatives have been produced and investigated in animal models of cancer and clinical studies

considered for the development of targeted biopharmaceuticals. Many of these strategies have been experimentally implemented with the L19 antibody, specific to the EDB domain of fibronectin, thus allowing a direct comparison of the relative advantages and drawbacks of the different strategies. Such strategies are described in detail elsewhere (Rybak et al. 2007b; Schliemann and Neri 2007) and will only be briefly analyzed here.

Radiolabeled antibodies for cancer radioimmunotherapy represent a class of therapeutic agents of special interest, in light of the fact that their performance can be predicted on the basis of biodistribution and/or imaging data. It is generally believed that solid tumors may be cured if they receive a radiation dose of at least 50 Gy delivered by the radionuclide ^{131}I, while the bone marrow can tolerate at most 2.5 Gy. A systematic analysis of various antibody formats revealed that mini-antibodies are ideally suited for radioimmunotherapeutic applications (Berndorff et al. 2005; Hu et al. 1996; Tijink et al. 2006). By contrast, smaller fragments (e.g., scFv fragments) are rapidly cleared via the renal route and deliver excessive radiation doses to the kidneys, while the performance of radiolabeled IgG is often suboptimal, due to their long circulation time in the blood. The L19 antibody, in mini-antibody format and labeled with ^{131}I, is currently being investigated in Phase I/II clinical trials for the radioimmunotherapy of cancer. In animal models, this agent has shown a therapeutic activity both in monotherapy and in combination with Erbitux (Tijink et al. 2006).

Immunocytokines represent a second class of considerable therapeutic potential. The targeted delivery of certain proinflammatory cytokines (e.g., IL-2, TNF, IL-12, IL-15, GM-CSF) has been shown to mediate superior therapeutic effects compared to the nontargeted version of the same cytokine (Borsi et al. 2003; Carnemolla et al. 2002; Ebbinghaus et al. 2005; Halin et al. 2002b, 2003; Kaspar et al. 2007). Indeed, L19-IL2 and L19-TNF are currently being investigated in clinical trials in patients with cancer. It is worth mentioning that, upon fusion to certain cytokines or growth factors, vascular targeting antibodies may display a reduced tumor uptake. For example, fusion to interferon-γ was shown to reduce the tumor targeting performance of the L19 antibody. However, the tumor targeting potential could be restored in mice in which the interferon-γ receptor had been knocked out (Ebbinghaus et al. 2005). Similarly, fusion of the L19 antibody to murine VEGF-164 (but not VEGF-120) or to other highly charged polypeptides abrogates tumor targeting (Halin et al. 2002a; Melkko et al. 2002; Niesner et al. 2002). While our group has always preferred to construct immunocytokines by sequential gene fusion with scFv fragments, other groups have favored to append cytokines at the C-terminal end of antibodies in IgG format (Dela Cruz et al. 2004; Schrama et al. 2006).

A third class of therapeutic antibody derivatives of particular interest is represented by antibody-drug conjugates with cleavable linkers (Chari 2008; Doronina et al. 2003). Most groups have so far used this technology with antibodies capable of selective internalization on tumor cells, but it would be conceivable to deliver potent drugs to the tumor neovasculature by means of antibodies which remain in the extracellular space and slowly release a drug as a consequence of hydrolytic processes. Considering the difference in molecular weight between antibodies and cytotoxic drugs, the availability of chemotherapeutic agents which are active at nano- or picomolar concentration and which can be coupled to antibodies will greatly facilitate progress in this area, thus leading to a new generation of armed monoclonal antibodies.

Finally, it is worth mentioning that intact IgGs continue to represent an important segment of pharmaceutical biotechnology. In general, they display a low toxicity profile which makes them ideally suited for combination therapy. It is becoming increasingly clear that even IgGs specific to tumor cell antigens are often confined to the perivascular space, as a result of the high interstitial pressure in the tumor environment

12

and of capture by antigen in stoichiometric excess immediately after extravasation (Adams et al. 2001; Dennis et al. 2007). Modern research in protein engineering aims at potentiating the IgG-mediated cytotoxic activity (ADCC) by increasing the affinity between the antibody Fc portion and the corresponding FcγRIII receptor, either by glycosylation engineering (Umana et al. 1999) or by introducing mutations in the Fc fragment (Lazar et al. 2006).

Acknowledgments Financial support from the Swiss National Science Foundation, the Gebert-Ruef Foundation, the Schweizer Krebsliga, the ETH Zurich and the European Union projects STROMA, FLUORMMPI and IMMUNOPDT is gratefully acknowledged. C.S. is recipient of a postdoctoral scholarship from the Deutsche Krebshilfe.

References

Adams GP, Schier R, McCall AM, Simmons HH, Horak EM, Alpaugh RK, Marks JD, Weiner LM (2001) High affinity restricts the localization and tumor penetration of single-chain fv antibody molecules. Cancer Res 61:4750–4755

Adams GP, Tai MS, McCartney JE, Marks JD, Stafford WF 3rd, Houston LL, Huston JS, Weiner LM (2006) Avidity-mediated enhancement of in vivo tumor targeting by single-chain Fv dimers. Clin Cancer Res 12:1599–1605

Balza E, Castellani P, Zijlstra A, Neri D, Zardi L, Siri A (2001) Lack of specificity of endoglin expression for tumor blood vessels. Int J Cancer 94:579–585

Bander NH, Milowsky MI, Nanus DM, Kostakoglu L, Vallabhajosula S, Goldsmith SJ (2005) Phase I trial of 177lutetium-labeled J591, a monoclonal antibody to prostate-specific membrane antigen, in patients with androgen-independent prostate cancer. J Clin Oncol 23:4591–4601

Berndorff D, Borkowski S, Sieger S, Rother A, Friebe M, Viti F, Hilger CS, Cyr JE, Dinkelborg LM (2005) Radioimmunotherapy of solid tumors by targeting extra domain B fibronectin: identification of the best-suited radioimmunoconjugate. Clin Cancer Res 11:7053s–7063s

Birchler MT, Milisavlijevic D, Pfaltz M, Neri D, Odermatt B, Schmid S, Stoeckli SJ (2003) Expression of the extra domain B of fibronectin, a marker of angiogenesis, in head and neck tumors. Laryngoscope 113:1231–1237

Birchler MT, Thuerl C, Schmid D, Neri D, Waibel R, Schubiger A, Stoeckli SJ, Schmid S, Goerres GW (2007) Immunoscintigraphy of patients with head and neck carcinomas, with an anti-angiogenetic antibody fragment. Otolaryngol Head Neck Surg 136:543–548

Borsi L, Carnemolla B, Nicolo G, Spina B, Tanara G, Zardi L (1992) Expression of different tenascin isoforms in normal, hyperplastic and neoplastic human breast tissues. Int J Cancer 52:688–692

Borsi L, Balza E, Bestagno M, Castellani P, Carnemolla B, Biro A, Leprini A, Sepulveda J, Burrone O, Neri D, Zardi L (2002) Selective targeting of tumoral vasculature: comparison of different formats of an antibody (L19) to the ED-B domain of fibronectin. Int J Cancer 102: 75–85

Borsi L, Balza E, Carnemolla B, Sassi F, Castellani P, Berndt A, Kosmehl H, Biro A, Siri A, Orecchia P, Grassi J, Neri D, Zardi L (2003) Selective targeted delivery of TNFalpha to tumor blood vessels. Blood 102:4384–4392

Brack SS, Silacci M, Birchler M, Neri D (2006) Tumor-targeting properties of novel antibodies specific to the large isoform of tenascin-C. Clin Cancer Res 12:3200–3208

Bredow S, Lewin M, Hofmann B, Marecos E, Weissleder R (2000) Imaging of tumour neovasculature by targeting the TGF-beta binding receptor endoglin. Eur J Cancer 36:675–681

Bremer C, Ntziachristos V, Weissleder R (2003) Optical-based molecular imaging: contrast agents and potential medical applications. Eur Radiol 13:231–243

Burrows FJ, Thorpe PE (1993) Eradication of large solid tumors in mice with an immunotoxin directed against tumor vasculature. Proc Natl Acad Sci USA 90:8996–9000

Burrows FJ, Derbyshire EJ, Tazzari PL, Amlot P, Gazdar AF, King SW, Letarte M, Vitetta ES, Thorpe PE (1995) Up-regulation of endoglin on vascular endothelial cells in human solid tumors: implications for diagnosis and therapy. Clin Cancer Res 1:1623–1634

Cai W, Wu Y, Chen K, Cao Q, Tice DA, Chen X (2006) In vitro and in vivo characterization of 64cu-labeled abegrintm, a humanized monoclonal antibody against integrin {alpha}v{beta}3. Cancer Res 66:9673–9681

Carnemolla B, Balza E, Siri A, Zardi L, Nicotra MR, Bigotti A, Natali PG (1989) A tumor-associated fibronectin isoform generated by alternative splicing of messenger RNA precursors. J Cell Biol 108:1139–1148

Carnemolla B, Neri D, Castellani P, Leprini A, Neri G, Pini A, Winter G, Zardi L (1996) Phage antibodies with pan-species recognition of the oncofoetal angiogenesis marker fibronectin ED-B domain. Int J Cancer 68:397–405

Carnemolla B, Borsi L, Balza E, Castellani P, Meazza R, Berndt A, Ferrini S, Kosmehl H, Neri D, Zardi L (2002) Enhancement of the antitumor properties of interleukin-2 by its targeted delivery to the tumor blood vessel extracellular matrix. Blood 99:1659–1665

Castellani P, Viale G, Dorcaratto A, Nicolo G, Kaczmarek J, Querze G, Zardi L (1994) The fibronectin isoform containing the ED-B oncofetal domain: a marker of angiogenesis. Int J Cancer 59:612–618

Castronovo V, Waltregny D, Kischel P, Roesli C, Elia G, Rybak JN, Neri D (2006) A chemical proteomics approach for the identification of accessible antigens expressed in human kidney cancer. Mol Cell Proteomics 5:2083–2091

Chang SS, O'Keefe DS, Bacich DJ, Reuter VE, Heston WD, Gaudin PB (1999) Prostate-specific membrane antigen is produced in tumor-associated neovasculature. Clin Cancer Res 5: 2674–2681

Chari RV (2008) Targeted cancer therapy: conferring specificity to cytotoxic drugs. Acc Chem Res 41:98–107

Christian S, Pilch J, Akerman ME, Porkka K, Laakkonen P, Ruoslahti E (2003) Nucleolin expressed at the cell surface is a marker of endothelial cells in angiogenic blood vessels. J Cell Biol 163:871–878

Cohen J (1995) IL-12 deaths: explanation and a puzzle. Science 270:908

Cooke SP, Boxer GM, Lawrence L, Pedley RB, Spencer DI, Begent RH, Chester KA (2001) A strategy for antitumor vascular therapy by targeting the vascular endothelial growth factor: receptor complex. Cancer Res 61:3653–3659

Dela Cruz JS, Huang TH, Penichet ML, Morrison SL (2004) Antibody-cytokine fusion proteins: innovative weapons in the war against cancer. Clin Exp Med 4:57–64

Dennis MS, Jin H, Dugger D, Yang R, McFarland L, Ogasawara A, Williams S, Cole MJ, Ross S, Schwall R (2007) Imaging tumors with an albumin-binding Fab, a novel tumor-targeting agent. Cancer Res 67:254–261

Doronina SO, Toki BE, Torgov MY, Mendelsohn BA, Cerveny CG, Chace DF, DeBlanc RL, Gearing RP, Bovee TD, Siegall CB, Francisco JA, Wahl AF, Meyer DL, Senter PD (2003) Development of potent monoclonal antibody auristatin conjugates for cancer therapy. Nat Biotechnol 21:778–784

Dumelin CE, Trüssel S, Buller F, Trachsel E, Bootz F, Zhang Y, Manocci L, Beck SC, Drumea-Mirancea M, Seeliger MWP, Baltes C, Müggler TP, Kranz FP, Rudin MP, Melkko S, Scheuermann JP, Neri D (2008) Discovery and applications of a portable albumin binder from a DNA-encoded chemical library. Angew Chem Int Ed Eng 47(17):3196–3201

Durr E, Yu J, Krasinska KM, Carver LA, Yates JR, Testa JE, Oh P, Schnitzer JE (2004) Direct proteomic mapping of the lung microvascular endothelial cell surface in vivo and in cell culture. Nat Biotechnol 22:985–992

Ebbinghaus C, Ronca R, Kaspar M, Grabulovski D, Berndt A, Kosmehl H, Zardi L, Neri D (2005) Engineered vascular-targeting antibody-interferon-gamma fusion protein for cancer therapy. Int J Cancer 116:304–313

Fonsatti E, Jekunen AP, Kairemo KJ, Coral S, Snellman M, Nicotra MR, Natali PG, Altomonte M, Maio M (2000) Endoglin is a suitable target for efficient imaging of solid tumors: in vivo evidence in a canine mammary carcinoma model. Clin Cancer Res 6:2037–2043

Gao X, Cui Y, Levenson RM, Chung LW, Nie S (2004) In vivo cancer targeting and imaging with semiconductor quantum dots. Nat Biotechnol 22:969–976

Halin C, Niesner U, Villani ME, Zardi L, Neri D (2002a) Tumor-targeting properties of antibody-vascular endothelial growth factor fusion proteins. Int J Cancer 102:109–116

Halin C, Rondini S, Nilsson F, Berndt A, Kosmehl H, Zardi L, Neri D (2002b) Enhancement of the antitumor activity of interleukin-12 by targeted delivery to neovasculature. Nat Biotechnol 20:264–269

Halin C, Gafner V, Villani ME, Borsi L, Berndt A, Kosmehl H, Zardi L, Neri D (2003) Synergistic therapeutic effects of a tumor targeting antibody fragment, fused to interleukin 12 and to tumor necrosis factor alpha. Cancer Res 63: 3202–3210

Heldin CH, Rubin K, Pietras K, Ostman A (2004) High interstitial fluid pressure - an obstacle in cancer therapy. Nat Rev Cancer 4:806–813

Hu S, Shively L, Raubitschek A, Sherman M, Williams LE, Wong JY, Shively JE, Wu AM (1996) Minibody: A novel engineered anti-carcinoembryonic antigen antibody fragment (single-chain Fv-CH3) which exhibits rapid, high-level targeting of xenografts. Cancer Res 56:3055–3061

Huang X, Bennett M, Thorpe PE (2005) A monoclonal antibody that binds anionic phospholipids on tumor blood vessels enhances the antitumor effect of docetaxel on human breast tumors in mice. Cancer Res 65:4408–4416

Huminiecki L, Bicknell R (2000) In silico cloning of novel endothelial-specific genes. Genome Res 10:1796–1806

Jacobson BS, Schnitzer JE, McCaffery M, Palade GE (1992) Isolation and partial characterization of the luminal plasmalemma of microvascular endothelium from rat lungs. Eur J Cell Biol 58: 296–306

Jain RK (1999) Transport of molecules, particles, and cells in solid tumors. Annu Rev Biomed Eng 1:241–263

Jayson GC, Zweit J, Jackson A, Mulatero C, Julyan P, Ranson M, Broughton L, Wagstaff J, Hakannson L, Groenewegen G, Bailey J, Smith N, Hastings D, Lawrance J, Haroon H, Ward T, McGown AT, Tang M, Levitt D, Marreaud S, Lehmann FF, Herold M, Zwierzina H (2002) Molecular imaging and biological evaluation of HuMV833 anti-VEGF antibody: implications for trial design of antiangiogenic antibodies. J Natl Cancer Inst 94: 1484–1493

Kaspar M, Trachsel E, Neri D (2007) The antibody-mediated targeted delivery of interleukin-15 and GM-CSF to the tumor neovasculature inhibits tumor growth and metastasis. Cancer Res 67: 4940–4948

Khan ZA, Caurtero J, Barbin YP, Chan BM, Uniyal S, Chakrabarti S (2005) ED-B fibronectin in non-small cell lung carcinoma. Exp Lung Res 31: 701–711

Korpanty G, Carbon JG, Grayburn PA, Fleming JB, Brekken RA (2007) Monitoring response to anti-cancer therapy by targeting microbubbles to tumor vasculature. Clin Cancer Res 13:323–330

Lazar GA, Dang W, Karki S, Vafa O, Peng JS, Hyun L, Chan C, Chung HS, Eivazi A, Yoder SC, Vielmetter J, Carmichael DF, Hayes RJ, Dahiyat BI (2006) Engineered antibody Fc variants with enhanced effector function. Proc Natl Acad Sci USA 103:4005–4010

Liu H, Moy P, Kim S, Xia Y, Rajasekaran A, Navarro V, Knudsen B, Bander NH (1997) Monoclonal antibodies to the extracellular domain of prostate-specific membrane antigen also react with tumor vascular endothelium. Cancer Res 57:3629–3634

Luster TA, He J, Huang X, Maiti SN, Schroit AJ, de Groot PG, Thorpe PE (2006) Plasma protein beta-2-glycoprotein 1 mediates interaction between the anti-tumor monoclonal antibody 3G4 and anionic phospholipids on endothelial cells. J Biol Chem 281:29863–29871

Matsuno F, Haruta Y, Kondo M, Tsai H, Barcos M, Seon BK (1999) Induction of lasting complete regression of preformed distinct solid tumors by targeting the tumor vasculature using two new anti-endoglin monoclonal antibodies. Clin Cancer Res 5:371–382

McNeel DG, Eickhoff J, Lee FT, King DM, Alberti D, Thomas JP, Friedl A, Kolesar J, Marnocha R, Volkman J, Zhang J, Hammershaimb L, Zwiebel JA, Wilding G (2005) Phase I trial of a monoclonal antibody specific for alphavbeta3 integrin (MEDI-522) in patients with advanced malignancies, including an assessment of effect on tumor perfusion. Clin Cancer Res 11:7851–7860

Melkko S, Halin C, Borsi L, Zardi L, Neri D (2002) An antibody-calmodulin fusion protein reveals a functional dependence between macromolecular isoelectric point and tumor targeting performance. Int J Radiat Oncol Biol Phys 54: 1485–1490

Menrad A, Menssen HD (2005) ED-B fibronectin as a target for antibody-based cancer treatments. Expert Opin Ther Targets 9:491–500

Milowsky MI, Nanus DM, Kostakoglu L, Sheehan CE, Vallabhajosula S, Goldsmith SJ, Ross JS, Bander NH (2007) Vascular targeted therapy with anti-prostate-specific membrane antigen monoclonal antibody J591 in advanced solid tumors. J Clin Oncol 25:540–547

Minhajat R, Mori D, Yamasaki F, Sugita Y, Satoh T, Tokunaga O (2006) Organ-specific endoglin (CD105) expression in the angiogenesis of human cancers. Pathol Int 56:717–723

Morris MJ, Pandit-Taskar N, Divgi CR, Bender S, O'Donoghue JA, Nacca A, Smith-Jones P,

Schwartz L, Slovin S, Finn R, Larson S, Scher HI (2007) Phase I evaluation of J591 as a vascular targeting agent in progressive solid tumors. Clin Cancer Res 13:2707–2713

Mulgrew K, Kinneer K, Yao XT, Ward BK, Damschroder MM, Walsh B, Mao SY, Gao C, Kiener PA, Coats S, Kinch MS, Tice DA (2006) Direct targeting of alphavbeta3 integrin on tumor cells with a monoclonal antibody, Abegrin. Mol Cancer Ther 5:3122–3129

Neri D, Carnemolla B, Nissim A, Leprini A, Querze G, Balza E, Pini A, Tarli L, Halin C, Neri P, Zardi L, Winter G (1997) Targeting by affinity-matured recombinant antibody fragments of an angiogenesis associated fibronectin isoform. Nat Biotechnol 15:1271–1275

Neri D, Bicknell R (2005) Tumour vascular targeting. Nat Rev Cancer 5:436–446

Niesner U, Halin C, Lozzi L, Gunthert M, Neri P, Wunderli-Allenspach H, Zardi L, Neri D (2002) Quantitation of the tumor-targeting properties of antibody fragments conjugated to cell-permeating HIV-1 TAT peptides. Bioconjug Chem 13:729–736

Oh P, Li Y, Yu J, Durr E, Krasinska KM, Carver LA, Testa JE, Schnitzer JE (2004) Subtractive proteomic mapping of the endothelial surface in lung and solid tumours for tissue-specific therapy. Nature 429:629–635

Paganelli G, Grana C, Chinol M, Cremonesi M, De Cicco C, De Braud F, Robertson C, Zurrida S, Casadio C, Zoboli S, Siccardi AG, Veronesi U (1999) Antibody-guided three-step therapy for high grade glioma with yttrium-90 biotin. Eur J Nucl Med 26:348–357

Pasqualini R, Koivunen E, Ruoslahti E (1997) Alpha v integrins as receptors for tumor targeting by circulating ligands. Nat Biotechnol 15:542–546

Pelegrin A, Folli S, Buchegger F, Mach JP, Wagnieres G, van den Bergh H (1991) Antibody-fluorescein conjugates for photoimmunodiagnosis of human colon carcinoma in nude mice. Cancer 67:2529–2537

Porkka K, Laakkonen P, Hoffman JA, Bernasconi M, Ruoslahti E (2002) A fragment of the HMGN2 protein homes to the nuclei of tumor cells and tumor endothelial cells in vivo. Proc Natl Acad Sci USA 99:7444–7449

Ran S, Downes A, Thorpe PE (2002) Increased exposure of anionic phospholipids on the surface of tumor blood vessels. Cancer Res 62:6132–6140

Ran S, He J, Huang X, Soares M, Scothorn D, Thorpe PE (2005) Antitumor effects of a monoclonal antibody that binds anionic phospholipids on the surface of tumor blood vessels in mice. Clin Cancer Res 11:1551–1562

Reardon DA, Akabani G, Coleman RE, Friedman AH, Friedman HS, Herndon JE 2nd, McLendon RE, Pegram CN, Provenzale JM, Quinn JA, Rich JN, Vredenburgh JJ, Desjardins A, Gururangan S, Badruddoja M, Dowell JM, Wong TZ, Zhao XG, Zalutsky MR, Bigner DD (2006) Salvage radioimmunotherapy with murine iodine-131-labeled antitenascin monoclonal antibody 81C6 for patients with recurrent primary and metastatic malignant brain tumors: phase II study results. J Clin Oncol 24:115–122

Riva P, Franceschi G, Frattarelli M, Lazzari S, Riva N, Giuliani G, Casi M, Sarti G, Guiducci G, Giorgetti G, Gentile R, Santimaria M, Jermann E, Maeke HR (1999) Loco-regional radioimmunotherapy of high-grade malignant gliomas using specific monoclonal antibodies labeled with 90Y: a phase I study. Clin Cancer Res 5:3275s–3280s

Roesli C, Neri D, Rybak JN (2006) In vivo protein biotinylation and sample preparation for the proteomic identification of organ- and disease-specific antigens accessible from the vasculature. Nat Protoc 1:192–199

Rybak JN, Ettorre A, Kaissling B, Giavazzi R, Neri D, Elia G (2005) In vivo protein biotinylation for identification of organ-specific antigens accessible from the vasculature. Nat Methods 2:291–298

Rybak JN, Roesli C, Kaspar M, Villa A, Neri D (2007a) The extra-domain A of fibronectin is a vascular marker of solid tumors and metastases. Cancer Res 67:10948–10957

Rybak JN, Trachsel E, Scheuermann J, Neri D (2007b) Ligand-based vascular targeting of disease. ChemMedChem 2:22–40

Santimaria M, Moscatelli G, Viale GL, Giovannoni L, Neri G, Viti F, Leprini A, Borsi L, Castellani P, Zardi L, Neri D, Riva P (2003) Immunoscintigraphic detection of the ED-B domain of fibronectin, a marker of angiogenesis, in patients with cancer. Clin Cancer Res 9:571–579

Schliemann C, Neri D (2007) Antibody-based targeting of the tumor vasculature. Biochim Biophys Acta 1776:175–192

Schrama D, Reisfeld RA, Becker JC (2006) Antibody targeted drugs as cancer therapeutics. Nat Rev Drug Discov 5:147–159

12

Seaman S, Stevens J, Yang MY, Logsdon D, Graff-Cherry C, St Croix B (2007) Genes that Distinguish Physiological and Pathological Angiogenesis. Cancer Cell 11:539–554

Silacci M, Brack SS, Spath N, Buck A, Hillinger S, Arni S, Weder W, Zardi L, Neri D (2006) Human monoclonal antibodies to domain C of tenascin-C selectively target solid tumors in vivo. Protein Eng Des Sel 19:471–478

Silver DA, Pellicer I, Fair WR, Heston WD, Cordon-Cardo C (1997) Prostate-specific membrane antigen expression in normal and malignant human tissues. Clin Cancer Res 3:81–85

Singh Jaggi J, Henke E, Seshan SV, Kappel BJ, Chattopadhyay D, May C, McDevitt MR, Nolan D, Mittal V, Benezra R, Scheinberg DA (2007) Selective alpha-particle mediated depletion of tumor vasculature with vascular normalization. PLoS ONE 2:e267

Sipkins DA, Cheresh DA, Kazemi MR, Nevin LM, Bednarski MD, Li KC (1998) Detection of tumor angiogenesis in vivo by alphaVbeta3-targeted magnetic resonance imaging. Nat Med 4:623–626

Siri A, Carnemolla B, Saginati M, Leprini A, Casari G, Baralle F, Zardi L (1991) Human tenascin: primary structure, pre-mRNA splicing patterns and localization of the epitopes recognized by two monoclonal antibodies. Nucleic Acids Res 19:525–531

St Croix B, Rago C, Velculescu V, Traverso G, Romans KE, Montgomery E, Lal A, Riggins GJ, Lengauer C, Vogelstein B, Kinzler KW (2000) Genes expressed in human tumor endothelium. Science 289:1197–1202

Stollman TH, Scheer MGW, Leenders WPJ, Verrijp CN, Soede AC, Oyen WJG, Ruers TJM, Boerman OC (2008) Specific imaging of VEFG-A expression with radiolabeled anti-VEGF monoclonal antibody. Int J Cancer 122(10):2310–2314

Tarli L, Balza E, Viti F, Borsi L, Castellani P, Berndorff D, Dinkelborg L, Neri D, Zardi L (1999) A high-affinity human antibody that targets tumoral blood vessels. Blood 94:192–198

Temming K, Schiffelers RM, Molema G, Kok RJ (2005) RGD-based strategies for selective delivery of therapeutics and imaging agents to the tumour vasculature. Drug Resist Updat 8:381–402

Tijink BM, Neri D, Leemans CR, Budde M, Dinkelborg LM, Stigter-van Walsum M, Zardi L, van Dongen GA (2006) Radioimmunotherapy of head and neck cancer xenografts using 131I-labeled antibody L19-SIP for selective targeting of tumor vasculature. J Nucl Med 47:1127–1135

Umana P, Jean-Mairet J, Moudry R, Amstutz H, Bailey JE (1999) Engineered glycoforms of an antineuroblastoma IgG1 with optimized antibody-dependent cellular cytotoxic activity. Nat Biotechnol 17:176–180

Velculescu VE, Zhang L, Vogelstein B, Kinzler KW (1995) Serial analysis of gene expression. Science 270:484–487

Verel I, Visser GW, van Dongen GA (2005) The promise of immuno-PET in radioimmunotherapy. J Nucl Med 46(Suppl 1):164S–171S

Villa A, Trachsel E, Kaspar M, Schliemann C, Sommavilla R, Rybak J, Rösli C, Borsi L, Zardi L, Neri D (2008) A high-affinity human monoclonal antibody specific to the alternatively-spliced EDA domain of fibronectin efficiently targets tumor neo-vasculature in vivo. Int J Cancer 122:2405–2413

Wang JM, Kumar S, Pye D, van Agthoven AJ, Krupinski J, Hunter RD (1993) A monoclonal antibody detects heterogeneity in vascular endothelium of tumours and normal tissues. Int J Cancer 54:363–370

Wu AM, Senter PD (2005) Arming antibodies: prospects and challenges for immunoconjugates. Nat Biotechnol 23:1137–1146

Zardi L, Carnemolla B, Siri A, Petersen TE, Paolella G, Sebastio G, Baralle FE (1987) Transformed human cells produce a new fibronectin isoform by preferential alternative splicing of a previously unobserved exon. Embo J 6:2337–2342

Caveolae and Cancer

13

Kerri A. Massey and Jan E. Schnitzer

Abstract All blood vessels are lined by a layer of endothelial cells that help to control vascular permeability. The luminal surface of vascular endothelial cells is studded with transport vesicles called caveolae that are directly in contact with the blood and can transport molecules into and across the endothelium. The vasculature within distinct tissue types expresses a unique array of proteins that can be used to target intravenously injected antibodies directly to that tissue. When the tissue-specific proteins are concentrated in caveolae, the antibodies can be rapidly pumped out of the blood and into the tissue. Tumors appear to be a distinct tissue type with their own unique marker proteins. Targeting accessible proteins at the surface of tumor vasculature with radiolabeled antibodies destroys tumors and drastically increases animal survival. One day, it may be possible to specifically pump targeted molecules into tumors. This could increase therapeutic efficacy and decrease side effects because most of the drug would accumulate specifically in the tumor. Thus, targeting caveolae may provide a universal portal to pump drugs, imaging agents, and gene vectors out of the blood and into underlying tissue.

J. E. Schnitzer (✉)
Proteogenomics Research Institute for Systems Medicine, 11107 Roselle St, San Diego, CA 92121, USA
e-mail: jschnitzer@prism-sd.org

13.1 Vascular Endothelium

All blood vessels are lined by a monolayer of endothelial cells called the endothelium that helps to control vascular permeability. To serve the specific needs of the underlying organs, vascular endothelial cells show molecular and functional variation, depending on their location in the body (Gumkowski et al. 1987; Janzer and Raff 1987; Aird et al. 1997). Three major types of endothelium have been identified based on structural differences. Sinusoidal endothelium lacks a basement membrane and is characterized by large intercellular gaps between endothelial cells. Thus, this endothelium is minimally restrictive and allows rapid and relatively nonselective flow from the blood into the tissue. Liver, spleen, and bone marrow all have sinusoidal endothelia. Fenestrated endothelium exhibits fenestrae, 60–80 nm circular transcellular openings. This endothelium is generally found in organs that need to rapidly exchange small molecules, such as the kidney, endocrine glands, and intestine. Continuous endothelium forms the most restrictive barrier via a monolayer of attenuated cells linked by intercellular junctions with various degrees of tightness (Jennings and Florey 1967).

Molecules can pass through the endothelial barrier via both passive and active mechanisms.

R. Liersch et al. (eds.), *Angiogenesis Inhibition,* Recent Results in Cancer Research,
DOI: 10.1007/978-3-540-78281-0_13,

Generally, water, solutes, and other small molecules may be passively transported by diffusion and convection through intracellular junctions, fenestrae, or transendothelial channels (Wagner and Chen 1991). Larger molecules may require active transport to move into the endothelial cell (endocytosis) or across the endothelial cell barrier (transcytosis).

13.2 Caveolae Structure

Two major forms of active transport are clathrin-coated vesicles and caveolae. Caveolae are 60 nm omega-shaped invaginations found at the plasma membrane in most continuous endothelia that may mediate both endocytosis and transcytosis (Palade 1953; Ghitescu et al. 1986; Milici et al. 1987; Ghitescu and Bendayan 1992; Ghinea et al. 1994; Schnitzer et al. 1994; Jacobson et al. 1996). Caveolae are abundant structures at the endothelial surface, occupying up to 50–70% of the surface plasma membrane and 10–15% of the total cell volume (about 500–600 vesicles/μm^3) (Bruns and Palade 1968; Simionescu et al. 1974; Johansson 1979). Caveolae are most abundant in the microvascular endothelia of the lung, skeletal muscle, and heart; relatively rare in the highly restrictive microvascular endothelia of brain, retina, and testes; and largely absent in passively leaky vessels with sinusoidal endothelia (Ogi et al. 2003), such as in liver.

Electron microscopy reveals that caveolae are structurally distinct from clathrin-coated vesicles, which have a thick, electron-dense coat. Instead, caveolae have bipolar oriented, thin striations that are formed by the oligomerization of the structural coat protein caveolin (Peters et al. 1985; Rothberg et al. 1992). The mammalian caveolin gene family has three members. Caveolin-1 is a 21 kDa integral membrane protein with two isoforms produced by alternative initiation, α and β, and which oligomerize to form the structural coat of the caveolar bulb (Monier et al. 1995; Sargiacomo et al. 1995). Caveolin-1 is both necessary and apparently sufficient to drive formation of caveolae in vitro and in vivo (Fra et al. 1994; Parolini et al. 1999; Drab et al. 2001; Razani et al. 2002a). Additionally, caveolae are lost from the cell surface when caveolin-1 mRNA expression is reduced with antisense oligonucleotides (Griffoni et al. 2000). Caveolin-2 is a 20 kDa protein that can form stable hetero-oligomeric complexes with caveolin-1 (Scherer et al. 1997) and is co-expressed with caveolin-1 in some endothelial cells, adipocytes, epithelial cells, smooth muscle cells, and fibroblasts (Scherer et al. 1997). Caveolin-2 requires caveolin-1 for proper membrane targeting and protein stability (Mora et al. 1999; Parolini et al. 1999), but caveolin-1 appears to be able to localize to the plasma membrane and influence caveolae formation without caveolin-2. Yet, the co-expression of both caveolin-1 and caveolin-2 appears necessary for the formation of stable, deep, plasma membrane-attached caveolae (Razani et al. 2002b; Sowa et al. 2003). Caveolin-3 appears to be expressed mainly in muscle cells, including smooth, skeletal, and cardiac myocytes (Tang et al. 1996).

13.3 Isolation of Caveolae

Early attempts to isolate caveolae relied on detergent-resistance and/or buoyant density after cell fragmentation. These isolates were often contaminated with significant amounts of low-density, detergent-resistant membranes derived from other intracellular organelles, such as nuclei, Golgi, and endoplasmic reticulum, as well as other membrane domains, such as lipid rafts (Smart et al. 1995; Oh and Schnitzer 1999). Alternative methods to isolate caveolae, especially in vivo, have been recently developed to isolate purer populations. In one method, a solution of colloidal silica nanoparticles is perfused through the blood vessels to selectively coat the luminal surface of endothelial cells. After tissue homogenization, the denser, silica-coated plasma membranes can be isolated away from the rest of the tissue by ultracentrifugation through a high-density media gradient. This effectively isolates luminal plasma membranes of endothelial cells, as can be seen by electron microscopy and western analysis. Known endothelial cell surface markers are highly enriched (>15-fold) while markers of blood, other tissue cells, and subcellular organelles are markedly depleted (15-fold).

The silica coat stabilizes the surface membrane but silica nanoparticles are too large to readily enter the caveolae. Caveolae can be separated from endothelium by mechanical force (Schnitzer et al. 1995c). GTP can also cause caveolae to bud through activation of dynamin (Schnitzer et al. 1996; Oh and Schnitzer 1998), allowing a more physiologically induced separation for isolation. Once separated from the endothelial cell membrane, caveolae can be isolated by flotation using a sucrose density gradient. Electron micrographs of the isolated membranes showed a homogeneous population of 60–80 nm vesicles. Caveolae markers such as caveolin are highly enriched whereas markers for other subcellular organelles are markedly depleted. Additionally, using beads conjugated to caveolin antibodies to further isolate caveolae showed that the population was highly pure (>95%) (Oh and Schnitzer 1999). These methods are especially valuable to separate caveolae from lipid rafts. Though lipid rafts are functionally distinct, they are difficult to isolate away from caveolae because both domains have a similar density. As lipid rafts are flat domains at the surface, they are coated by silica and retained with the rest of the plasma membrane when caveolae are separated (Schnitzer et al. 1995c). The proportion of lipid rafts to caveolae appears quite low in vivo, unlike in vitro where caveolae abundance decreases 50–100-fold in cultured endothelial cells and lipid rafts appear far more prevalent in the isolated detergent-resistant membrane.

13.4 Caveolae in Signal Transduction

By selectively isolating caveolae, the molecular and functional aspects of these structures can be studied with greater confidence. In the past few decades, significant research has accumulated showing that caveolae participate in signal transduction, either by directly transducing signals themselves or by concentrating and organizing signaling complexes (Carver and Schnitzer 2007b). The vascular endothelium is directly exposed to the blood and constantly subjected to mechanical forces, including shear forces and pressure. One of the major roles of the endothelium is to rapidly respond to changes in mechanical stressors to prevent damage. Caveolae themselves may be acute mechanosensing organelles (Oh and Schnitzer 1996; Liu et al. 1997; Rizzo et al. 1998b; Rizzo et al. 1998a; Oh and Schnitzer 2001).

Caveolae are responsive to changes in pressure or shear stress both in vitro and in vivo. In cultured endothelial cells, increasing flow rates increases the amount of caveolin and the number of caveolae at the luminal cell surface (Park et al. 2000; Boyd et al. 2003; Rizzo et al. 2003). In high-pressure conditions in vivo (Lee and Schmid-Schonbein 1995), caveolae are distorted and can even disappear or "pop." Caveolin may play a central role in signal transduction through caveolae. Caveolin oligomerizes to form a shell around caveolae that may allow these structures to directly transduce changes in mechanical stress by acting as tension-bearing springs (Rizzo et al. 1998a). Caveolin may also serve as a mechanosensitive scaffold, concentrating and inhibiting key signaling molecules in caveolae. Molecular mapping studies show that caveolae are enriched in various signaling molecules including specific

G-proteins, select nonreceptor tyrosine kinases, Ras, Raf, and eNOS (Rizzo et al. 1998b; Rizzo et al. 1998a; Oh and Schnitzer 2001; Rizzo et al. 2003). Many of these are enriched in caveolae under basal conditions and may be inhibited by interaction with caveolin (Li et al. 1995; Li et al. 1996; Song et al. 1996). Increasing hemodynamic stressors rapidly activates signaling pathways. Specific pathways, such as ERK, are dependent on both cholesterol and caveolin-1 for activation (Park et al. 1998; Park et al. 2000; Boyd et al. 2003). Proteins concentrated within caveolae are often tyrosine-phosphorylated in responses to changes in mechanical stress (Rizzo et al. 1998a), which can alter functional interactions. Caveolin interacts with eNOS and inhibits activity. Increased flow in situ rapidly dissociates eNOS from caveolin, freeing eNOS to associate with positive modulators such as calmodulin (Rizzo et al. 1998b; Feron and Balligand 2006). Conversely, overexpression of caveolin decreases activation of select mechanotransduction pathways, including the p42/44 MAPK pathway (Engelman et al. 1998). Also, mice lacking caveolin-1 have impaired mechanotransduction, showing a decreased ability to regulate blood vessel diameter in response to changes in flow rates, as well as a decreased activation of eNOS (Yu et al. 2006).

13.5 Caveolae as Active Transport Vesicles

Since caveolae were first identified in 1953 (Palade 1953); researchers have debated over whether these membrane invaginations might play a role in transport (Severs 1988). Over 50 years of evidence has accumulated to suggest that caveolae can indeed function as active transport vesicles. Cultured endothelial cells have been used to show that caveolae are dynamic vesicular carriers. Caveolae appear to traffic select ligands, such as cholera toxin and albumin-gold complexes, to specific locations within the cell, such as endosomes and lysosomes (Tran et al. 1987; Schnitzer et al. 1988a; Parton et al. 1994). Caveolae may also provide a route of entry for SV40 (Norkin 1999; Pelkmans et al. 2001), ebolavirus (Empig and Goldsmith 2002), and polyomavirus (Mackay and Consigli 1976; Richterova et al. 2001). Furthermore, cholesterol-binding agents, such as filipin, reduce caveolae number and significantly decrease caveolae-mediated cellular trafficking of such molecules as albumin (Schnitzer and Oh 1994; Orlandi and Fishman 1998).

The discovery that caveolae contain proteins classically associated with transport vesicles, including v-SNARES, NSF, and SNAP, suggested that caveolae might function as transport vesicles. Additionally, several GTPases known to play roles in vesicle budding have been found within caveolae (Schnitzer et al. 1995a). These proteins are found in caveolae under basal conditions; no activation is necessary to translocate the necessary machinery to the caveolae. This suggests that caveolae are ready to bud under basal conditions and may be primed for rapid transport. Like other vesicular pathways, caveolae-mediated endocytosis is sensitive to *N*-ethylmaleimide (NEM), a thioalkylating agent that inhibits the fusion of vesicles to target membranes (Goda and Pfeffer 1991; Schnitzer et al. 1995b).

More recently, isolated endothelial cell plasma membranes were used to show that caveolae can bud and form free vesicles. When GTP and ATP are added to isolated plasma membranes, caveolae budding is induced. Caveolae separate from the membrane and the budded caveolae can be isolated. This reconstituted, cell-free, in vitro assay was used to identify dynamin as the GTPase mediating this fission. Dynamin forms a ring around the neck of caveolae, likely acting as a pinchase to form free vesicles (Oh and Schnitzer 1996; Oh et al. 1998) This was subsequently confirmed in hepatocytes (Henley et al. 1998) which have readily apparent caveolae in cell culture but interestingly, have very few to no caveolae natively in liver tissue in vivo.

Caveolae appear to function in vesicular transport in vivo as well. Normally, albumin can be endo- or transcytosed by caveolae through interaction with caveolar proteins, even when conjugated to gold particles (Ghitescu et al. 1986; Milici et al. 1987; Schnitzer et al. 1988b; Schnitzer et al. 1992). In caveolin-1 knockout mice, the caveolae in microvascular endothelium are absent and this transport pathway is lost (Razani et al. 2001). Although albumin-gold particles bound to the endothelial cell surface in vivo, they were not transported into or across endothelial cells. Because caveolin-knockout mice are viable, other mechanisms must mediate the transport of essential nutrients and other molecules to underlying tissue cells. Indeed, these animals demonstrate increased paracellular transport. They have an overall increased microvascular permeability in vivo (Drab et al. 2001; Razani et al. 2001), resulting in rapid, nonselective transvascular transport of both large and small molecules from the bloodstream, apparently due to significant changes to intercellular junctions between the endothelial cells (Schubert et al. 2002).

13.6 Vascular Targeting

Caveolae are found at the luminal surface of most endothelium and may underlie transport to many different organs and even solid tumors. Many tumors, especially malignant ones, are highly vascularized. Without the ability to rapidly recruit new blood vessels, tumors must rely on passive diffusion to receive nutrients and are thus limited in size (1–2 mm) and localized to their primary site (Nicolson 1988; Blood and Zetter 1990). Tumor blood vessels differ significantly from blood vessels in normal tissue. Tumor blood vessels are usually disorganized and dilated with reduced basement membranes (Workman 2001; Anzick and Trent 2002). They also lack some normal endothelial cell markers, suggesting that they may express a unique array of proteins (Schlingemann et al. 1991). Because tumor growth depends on neovascularization, many investigators have suggested that both the process of angiogenesis and the vasculature itself are potential targets for tumor therapy (Dvorak et al. 1991; Drews 2000; Lindsay 2003).

A major part of recent anti-cancer research has focused on using antibodies to target treatments to the tumor cells themselves. These treatments have been successful in vitro, but the vast majority has failed when used in humans, probably because the endothelium limits movement into the tumors (Dvorak et al. 1991; Huang et al. 1997). Unlike antibodies, chemotherapeutic drugs are small molecules that can readily enter all tissues. As a result, these agents are rapidly diluted, cleared from the blood, and excreted. For both large antibodies and small chemotherapeutics, it appears that only a small portion of the injected dose actually reaches the inside of the tumor where it can be effective. Thus, higher doses must be administered to reach effective levels within the tumor, often leading to severe systemic side effects (Vitetta 2000). The vascular surface and its caveolae are a promising alternative target. Though targeting antibodies passively cross the endothelium of many organs very poorly, they may be transported more readily and rapidly across the endothelial cell barrier via caveolae.

To be effective, vascular targeting depends on the specific and unique expression of target proteins in different tissues and disease states. Multiple methods have been developed over the years to identify differential gene and protein expression. Initial work was performed in vitro, where large quantities of endothelial cells could be grown and analyzed. These early studies in culture revolutionized the study of vascular biology by providing both a pure population of cells to study and by identifying endothelial specific markers (for review see Jaffe 1987). Even in culture, endothelial cells are responsive to components of the environment, including mechanical forces such as shear stress and chemical factors such as chemokines (Malek and Izumo 1995), suggesting that it is vital to study these cells in the native environment.

Both in vitro and in vivo, endothelial cells from different vascular beds are unique (Auerbach et al. 1985; Kallmann et al. 2002; Durr et al. 2004; Oh et al. 2007). However, once in culture, endothelial cells rapidly de-differentiate into a more common phenotype (Madri and Williams 1983; Schnitzer 1997; Thum et al. 2000). Many tissue-specific proteins are no longer expressed and the number of caveolae decreases up to 100-fold (Schnitzer 1997). In spite of these changes, endothelial cells derived from different organs express different genes and proteins. Differences between different vascular beds and the rapid de-differentiation seen in culture strongly suggest that tissue microenvironment can profoundly influence the structure and function of endothelial cells. Recent mass spectrometry analysis shows that approximately 40% of the proteins expressed in vivo are not found in cultured endothelial cells (Durr et al. 2004). Cultured cells lack a normal microenvironment, including circulating blood, the basement membrane, perivascular cells, the tissue parenchyma, and hemodynamic forces (Rizzo et al. 2003), all of which can alter protein expression, structure, and function of endothelial cells. Therefore, experiments seeking to identify tissue-specific vascular targets must be performed, or at the very least, validated in vivo.

13.7 Phage Display Libraries

The idea of phage display libraries was first introduced by George Smith in 1985 (Smith 1985). He suggested that filamentous bacteriophages could be used to display proteins or antibody fragments by fusing a protein of interest to the coat protein of the bacteriophage. In 1991, he showed that these phage could be used to display vast amounts of short peptides (Smith 1991). These peptides were expressed on the surface of the bacteriophage and could bind to antibodies or other proteins. It is also possible to express larger proteins, such as antibody fragments, which are expressed in their native configuration on the outer surface of the phage. Because each bacteriophage expresses one protein of interest, huge libraries of random peptides can be rapidly screened for the ability to bind proteins, antibodies, or even tissue. Because the approach can use a large, random library, it is unbiased and unknown targets can be identified. In a process called panning, unbound phage are washed away, and the bound phage are isolated and amplified. This process is repeated until the phage that bind tightly are separated from those that bind non-specifically. Phage that bind to available proteins can be purified and used as probes themselves to isolate the binding partner for identification (Pasqualini and Ruoslahti 1996; Rajotte et al. 1998).

Phage can also be injected intravenously. Presumably, these phage circulate and bind to the endothelial surface in vivo if the protein targets are available. Then they can be isolated from each organ or tissue of interest. Several iterations create the opportunity for selection of specific peptides or antibodies with defined tissue tropism. However, phage are rapidly scavenged from the blood by the liver and spleen, preventing sufficient equilibrium to bind to endothelial cell surface proteins in vivo. Additionally, short peptides can lack specificity and may bind a large range of proteins in a multitude of organs, requiring additional ex vivo validation. Problems with in vivo targeting can be partially overcome by using phage that recognize specific proteins on endothelial cell extracts to create antibody-like fusion proteins. These can successfully immunotarget in vivo (Valadon et al. 1998). Though phage display libraries have revealed some promising targets, it seems particularly challenging for this approach on its own to be used in a high throughput manner to identify selective tissue-targeting probes, as well as their molecular targets.

13.8 Large-Scale Approaches

Comprehensively defining all the genes or proteins in an organ, cell type, or disease state can help to define the function of these cells, as well as identify therapeutic targets and biomarkers. Additionally, diseases such as cancer are extremely heterogeneous; tumors can differ widely within the same patient or even within the same tumor. Accordingly, tumors show marked variability in invasiveness, metastatic potential, and response to therapy. Comprehensively identifying the changes in gene or protein expression in an individual tumor may better predict the clinical outcome and allow more effective, personalized therapy. It is likely that hundreds of genes or proteins must be identified in order to successfully classify tumors, which demands rapid, high throughput methods.

Genomic approaches theoretically provide a means to identify gene expression in tissues or disease states and identify differences among samples in a relatively rapid manner (Huber 2003; Lindsay 2003). Thus genomic analysis can be used to compare global changes in gene expression. Large changes are needed to detect differences and to differentiate real changes. Even so, thousands of possible targets are often identified, requiring laborious in vivo validation. Additionally, changes in gene expression do not always correlate with changes in protein expression and proteins can be altered in subtler ways. Moving from the cell membrane to anintracellular compartment can render a protein at the endothelial cell surface inaccessible. Additionally, posttranslational modifications can rapidly alter protein function. To truly define the proteins present at the endothelial cell luminal surface, protein expression itself must be characterized.

Several methods allow for identification of proteins within a sample. Two-dimensional (2D) gels are a simple and rapid way to visualize differences between samples. By separating proteins based on multiple characteristics, these gels provide better separation between proteins. Spots that are unique to one tissue can be isolated; known proteins can be identified with antibodies and unknown proteins can be identified with mass spectrometry. For these approaches, successful identification of proteins requires that the proteins migrate onto the gel. Many proteins, especially integral membrane proteins, simply do not separate well on such gels and can be underrepresented or lost altogether. Mass spectrometry-based techniques can identify proteins based on the presence of digested peptides. Similar to genomics approaches, mass spectrometry allows relatively rapid analysis of large numbers of proteins. Because highly complex samples are difficult to separate, samples are often prefractionated before analysis. This has traditionally been done by 2D gels; however, analyzing each distinct spot can be prohibitively time consuming. An attractive alternative uses 2D liquid chromatography to further separate proteins before they are analyzed by the mass spectrometer (Washburn et al. 2001). Samples are separated on a column and directly fed into the mass spectrometer, decreasing handling time. A third alternative, protein arrays, uses antibodies or peptides to identify the proteins present in the sample, but is limited by affinity of the probes and the complexity of the sample. A detailed description of this field has recently been reported (Carver and Schnitzer 2007a).

13.9 Reducing Complexity

Each of these methods is limited by the complexity of the starting sample. Sample complexity can be reduced by focusing on subsets of cells or even subdomains of cells. Proteins at the surface of endothelial cells are directly exposed to the blood and can be labeled by perfusion with radiolabeled or biotinylated compounds. Radiolabeling has most often been used to verify the presence of known proteins because the fact that there is no simple way to separate and identify radiolabeled proteins significantly limited the utility of this approach. In contrast, in vivo biotinylation chemically labels proteins at the luminal surface of vascular endothelial cells and the strong interaction between biotin and avidin can be used to purify biotinylated proteins which can be identified with mass spectrometry (Rybak et al. 2005; Scheurer et al. 2005) or antibodies (Sargiacomo et al. 1989; Fujimoto et al. 1992). Though this method indeed labels a subset of endothelial cell-surface proteins (De La Fuente et al. 1997), some surface proteins may be missed or the small biotin compounds may permeate throughout the tissue and identify proteins beyond the endothelial surface. Labeling other cell types can effectively dilute the pool and increase the false-positive discovery rate of endothelial surface targets considerably.

As discussed earlier, using silica-based nanoparticles can selectively coat the luminal surface of endothelial cells in vivo, allowing this surface to be isolated from the rest of the tissue and further subfractionated to yield a pure population of caveolae. Though far simpler than total tissue homogenate, the membrane isolate is still a complex mixture of proteins. Further separation can be provided by linking 2D chromatography to mass-spectrometry (MudPIT). In MudPIT, proteins are solubilized and digested, then separated by both hydrophobicity and charge. Even with these extra separation steps, each mass spectrometry measurement only identifies a portion of the proteins present in a sample. Identifying new tissue-specific proteins requires comprehensive analysis of the proteins present in different tissues. Five to ten replicates are needed to identify approximately 95% of the proteins identifiable by a single method (Durr et al. 2004).

Additionally, combining multiple mass spectrometry-based methods can increase the number of proteins identified. Recently, traditional 2D mass spectrometry methods such as MudPIT were compared with first separating peptides by size on SDS-PAGE gels followed by analysis by mass spectrometry. These experiments showed that gel prefractionation preserved many membrane proteins that do not re-solubilize after the sample preparation steps required for traditional mass spectrometry. Each technique identified unique peptides; therefore, combining multiple techniques dramatically increased sensitivity, especially for integral membrane proteins. Previous analysis of the plasma membranes identified 450 proteins (Durr et al. 2004). Using the combination of methodologies described earlier identified 1834 proteins were (Y. Li et al. 2009).

Though replicate measurements and multiple methods appear necessary to comprehensively map all proteins present in a sample, intrinsic variability between measurements and methodologies makes it difficult to compare the levels of peptides found with different techniques. New, label-free methods offer a way to overcome these limitations by normalizing and quantifying mass spectrometry data using intrinsic properties of the data. By normalizing data around a Spectral Index that takes peptide number, spectral count, peak precursor ion intensities, and protein length into account, this method reduces the variance between replicates and across a dynamic range of protein loads. Such quantification and normalization of the data is essential for mapping the proteome of endothelium and its caveolae and to identifying tissue or disease-specific targets.

13.10 Tissue-Specific Targets

When samples of the luminal surface of vascular endothelial cells from the lung were analyzed by mass spectrometry, nearly 2000 proteins were identified (Y. Li et al. 2009). Though further analysis must be undertaken to fully map proteins found within subdomains such as the caveolae, this analysis provides the first step in identifying tissue-specific targets.

Endothelial cells depend on the tissue microenvironment to maintain both structure and protein expression. Different vascular beds or even diseases such as cancer can lead to changes in the structure, function, and protein complement of the endothelial cells. Therefore, proteins that are expressed both in vivo and in culture may also be expressed universally across different vascular beds or disease states. Similarly, if protein expression is lost when endothelial cells are grown in culture, this could indicate that expression is dependent upon a specific tissue microenvironment. Thus, eliminating proteins found in culture focuses attention on those proteins that might be more selectively expressed. Only endothelial cell surface proteins that extend into the blood are readily accessible to circulating antibodies. By analyzing the sequences of identified proteins, those likely to have extracellular domains can be identified. Of the 450 proteins identified at the luminal surface of lung endothelium at that time, and of the 187 proteins that were not detected in lung endothelial cells grown in culture, only APP and OX-45 were both specific to lung and likely to extend into the luminal space (Durr et al. 2004; Oh et al. 2004).

Further analysis showed that APP is concentrated in caveolae and accessible to circulating antibodies (Oh et al. 2007). Electron microscopy studies showed that antibodies against APP collected in endothelial caveolae in lung tissue and were internalized and transcytosed across the endothelial cell layer (McIntosh et al. 2002; Oh et al. 2007). When APP antibodies were imaged with dynamic intravital microscopy, this trafficking proved to be extraordinarily rapid. Fluorescently labeled APP antibodies bound to the lung microvascular endothelium within 10 s after intravenous injection and were detected within 15 s outside the endothelium in the perivascular space and interstitium of the tissue. Within minutes, the antibody was cleared from the blood (>80%) as it rapidly accumulated in the lungs. This transcytotic trafficking was specific, active, and dependent on caveolae. Antibodies were actually pumped out of the blood and across the endothelial cell barrier to accumulate at higher concentration in the tissue than the blood. The antibody rapidly filled the entire lung tissue but did not extend beyond this tissue, nor did fluorescent control IgG leak from the vasculature into the tissue (Oh et al. 2004).

Target enrichment in caveolae may be necessary for rapid transport. Antibodies targeted against proteins found outside of the caveolae still bound to the vasculature but were not pumped into the tissue. If caveolae were depleted by reducing expression levels of the structural protein caveolin, APP antibodies could still bind to the endothelium but were not transported out of the vessels and into tissue. Whole-body imaging as well as biodistribution analysis showed that APP antibodies also target the lungs within minutes in the context of the whole animal. Radiolabeled antibody rapidly accumulated in the lungs and was maintained in the tissue for several days (Oh et al. 2004; Oh et al. 2007).

13.11 Tumor-Specific Targets

Though APP antibodies readily traffic to the lungs, these antibodies do not target lung tumors. When injected into rats bearing lung tumors, APP antibodies were concentrated in the tumor-free lung tissue. When the luminal endothelial surface of vasculature from lung tumors was isolated and run on a 2D blot, a distinct pattern of proteins was seen, suggesting that the solid tumors might form a distinct type of tissue. Analyzing this extract with mass spectrometry confirmed that APP expression was lost in tumor vasculature. Instead, several known cancer markers were upregulated. Surprisingly, a novel protein was induced at the endothelial cell surface. AnnexinA1 (AnnA1) is reported to be expressed in select cells, normally intracellularly; but AnnA1 could be detected at the luminal endothelial cell surface in tumor tissue. AnnA1 expression is also found in blood vessels of many types of human solid tumors (prostate, liver, breast, lung), but is lacking from healthy tissue (Oh et al. 2004).

The AnnA1 found on vascular endothelial cells in tumors was accessible to the blood. Intravenously injected AnnA1 antibodies specifically targeted tumor vasculature and provided excellent imaging with single photon emission computed tomography (SPECT) of lung tumors in the rat. Tumor-bearing rats that received injections of radiolabeled IgG died several days after the injection. When rats were instead injected with radiolabeled AnnA1 antibodies, the vast majority survived, even with just one treatment (Oh et al. 2004). It still remains to be determined which, if any, tumor-induced endothelial proteins exist concentrated in caveolae.

13.12 Clinical Implications

Targeting drugs directly to the caveolae may provide a universal route into underlying tissue. Tumor-specific delivery and transcytosis of drugs and imaging agents could increase efficacy and decrease harmful side by effectively concentrating drugs in the target tissue. Active pumping of antibodies across the endothelial cell layer and into tissue may increase the therapeutic potential (Oh et al. 2007; Red-Horse and Ferrara 2007). Additionally, targeted anti-angiogenic compounds can be used to specifically destroy vasculature, effectively destroying all the cells fed by that vasculature. Such targeting could also revitalize older drugs that failed in clinical testing due to severe side effects. These drugs could be retargeted to the diseased tissues, thus significantly decreasing systemic side effects.

Comprehensive analysis of the vascular proteome is absolutely essential to identify tissue-specific protein expression and to identify differences between normal and diseased tissue. Identifying unique markers may allow the targeting of gene therapy, drugs, and imaging agents. Comprehensive mapping of the proteins in both healthy and tumor tissue may identify additional targets and extend the utility of targeted delivery. Drugs could theoretically be targeted to the endothelial surface, to the endothelial cell itself, or to the underlying tissue, depending on the nature of the target and the processing of the antibody once bound. Additionally, understanding the functional changes in the endothelial cell plasma membrane between tissues and between healthy tissue and disease states provides insight into the needs of each tissue and the changes that develop with disease.

Developing animal models of tumors that better represent human disease is essential not only for identifying targets, but also for testing the efficacy of targeted drugs. Most current models rely on subcutaneous tumors grown directly on the skin. These tumors lack the native tissue microenvironment and may differ from tumors grown on orthotopic tissue. Indeed, most new drugs are tested in subcutaneous tumor models. Efficacy in these models rarely reflects efficacy in human trials. Many genetic models of tumors currently exist. However, these spontaneous tumors do not, so far, fully recapitulation human disease, are often difficult to image, and are rarely used for preclinical testing. Clearly, reliable models are needed to bridge the gap between laboratory experiments and success in human patients.

The possibilities of caveolar targeting go well beyond the delivery of drugs to cancer cells. Tissue-specific markers for the lung itself have been identified and validated in vivo (Oh et al. 2007). Such markers could target drugs, imaging agents, nanoparticles, or even genetic material to a specific organ. Additionally, caveolae are rich in signaling molecules, and targeted small molecules, siRNAs, peptides, or nanoparticles could be used to activate or inhibit specific pathways. Pumping agents into a specific tissue may open the door not only to new molecular therapies but also to more effective experimentation in vivo, including molecular and functional imaging.

References

Aird WC, Edelberg JM, Weiler-Guettler H, Simmons WW, Smith TW, Rosenberg RD (1997) Vascular bed-specific expression of an endothelial cell gene is programmed by the tissue microenvironment. J Cell Biol 138:1117–1124

Anzick SL, Trent JM (2002) Role of genomics in identifying new targets for cancer therapy. Oncology (Huntingt) 16:7–13

Auerbach R, Alby L, Morrissey LW, Tu M, Joseph J (1985) Expression of organ-specific antigens on capillary endothelial cells. Microvasc Res 29:401–411

Blood CH, Zetter BR (1990) Tumor interaction with the vasculature: angiogenesis and tumor metastasis. Biochim Biophys Acta 1032:89–118

Boyd NL, Park H, Yi H, Boo YC, Sorescu GP, Sykes M, Jo H (2003) Chronic shear induces caveolae formation and alters ERK and Akt responses in endothelial cells. Am J Physiol Heart Circ Physiol 285:H1113–H1122

Bruns RR, Palade GE (1968) Studies on blood capillaries. I. General organization of blood capillaries in muscle. J Cell Biol 37:244–276

Carver LA, Schnitzer JE (2007a) Proteomic mapping of endothelium and vascular targeting in vivo. In: Aird WC (ed) Endothelial biomedicine. Cambridge University Press, New york, pp 881–898

Carver LA, Schnitzer JE (2007b) Multiple functions and clinical uses of caveolae in endothelium. In: Aird WC (ed) Endothelial biomedicine. Cambridge University Press, New york, pp 664–678

De La Fuente EK, Dawson CA, Nelin LD, Bongard RD, McAuliffe TL, Merker MP (1997) Biotinylation of membrane proteins accessible via the pulmonary circulation in normal and hyperoxic rats. Am J Physiol 272:L461–L470

Drab M, Verkade P, Elger M, Kasper M, Lohn M, Lauterbach B, Menne J, Lindschau C, Mende F, Luft FC, Schedl A, Haller H, Kurzchalia TV (2001) Loss of caveolae, vascular dysfunction, and pulmonary defects in caveolin-1 gene-disrupted mice. Science 293:2449–2452

Drews J (2000) Drug discovery: a historical perspective. Science 287:1960–1964

Durr E, Yu J, Krasinska KM, Carver LA, Yates JRI, Testa JE, Oh P, Schnitzer JE (2004) Direct proteomic mapping of the lung microvascular endothelial cell surface in vivo and in cell culture. Nat Biotechnol 22:985–992

Dvorak HF, Nagy JA, Dvorak AM (1991) Structure of solid tumors and their vasculature: implications for therapy with monoclonal antibodies. Cancer Cells 3:77–85

Empig CJ, Goldsmith MA (2002) Association of the caveola vesicular system with cellular entry by filoviruses. J Virol 76:5266–5270

Engelman JA, Chu C, Lin A, Jo H, Ikezu T, Okamoto T, Kohtz DS, Lisanti MP (1998) Caveolin-mediated regulation of signaling along the p42/44 MAP kinase cascade in vivo. A role for the caveolin-scaffolding domain. FEBS Lett 428:205–211

Feron O, Balligand JL (2006) Caveolins and the regulation of endothelial nitric oxide synthase in the heart. Cardiovasc Res 69:788–797

Fra AM, Williamson E, Simons K, Parton RG (1994) Detergent-insoluble glycolipid microdomains in lymphocytes in the absence of caveolae. J Biol Chem 269:30745–30748

Fujimoto T, Nakade S, Miyawaki A, Mikoshiba K, Ogawa K (1992) Localization of inositol 1, 4, 5-trisphosphate receptor-like protein in plasmalemmal caveolae. J Cell Biol 119:1507–1513

Ghinea N, Mai TV, Groyer-Picard MT, Milgrom E (1994) How protein hormones reach their target cells. Receptor-mediated transcytosis of hCG through endothelial cells. J Cell Biol 125:87–97

Ghitescu L, Bendayan M (1992) Transendothelial transport of serum albumin: a quantitative immunocytochemical study. J Cell Biol 117:745–755

Ghitescu L, Fixman A, Simionescu M, Simionescu N (1986) Specific binding sites for albumin restricted to plasmalemmal vesicles of continuous capillary endothelium: receptor-mediated transcytosis. J Cell Biol 102:1304–1311

Goda Y, Pfeffer SR (1991) Identification of a novel, *N*-ethylmaleimide-sensitive cytosolic factor required for vesicular transport from endosomes to the trans-golgi network in vitro. J Cell Biol 112:823–831

Griffoni C, Spisni E, Santi S, Riccio M, Guarnieri T, Tomasi V (2000) Knockdown of caveolin-1 by antisense oligonucleotides impairs angiogenesis in vitro and in vivo. Biochem Biophys Res Commun 276:756–761

Gumkowski F, Kaminska G, Kaminski M, Morrissey LW, Auerbach R (1987) Heterogeneity of mouse vascular endothelium. Blood Vessels 24:11–23

Henley JR, Krueger EW, Oswald BJ, McNiven MA (1998) Dynamin-mediated internalization of caveolae. J Cell Biol 141:85–99

Huang X, Molema G, King S, Watkins L, Edgington TS, Thorpe PE (1997) Tumor infraction in mice by antibody-directed targeting of tissue factor to tumor vasculature. Science 275:547–550

Huber LA (2003) Is proteomics heading in the wrong direction? Nat Rev Mol Cell Biol 4:74–80

Jacobson BS, Stolz DB, Schnitzer JE (1996) Identification of endothelial cell-surface proteins as targets for diagnosis and treatment of disease. Nat Med 2:482–484

Jaffe EA (1987) Cell biology of endothelial cells. Hum Pathol 18:234–239

Janzer RC, Raff MC (1987) Astrocytes induce blood-brain barrier properties in endothelial cells. Nature 325:253–257

Jennings MA, Florey L (1967) An investigation of some properties of endothelium related to capillary permeability. Proc R Soc Lond B Biol Sci 167:39–63

Johansson BR (1979) Size and distribution of endothelial plasmalemmal vesicles in consecutive segments of the microvasculature in cat skeletal muscle. Microvasc Res 17:107–117

Kallmann BA, Wagner S, Hummel V, Buttmann M, Bayas A, Tonn JC, Rieckmann P (2002) Characteristic gene expression profile of primary human cerebral endothelial cells. FASEB J 16:589–591

Lee J, Schmid-Schonbein GW (1995) Biomechanics of skeletal muscle capillaries: hemodynamic resistance, endothelial distensibility and pseudopod formation. Ann Biomed Eng 23:226–246

Li S, Okamoto T, Chun M, Sargiacomo M, Casanova JE, Hansen SH, Nishimoto I, Lisanti MP (1995) Evidence for a regulated interaction between heterotrimeric G proteins and caveolin. J Biol Chem 270:15693–15701

Li S, Seitz R, Lisanti MP (1996) Phosphorylation of caveolin by src tyrosine kinases. The alpha-isoform of caveolin is selectively phosphorylated by v-Src in vivo. J Biol Chem 271:3863–3868

Li Y, Yu J, Wang YZ, Griffin NM, Long F, Shore S, Oh P, Schnitzer JE (2009) Enhancing identifications of lipid-embedded proteins by mass spectrometry for improved mapping of endothelial plasma membranes in vivo. Mol Cell Proteomics 8(6):1219–1235

Lindsay MA (2003) Target discovery. Nat Rev Drug Discov 2:831–838

Liu J, Oh P, Horner T, Rogers RA, Schnitzer J (1997) Organized cell surface signal transduction in caveolae distinct from GPI-anchored protein microdomains. J Biol Chem 272:7211–7222

Mackay RL, Consigli RA (1976) Early events in polyoma virus infection: attachment, penetration, and nuclear entry. J Virol 19:620–636

Madri JA, Williams SK (1983) Capillary endothelial cell culture: phenotype modulation by matrix components. J Cell Biol 97:153–165

Malek AM, Izumo S (1995) Control of endothelial cell gene expression by flow. J Biomech 28: 1515–1528

McIntosh DP, Tan X-Y, Oh P, Schnitzer JE (2002) Targeting endothelium and its dynamic caveolae for tissue-specific transcytosis in vivo: a pathway to overcome cell barriers to drug and gene delivery. Proc Natl Acad Sci USA 99:1996–2001

Milici AJ, Watrous NE, Stukenbrok H, Palade GE (1987) Transcytosis of albumin in capillary endothelium. J Cell Biol 105:2603–2612

Monier S, Parton RG, Vogel F, Behlke J, Henske A, Kurzchalia TV (1995) VIP21-caveolin, a membrane protein constituent of the caveolar coat, oligomerizes in vivo and in vitro. Mol Biol Cell 6:911–927

Mora R, Bonilha VL, Marmorstein A, Scherer PE, Brown D, Lisanti MP, Rodriguez-Boulan E (1999) Caveolin-2 localizes to the golgi complex but redistributes to plasma membrane, caveolae, and rafts when co-expressed with caveolin-1. J Biol Chem 274:25708–25717

Nicolson GL (1988) Cancer metastasis: tumor cell and host organ properties important in metastasis to specific secondary sites. Biochim Biophys Acta 948:175–224

Norkin LC (1999) Simian virus 40 infection via MHC class I molecules and caveolae. Immunol Rev 168:13–22

Ogi M, Yokomori H, Oda M, Yoshimura K, Nomura M, Ohshima S, Akita M, Toda K, Ishii H (2003) Distribution and localization of caveolin-1 in sinusoidal cells in rat liver. Med Electron Microsc 36:33–40

Oh P, Schnitzer JE (1996) Dynamin-mediated fission of caveolae from plasma membranes. Mol Biol Cell 7:83a

Oh P, Schnitzer JE (1998) solation and subfractionation of plasma membranes to purify caveolae separately from glycosyl-phospatidylinositol-anchored protein microdomains. In: Celis J (ed) Cell biology: a laboratory handbook. Academic Press, New York, pp 34–46

Oh P, Schnitzer JE (1999) Immunoisolation of caveolae with high affinity antibody binding to the oligomeric caveolin cage. Toward understanding the basis of purification. J Biol Chem 274: 23144–23154

Oh P, Schnitzer JE (2001) Segregation of heterotrimeric G proteins in cell surface microdomains: Gq binds caveolin to concentrate in caveolae whereas Gi and Gs target lipid rafts by default. Mol Biol Cell 12:685–698

Oh P, McIntosh DP, Schnitzer JE (1998) Dynamin at the neck of caveolae mediates their budding to form transport vesicles by GTP-driven fission from the plasma membrane of endothelium. J Cell Biol 141:101–114

Oh P, Li Y, Yu J, Durr E, Krasinska KM, Carver LA, Testa JE, Schnitzer JE (2004) Subtractive proteomic mapping of the endothelial surface in lung and solid tumours for tissue-specific therapy. Nature 429:629–635

Oh P, Borgstrom P, Witkiewicz H, Li Y, Borgstrom BJ, Chrastina A, Iwata K, Zinn KR, Baldwin R, Testa JE, Schnitzer JE (2007) Live dynamic imaging of caveolae pumping targeted antibody rapidly and specifically across endothelium in the lung. Nat Biotechnol 25:327–337

Orlandi PA, Fishman PH (1998) Filipin-dependent inhibition of cholera toxin: evidence for toxin internalization and activation through caveolae-like domains. J Cell Biol 141:905–915

Palade GE (1953) Fine structureof blood capillaries. J Appl Phys 24:1424

Park H, Go YM, St John PL, Maland MC, Lisanti MP, Abrahamson DR, Jo H (1998) Plasma membrane cholesterol is a key molecule in shear stress-dependent activation of extracellular signal-regulated kinase. J Biol Chem 273: 32304–32311

Park H, Go YM, Darji R, Choi JW, Lisanti MP, Maland MC, Jo H (2000) Caveolin-1 regulates shear stress-dependent activation of extracellular signal-regulated kinase. Am J Physiol Heart Circ Physiol 278:H1285–H1293

Parolini I, Topa S, Sorice M, Pace A, Ceddia P, Montesoro E, Pavan A, Lisanti MP, Peschle C, Sargiacomo M (1999) Phorbol ester-induced disruption of the CD4-Lck complex occurs within a detergent-resistant microdomain of the plasma membrane. Involvement of the translocation of activated protein kinase C isoforms. J Biol Chem 274:14176–14187

Parton RG, Joggerst B, Simons K (1994) Regulated internalization of caveolae. J Cell Biol 127: 1199–1215

Pasqualini R, Ruoslahti E (1996) Organ targeting in vivo using phage display peptide libraries. Nature 380:364–366

Pelkmans L, Kartenback J, Helenius A (2001) Caveolar endocytosis of Simian virus 40 reveals a novel two-step vesicular transport pathway to the ER. Nat Cell Biol 3:473–483

Peters KR, Carley WW, Palade GE (1985) Endothelial plasmalemmal vesicles have a characteristic striped bipolar surface structure. J Cell Biol 101:2233–2238

Rajotte D, Arap W, Hagedorn M, Koivunen E, Pasqualini R, Ruoslahti E (1998) Molecular heterogeneity of the vascular endothelium revealed by in vivo phage display. J Clin Invest 102: 430–437

Razani B, Engelman JA, Wang XB, Schubert W, Zhang XL, Marks CB, Macaluso F, Russell RG, Li M, Pestell RG, Di Vizio D, Hou H Jr, Kneitz B, Lagaud G, Christ GJ, Edelmann W, Lisanti MP (2001) Caveolin-1 null mice are viable but show evidence of hyperproliferative and vascular abnormalities. J Biol Chem 276:38121–38138

Razani B, Woodman SE, Lisanti MP (2002a) Caveolae: from cell biology to animal physiology. Pharmacol Rev 54:431–467

Razani B, Wang XB, Engelman JA, Battista M, Lagaud G, Zhang XL, Kneitz B, Hou H Jr, Christ GJ, Edelmann W, Lisanti MP (2002b) Caveolin-2-deficient mice show evidence of severe pulmonary dysfunction without disruption of caveolae. Mol Cell Biol 22:2329–2344

Red-Horse K, Ferrara N (2007) Vascular targeting via caveolae. Nat Biotechnol 25:431–432

Richterova Z, Liebl D, Horak M, Palkova Z, Stokrova J, Hozak P, Korb J, Forstova J (2001) Caveolae are involved in the trafficking of mouse polyomavirus virions and artificial VP1 pseudocapsids toward cell nuclei. J Virol 75:10880–10891

Rizzo V, Sung A, Oh P, Schnitzer JE (1998a) Rapid mechanotransduction in situ at the luminal cell surface of vascular endothelium and its caveolae. J Biol Chem 273:26323–26329

Rizzo V, McIntosh DP, Oh P, Schnitzer JE (1998b) In situ flow activates endothelial nitric oxide

13

synthase in luminal caveolae of endothelium with rapid caveolin dissociation and calmodulin association. J Biol Chem 273:34724–34729

Rizzo V, Morton C, DePaola N, Schnitzer JE, Davies PF (2003) Recruitment of endothelial caveolae into mechanotransduction pathways by flow conditioning in vitro. Am J Physiol Heart Circ Physiol 285:H1720–H1729

Rothberg KG, Heuser JE, Donzell WC, Ying YS, Glenney JR, Anderson RG (1992) Caveolin, a protein component of caveolae membrane coats. Cell 68:673–682

Rybak JN, Ettorre A, Kaissling B, Giavazzi R, Neri D, Elia G (2005) In vivo protein biotinylation for identification of organ-specific antigens accessible from the vasculature. Nat Methods 2:291–298

Sargiacomo M, Lisanti M, Graeve L, Le Bivic A, Rodriguez-Boulan E (1989) Integral and peripheral protein composition of the apical and basolateral membrane domains in MDCK cells. J Membr Biol 107:277–286

Sargiacomo M, Scherer PE, Tang Z, Kubler E, Song KS, Sanders MC, Lisanti MP (1995) Oligomeric structure of caveolin: implications for caveolae membrane organization. Proc Natl Acad Sci U S A 92:9407–9411

Scherer PE, Lewis RY, Volonte D, Engelman JA, Galbiati F, Couet J, Kohtz DS, van Donselaar E, Peters P, Lisanti MP (1997) Cell-type and tissue-specific expression of caveolin-2. Caveolins 1 and 2 co-localize and form a stable hetero-oligomeric complex in vivo. J Biol Chem 272: 29337–29346

Scheurer SB, Roesli C, Neri D, Elia G (2005) A comparison of different biotinylation reagents, tryptic digestion procedures, and mass spectrometric techniques for 2-D peptide mapping of membrane proteins. Proteomics 5:3035–3039

Schlingemann RO, Rietveld FJ, Kwaspen F, van de Kerkhof PC, de Waal RM, Ruiter DJ (1991) Differential expression of markers for endothelial cells, pericytes, and basal lamina in the microvasculature of tumors and granulation tissue. Am J Pathol 138:1335–1347

Schnitzer JE (1997) Vascular endothelium: physiology, pathology and therapeutic opportunities. In: Born GVR, Schwartz CJ (eds) The endothelial cell surface and caveolae in health and disease. Schattauer, Stuttgart, pp 77–95

Schnitzer JE, Oh P (1994) Albondin-mediated capillary permeability to albumin. Differential role of receptors in endothelial transcytosis and endocytosis of native and modified albumins. J Biol Chem 269: 6072–6082

Schnitzer JE, Carley WW, Palade GE (1988a) Specific albumin binding to microvascular endothelium in culture. Am J Physiol 254:H425–H437

Schnitzer JE, Carley WW, Palade GE (1988b) Albumin interacts specifically with a 60-kDa microvascular endothelial glycoprotein. Proc Natl Acad Sci U S A 85:6773–6777

Schnitzer JE, Bravo J, Sung A, Pinney E (1992) Non-coated caveolae-mediated endocytosis of modified proteins via novel scavenger receptors, gp30 and gp18. Mol Biol Cell 3:59a

Schnitzer JE, Oh P, Jacobson BS, Dvorak AM (1994) Caveolin-enriched caveolae purified from endothelium in situ are transport vesicles for albondin-mediateed transcytosis of albumin. Mol Biol Cell 5:A75

Schnitzer JE, Liu J, Oh P (1995a) Endothelial caveolae have the molecular transport machinery for vesicle budding, docking, and fusion including VAMP, NSF, SNAP, annexins, and GTPases. J Biol Chem 270:14399–14404

Schnitzer JE, Allard J, Oh P (1995b) NEM inhibits transcytosis, endocytosis, and capillary permeability: implication of caveolae fusion in endothelia. Am J Physiol 268:H48–H55

Schnitzer JE, McIntosh DP, Dvorak AM, Liu J, Oh P (1995c) Separation of caveolae from associated microdomains of GPI-anchored proteins [see comments]. Science 269:1435–1439

Schnitzer JE, Oh P, McIntosh DP (1996) Role of GTP hydrolysis in fission of caveolae directly from plasma membranes [publisher's erratum appears in Science 1996 Nov 15;274(5290):1069]. Science 274:239–242

Schubert W, Frank PG, Woodman SE, Hyogo H, Cohen DE, Chow CW, Lisanti MP (2002) Microvascular hyperpermeability in caveolin-1 (-/-) knock-out mice. Treatment with a specific nitric-oxide synthase inhibitor, L-name, restores normal microvascular permeability in Cav-1 null mice. J Biol Chem 277:40091–40098

Severs NJ (1988) Caveolae: static inpocketings of the plasma membrane, dynamic vesicles or plain artifact? J Cell Sci 90:341–348

Simionescu M, Simionescu N, Palade GE (1974) Morphometric data on the endothelium of blood capillaries. J Cell Biol 60:128–152

Smart EJ, Ying YS, Mineo C, Anderson RG (1995) A detergent-free method for purifying caveolae

membrane from tissue culture cells. Proc Natl Acad Sci U S A 92:10104–10108
Smith GP (1985) Filamentous fusion phage: novel expression vectors that display cloned antigens on the virion surface. Science 228:1315–1317
Smith GP (1991) Surface presentation of protein epitopes using bacteriophage expression systems. Curr Opin Biotechnol 2:668–673
Song KS, Li S, Okamoto T, Quilliam LA, Sargiacomo M, Lisanti MP (1996) Co-purification and direct interaction of Ras with caveolin, an integral membrane protein of caveolae microdomains. Detergent-free purification of caveolae microdomains. J Biol Chem 271:9690–9697
Sowa G, Pypaert M, Fulton D, Sessa WC (2003) The phosphorylation of caveolin-2 on serines 23 and 36 modulates caveolin-1-dependent caveolae formation. Proc Natl Acad Sci U S A 100: 6511–6516
Tang Z, Scherer PE, Okamoto T, Song K, Chu C, Kohtz DS, Nishimoto I, Lodish HF, Lisanti MP (1996) Molecular cloning of caveolin-3, a novel member of the caveolin gene family expressed predominantly in muscle. J Biol Chem 271: 2255–2261
Thum T, Haverich A, Borlak J (2000) Cellular dedifferentiation of endothelium is linked to activation and silencing of certain nuclear transcription factors: implications for endothelial dysfunction and vascular biology. FASEB J 14:740–751
Tran D, Carpentier JL, Sawano F, Gorden P, Orci L (1987) Ligands internalized through coated or noncoated invaginations follow a common intracellular pathway. Proc Natl Acad Sci U S A 84: 7957–7961
Valadon P, Nussbaum G, Oh J, Scharff MD (1998) Aspects of antigen mimicry revealed by immunization with a peptide mimetic of *Cryptococcus neoformans* polysaccharide. J Immunol 161: 1829–1836
Vitetta ES (2000) Immunotoxins and vascular leak syndrome. Cancer J 6(Suppl 3):S218–S224
Wagner RC, Chen S-C (1991) Transcapillary transport of solute by the endothelial vesicular system: evidence from thin serial section analysis. Microvasc Res 42:139–150
Washburn MP, Wolters D, Yates JR III (2001) Large-scale analysis of the yeast proteome by multidimensional protein identification technology. Nat Biotechnol 19:242–247
Workman P (2001) New drug targets for genomic cancer therapy: successes, limitations, opportunities and future challenges. Curr Cancer Drug Targets 1:33–47
Yu J, Bergaya S, Murata T, Alp IF, Bauer MP, Lin MI, Drab M, Kurzchalia TV, Stan RV, Sessa WC (2006) Direct evidence for the role of caveolin-1 and caveolae in mechanotransduction and remodeling of blood vessels. J Clin Invest 116:1284–1291

MIX
Papier aus verantwortungsvollen Quellen
Paper from responsible sources
FSC® C105338

If you have any concerns about our products,
you can contact us on
ProductSafety@springernature.com

In case Publisher is established outside the EU,
the EU authorized representative is:
Springer Nature Customer Service Center GmbH
Europaplatz 3, 69115 Heidelberg, Germany

Printed by Libri Plureos GmbH
in Hamburg, Germany